Voices of Pineland

Eugenics, Social Reform, and the Legacy of "Feeblemindedness" in Maine

Voices of Pineland

Eugenics, Social Reform, and the Legacy of "Feeblemindedness" in Maine

by

Stephen T. Murphy
University of Southern Maine

IAP
INFORMATION AGE PUBLISHING, INC.
Charlotte, NC • www.infoagepub.com

Library of Congress Cataloging-in-Publication Data

Murphy, Stephen T.
Voices of Pineland : eugenics, social reform, and the legacy of "feeblemindedness" in Maine / by Stephen T. Murphy.
p. cm.
Includes bibliographical references.
ISBN 978-1-61735-414-4 (pbk.) -- ISBN 978-1-61735-415-1 (hbk.) -- ISBN 978-1-61735-416-8 (e-book)
1. Pineland Hospital and Training Center (New Gloucester, Me.)--History. 2. Mental retardation facilities--Maine--History. 3. People with mental disabilities--Institutional care--Maine--History. I. Title.
HV3006.M22P566 2011
362.3'850974191--dc22

2011010593

Printed in the United States of America

CONTENTS

ACKNOWLEDGMENTS

First and foremost, I would like to thank all of those who agreed to be interviewed for this research. Without their assistance and rich descriptions this book could not have been written. I have concealed the identities of all former Pineland residents and employees and family members whom I interviewed, giving them all fictitious names. The only exceptions are those who expressed a desire to be identified and gave me written permission to do so. I also included real names as they appeared in previously published newspaper or magazine articles.

I am also deeply indebted to all of the University of Southern Maine (USM) counseling students who served as graduate assistants on this project and assisted me in numerous ways, from conducting and analyzing interviews to searching the archives and literature. They include in alphabetical order, Kaitlyn Blackstone, Deidre Coltrera, Linda Dowell, Betsy Hopkins, Mary Kelly, Michelle Rancourt, and Beth Wallner.

Numerous individuals have been extremely helpful, generous and supportive over the years as I conducted and prepared this manuscript. Kevin Baack, Sandy Ellis, Norma Higgins, Rose Ricker, Ron Welch, and Neville Woodruff shared important materials and allowed me to interrupt their busy schedules for numerous follow-up interviews and questions. Betty True at the New Gloucester Historical Society, Lutz Kaelber, of the University of Vermont, and Bill Barry at the Maine Historical Society were wonderful resources for documents and information. Bill Barry, Allen Breed, Will Callendar, Kathy McInnis, Mary Kelly, Steve Taylor, Paul Tabor, Lance Tapley, and Wanda Whitten reviewed all or part of early manuscript drafts, offering constructive and insightful comments. Debra and Bill Barry, Anne Marie Bushhardt, John Kerry, Tom Jones, Kathy McInnis Michael Kamber, and Lance Tapley generously gave me permission to reproduce photos and cite their materials. Ben Pinault of USM's printing services was very helpful in preparing my photographs.

My wife Nancy deserves special thanks. She has endured years of messy cabinets and book shelves, all too frequent conversations about eugenics, publishing frustrations, and my frequent distractions. Nancy also patiently reviewed various versions of the manuscript and offered valuable technical assistance and personal support.

I would like to make a final comment about the language that I use in this book. In describing Pineland's history, and the accompanying local and national climate, I frequently use outdated terms to describe persons with disabilities. I understand that such terminology may offend some readers. My intention is not to disparage or affront, but characterize as accurately as possible the language of particular historical periods.

FOREWORD

Steven J. Taylor

Voices of Pineland: Eugenics, Social Reform, and the Legacy of "Feeblemindedness" in Maine by Stephen Murphy tells the story of the Maine School for the Feebleminded, later known as Pineland Hospital and Training Center. Based on an in depth analysis of annual institutional reports, newspaper clippings, legal documents, and other archival sources as well as interviews with former residents, their family members, and staff, Murphy traces the history of the Maine institution from its founding in 1908 to its eventual closure in 1996. Prior to 1908, Maine sent many of its citizens with intellectual and developmental disabilities to Massachusetts. When the state established the Maine School for the Feebleminded, it modeled it after an institution in Massachusetts that had been the first asylum for so-called "idiots" in the United States. Murphy shows the influences of both social forces and the personalities of superintendents, elected officials, and eventually lawyers, advocates, and court officials on Pineland's history.

In telling the story of Pineland, Murphy reveals fascinating details of both Maine's and the institution's history. Perhaps the most striking example is the story of Malaga Island off the coast of Maine, home to an interracial fishing community of 45 people. Many members of the community were reported to be descendants of a former African American slave, Benjamin Darling. Starting around 1900, newspaper stories started decrying the pauperism and presumed moral depravity of the residents of Malaga. Soon after his election in 1911, Governor Frederick Plaisted launched a campaign to evict residents from the island. State officials declared that the descendents of a resident of a nearby mainland town owned the island, paid them $400 for the property, and ordered the islanders off of Malaga. A number of the residents of the island were sent to the Maine School for the Feebleminded, and the bodies of people who had been buried on Malaga were moved to the cemetery for residents of the state school. Almost 90 years later a former state legislator and past president of Maine's chapter of the NAACP would call for an investigation of what had happened at Malaga and an apology to descendents of the island. Malaga's history shows the connection between race and disability in early twentieth century efforts to halt the spread of presumed defective genes among certain segments of the population.

Voices of Pineland is more than the story of Maine's institution for the feebleminded, though. It provides a lens through which to view the history of people with intellectual disabilities in twentieth century America. The founding of the Maine School for the Feebleminded was a product of the eugenics fervor that swept the country around the turn of the century and continued for several decades. The feebleminded were seen as a cause of a broad range of social problems and a threat to the social order. Like other states, Maine turned to the institution and later involuntary sterilization to prevent the feebleminded from spreading their alleged defective genes. The population of the Maine school steadily grew, and the institution soon became overcrowded and understaffed. As early as 1938, charges of abuse and neglect at the institution were reported in the press. This predated the flurry of exposes on state schools and mental hospitals in the national media, including *Life* magazine and *Reader's Digest,* in the post-World War II era.

By the 1950s, medical experiments were conducted on residents of the Maine school, now known as Pownal State School. Like hepatitis B experiments at Willowbrook State School in New York and radiation experiments at Fernald State School in Massachusetts, the Pownal experiments exposed residents to potential physical harm and were conducted without the informed consent of the residents or their families. The nation's prisons and institutions for the mentally ill and mentally retarded often provided a ready source of subjects in experiments that were seldom conducted on nonconfined persons.

In the 1960s and 70s, the Maine institution, which had been renamed Pineland Hospital and Training Center, was subjected to the same attacks on state institutions that occurred across the country. Newspapers exposed the squalid conditions at the institution: filth, nakedness, neglect, injuries, lack of treatment. Following widely publicized law suits against Willowbrook State School in New York and Partlow State School and Hospital in Alabama, Maine's Legal Services, later joined by the national Mental Health Law Project, filed a class action law suit, the *Wuori* case, against Pineland for its poor treatment of residents. Like other court cases, *Wuori* brought out tensions among the many persons who had a stake in the institution and Maine's treatment of people with intellectual disabilities. Parents and family members were divided in their views on the place of the institution in the state's system of care. Professionals and advocates had differing treatment philosophies, with some endorsing the principle of normalization that arose in the late 1960s and was fully developed by the early 1970s. Some Pineland employees regarded the lawsuit as a threat to their autonomy and even their jobs. Public officials differed on whether a federal court should be dictating how a state should care for its dependent citizens. Finally, in 1978, the state agreed to enter into a consent decree to improve institutional conditions and develop community services. Implementation of the decree was turned over to special masters appointed by the federal judge in the case.

Although active court oversight of Pineland ended in 1983, the law suit had set into motion forces that would eventually lead to the closure of the institution. The last resident left Pineland on April 22, 1996, and the official closure of the institution was marked at a ceremony on June 1 of that year. With the closure of Pineland, Maine became the fourth New England state that no longer operated a public institution for people with intellectual disabilities.

In his concluding chapter, Murphy argues that Pineland's history is relevant to the present and the future. In 2000, a Maine philanthropic organization proposed the creation of a new 125 person institution on the grounds of the former Pineland Hospital and Training Center and commissioned a book to honor Pineland's history. Then, in 2004, a hospital associated with Maine Medical Center announced the opening of a new psychiatric facility that would include a unit housing approximately 40 children, including those with autism or mental retardation. The rationale for this facility is reminiscent of the rhetoric surrounding the Maine School for the Feebleminded under its various names. The idea that people with intellectual disabilities need to be segregated from society is not dead yet. *Voices of Pineland* records a history that needs to be remembered.

Steven J. Taylor, PhD
Centennial Professor of Disability Studies
Syracuse University

CHAPTER 1

INTRODUCTION

Betty Thompson is 54 years old and lives in an apartment across from a nursing home in a central Maine city. She moved there several years ago to be closer to her husband who, after becoming ill, could no longer live at home. After her husband died, Betty kept her apartment and now volunteers at the nursing home, her church, and an advocacy group for persons with intellectual disabilities. She is not currently employed but reports having enough friends and activities "to keep busy and a part of things" (Thompson, personal communication, June 17, 2003).

Doreen Reynolds is 57 years old, divorced, and a mother and grandmother with three grown children and several grandchildren. She lives in her northern Maine home with a son and his family. Doreen enjoys playing bingo and gambling at local state fairs, and although she has worked sporadically over the years, is presently unemployed.

From the brief descriptions, the two women appear to be leading unremarkable lives that are typical of many other citizens. Closer inspection, however, reveals lived experiences that are far from ordinary or familiar to most people. As children, they were considered "mentally sub-normal" and sent to the Pineland Center, Maine's only large state institution for persons having mental retardation (a condition now called developmental and/or intellectual disability). Neither Ms. Thompson nor Ms. Reynolds fully understand why they were assigned or languished there for so long—the former for 12 years, the latter for 22. Both consider

Voices of Pineland: Eugenics, Social Reform, and the Legacy of "Feeblemindedness" in Maine, pp. 1–7

their institutionalization a terrible mistake for which they are still seeking answers.

These are two voices of Pineland. There are others, not only of former residents, but also of numerous other parties with diverse perspectives. In their own unique ways, all shaped Pineland's changing historical definitions, rationales, functions, and images. The varied voices may not be considered equally prominent or credible, but each needs to be carefully examined in order to understand Pineland's complex origin, ending, and legacy.

OPENING, EXPANDING, AND PERPETUATING THE MAINE SCHOOL FOR FEEBLE-MINDED

Opened in 1908 as the Maine School for Feeble-Minded, and for 88 years thereafter, Pineland housed thousands of the state's citizens who often were placed there for years, sometimes for life. The facility was built at the beginning of what many historians consider the peak period of eugenic persecution of persons identified as "mentally defective." Initially imbued with an aura of home and education, in practice the institution functioned as a repository for troublesome people who in their "amorality and fecundity were considered the most prominent cause of genetically transmitted social vices and whose control was an urgent necessity for preserving generations of human fitness and social order" (Ludmerer, 1972, pp. 140–141).

While the story of Pineland has many features and contours unique to Maine, it is not an isolated tale. Throughout the country, beginning in the mid nineteenth century and extending into the early decades of the twentieth century, many state institutions like Pineland were built and defended for decades as "best practice" for controlling and/or "treating" mental deficiency. Every state had at least one such facility and some had several. Like similar institutions, Pineland symbolizes the historical pursuit of a "noble vision" for societal improvement that inspired a national and international movement by society's elites, applying the laws of science to achieve greater human perfection (Gallagher, 1999, p. 2). Described in 1905 by its founder, Sir Francis Galton, as "a virile creed, full of hopefulness" (as cited in Nourse, 2008, p. 13), the eugenics movement illustrated how the fine line between "good intentions and malice aforethought" is easily crossed, as its most prominent solutions for achieving social and human progress soon became social weapons in a war against the "weak" (Gallagher, 1999, p. 2).

Educator, Burton Blatt (1981, p. 118), calls the institutionalization of persons with intellectual disabilities an "invented treatment" for an "invented disease," based on stories that were largely untrue. But even when the stories changed, the institution remained, even prospered. Shortly after Pineland was built and certainly by the time Mss. Thompson and Reynolds were admitted in the 1950s and 1960s, scientists had discredited much of the institution's eugenic rationales. As Rothman (1971) observed, however, once we began segregating and congregating people considered deficient, deviant, expensive, and/or unproductive, the practice became so efficient and appealing that it continued as a well—entrenched societal tradition "that would not be easily or quickly changed" (p. 294).

Important changes did eventually come—in Maine and elsewhere. On April 23, 1996, the headline in the *Portland Press Herald* read: "Pineland Center Stands Empty After 88 Years" (Hench, 1996b, p. A1). Reflecting on the event, local columnist Roberta Scruggs (1996) recalled visiting the facility and seeing people "with unendurable handicaps," never imagining that "community care would ever accommodate such needs. Now it has" (p. C5). In closing Pineland, Maine became one of nine states and the District of Columbia to have no state institution for persons with intellectual disabilities, although, like it's beginning, Pineland's end was not easily or quickly realized. As in other states, closing the facility was bitterly and vocally opposed by some, becoming one of the most contested and controversial social policies in Maine's history. Despite the protests, the decision to close the facility prevailed, reflecting a changing legal, economic, political, and professional landscape that already had begun elsewhere. In 1991, neighboring New Hampshire shuttered its only state facility for persons with intellectual disabilities. Nearby Rhode Island and Vermont would soon follow suit, enabling Maine officials to openly propose in 1992 what they could not even mention publically a decade earlier.

Changing our minds about mental deficiency is a recurring historical theme, reflecting the social character of this concept. Trent (1994, p. 4) concludes that the shifting definitions and meanings attached to intellectual disability is shaped both by societal decision makers who initiate and administer policies and programs, and by the surrounding societal forces to which policymakers respond. Over the years, state and Pineland officials frequently changed the image of residents and altered the primary functions of the facility, all in response to changing professional interests and/or internal and external factors, whether fiscal, political, legal, or professional.

A social lens, however, is not the one most frequently used to examine individuals with intellectual disabilities. These are individuals who may need varying degrees of assistance in daily living routines, do poorly on IQ tests, and are often considered incompetent, troublesome, unhealthy, and/or unproductive (Rapley, 2004, pp. 42, 205). To most people, intellectual/

developmental disabilities are considered a form of human pathology, biological in nature, emanating from neurological disorder and requiring specialized, clinical treatment. From this perspective, intellectual disability is an "absolute human condition" that people are deemed by certified experts to either have or not (Bogdan & Taylor, 1994, p. 8).

Social theorists like Michel Foucault (1973, 1976) argue, however, that there is nothing self-evident or essential in an individual's body, character, or behavior that predispose her/him to being a disabled or abnormal person. Rather, the genesis of disability emerges from linguistic, discursive and cultural practices. Becoming insane, abnormal or deviant (as well as sane and normal) are social designations conceived and assigned by those who have successfully claimed the knowledge and achieved the power and legitimacy to do so.

Shakespeare (1997, p. 658) points to recent historical accounts that also challenge fixed, objective conceptions of disability, illuminating its socially dynamic nature, and raising serious doubts about the psycho-biological explanations and transhistorical certainties that surround the concept. One of the most widely cited historical examples involves the American Association on Mental Retardation (AAMR), the primary source for officially defining what should be considered cognitive adequacy/inadequacy in our society (see Rapley, 2004, pp. 30–40). The AAMR, recently renamed the American Association on Intellectual and Developmental Disabilities (AAIDD), has changed its definition about 10 times, sometimes dramatically modifying the term's meaning, and radically changing the number of people affected (see also Switzky & Greenspan, 2003). Until the late 1950s, experts believed that 3% of the U.S. population was mentally deficient. In 1961, however, the AAMR expanded its definition to include a higher functioning category, termed borderline mental retardation, increasing the prevalence of this condition to 16%. In 1973 the organization again revised its definition, reverting to the 3% figure, declaring that sub average intelligence could only be declared if a person scored two or more standard deviations below the mean (IQ of 70). Citing this change as evidence that the term, mental retardation, is more social and bureaucratic than biological in nature, Blatt (1981) argues:

> With the figurative, and possibly literal stroke of … [a] pen, a committee sitting around a conference table reduced enormously the potential incidence of mental retardation, never having to see, or dose, or deal with a client, only having to say that, hereinafter, mental retardation is such and such rather than this or that. We cannot redefine measles, or cancer, or pregnancy with such external procedures.
>
> Sixteen percent of the population have IQs below 85; three percent … [score] below 75; but probably no more than one percent of the population are

> ever in their lifetimes administratively adjudicated as "mentally retarded." This is by way of saying that the incidence, prevalence, and characteristics of mental retardation depend upon such influences as definition and criteria, program supports, cultural value, social class, and other factors that have more to do with political and administrative, rather than biological or psychological, matters. This situation exists across all so-called disability areas and consequently, estimates of various categorical handicaps vary from study to study, from culture to culture, and from time to time. (pp. 227-228)

Reflected in Pineland's history are the many, diverse national themes surrounding our changing definitions and treatment of persons with intellectual disabilities throughout the twentieth century, ranging from menace to medicine and civil rights to civic inclusion. Some things, however, have changed less than we might imagine. More recent themes such as institutional scandals, legal advocacy, de-institutionalization, disability rights, and community integration served to modify, but not always eliminate, earlier themes like segregation, medicalization, and rights restrictions. In addition, regardless of what historical trends prevail at a given time, the primary problem has always been identified as the individual, who remains the target for interventions by professionals who alternately call for care and/or control depending on changing contextual circumstances (Trent, 1994, p. 4), and claim to have the prerequisite expert knowledge, clinical skills, and technical advantage over families and communities. Continually minimized or ignored are the social, political and economic inequities that have plagued persons who have been presented first and foremost as mentally deficient (Noll & Trent, 2004, p. 6).

The origins and nature of our technical and circumscribed definitions of intellectual disability should cause us to reflect on the causes we continually offer to account for complex social problems that threaten our security, prosperity, and/or quality of life; on the studies we commission to produce such knowledge; and on the solutions we subsequently endorse based on that research (Gallagher, 1999):

> We find ourselves somewhere between a past we condemn and a future in which we have invested tremendous resources in the collection of genetic data and its digestion in endless studies that define our humanity and predict our future health. As eugenic sentiments emerge, as they frequently do, our best safeguard against the injustices of the past rests with our willingness to confront our connection to this history before disowning it and with our recognition of the enduring power of research findings and the consensus of experts over our perceptions of other people's problems. (p. 8)

As part of a larger story, Pineland's history also illustrates the importance of institutional settings as prominent "cultural locations of disability" that, according to Snyder and Mitchell (2006, p. 3), might be more aptly termed "dis-locations" since they dramatically illustrate the extent to which persons classified as disabled have been actively excluded from the social participation and experiences afforded other citizens. Uncritically accepted as the pre-eminent public policy option for individuals with intellectual disabilities for most of the twentieth century, specialized institutions have continued to shape our perspectives and treatment approaches long after the institutions declined in use and despite the fact that the majority of people classified as mentally deficient never resided in them.

Despite the heightened attention recently directed toward disability studies, scholars have largely overlooked persons with intellectual disabilities and the specialized institutions to which many were relegated (for exceptions—see Carey, 2009; Ferguson, 1994; Noll, 1995; Noll & Trent, 2004; Trent, 1994; Wolfensberger, 1975). Even less historical attention has been paid to specific cases of institutional closure, a trend that began in a few states in the 1970s and 1980s, spearheading a national movement termed de-institutionalization that evolved into one of the most prominent, debated, and litigated social policies of the twentieth century. De-institutionalization has been studied from numerous angles, mostly by social scientists measuring its functional effects on released residents. Detailed accounts of institutional closings and other important aspects of that process remain largely unexamined, however. Rothman and Rothman's (1984) early study of the Willowbrook State School in New York City, while omitting the perspectives of important participants, still remains the classic, multifaceted case study of de-institutionalization. In addition, the collective, lived, and self-reported experiences of those integrally involved in the process are scarcely documented (for exceptions, see Johnson, 1998; Johnson & Traustadottir, 2005; Racino, 1993; Shoultz, Walker, Hulgin, Bogdan, & Taylor, 1999; Traustadottir, 2005).

The following account of Pineland's history includes numerous, compelling voices stemming from diverse and sometimes overlapping constituencies that have surrounded the facility, shaped its meanings, structures and functions, and illustrated the interactive roles played by single individuals, organized groups, and social events. Stories include not only those of former residents and their families, but also social reformers interested in improving society, professional administrators and practitioners seeking legitimacy and authority, politicians measuring pubic and fiscal pressures, media precariously balancing support and scrutiny, employees fearing for their livelihood, and disability and legal advocates focusing on human rights. Including such perspectives is essential for understanding the complex social phenomena we call institutionalization and de-institutionalization. Becker (1973, p. 183) argues that since specific instances of deviance involve the tacit or overt involvement of many people and groups to occur as they do, such phenomena cannot be fully understood without comprehending the actions and perspectives of all of the involved parties, including those considered deviant. The contributions of the latter group have proven especially valuable. Ferguson, Ferguson, and Taylor (1992, pp. 300–301) report, for example, that when individuals with disabilities have presented their personal accounts and experiences at public, legal, and/or legislative forums, they have often differed dramatically from the perspectives of professional experts and researchers, producing new insights and dramatic changes in disability definitions, institutional policies, and state and federal laws. Similarly, the activism of former Pineland residents who successfully escaped to live anonymous, community lives and later spoke out about their experiences; individuals who were discharged from Pineland and joined political and self-advocacy groups such as "People First of Maine" to protest their treatment; and residents, family members, dissident professionals and legal advocates who rejected institutionalization in favor of community alternatives, all illustrate how powerful cultural discourses, definitions, and images may be credibly and successfully challenged.

Over the years, national policy changes, supportive court decisions, revised social science research, heightened political action, and altered professional practices have offered convincing evidence that segregating persons with intellectual disabilities has lost public, legal, and professional support. We now declare that our policies, services, and proposals toward persons with intellectual/developmental disabilities are "community-based," implying that they are woven into the surrounding social fabric. The eugenics era, however, was a social catastrophe from which persons with disabilities have not fully recovered. Regardless of how proponents describe current policies and practices, they have evolved from, and retain, remnants of an institutional past that shapes, burdens, and obligates us, serving as a cautionary note. Obscured by ever-changing professional and technical language, is the continuing influence of eugenic ideology, illustrating a powerful but perhaps less obvious effect of the movement: the persistence of the rhetoric of biological, mental, and moral inferiority, legitimating continuing segregation and discrimination. Rothman's (1971) previously cited observation that our historical tendency to congregate "troublesome" people would prove too useful and efficient to be easily changed, captures well how exclusionary ideas, language, and practices can persist for so long and continue to be proposed, rationalized, and defended in numerous and subtle ways.

CHAPTER 2

NATIONAL CONTEXT SURROUNDING MAINE'S SCHOOL FOR "FEEBLEMINDED"

The construction, growth, and demise of what began as the *Maine School for Feeble-Minded* did not occur independently of broader social themes. Political, cultural, economic, professional, and religious factors in and outside of the state significantly influenced the history of this facility, affecting events like when the institution was built, who was admitted, who operated it, and when and how it grew, changed and eventually closed. Likewise, decisions and actions surrounding Maine's institution influenced perspectives and policies elsewhere in the region and country.

The chapter is intended as a brief historical overview that illuminates what was occurring in Maine during much of the twentieth century. For comprehensive national and local histories of persons with intellectual disabilities, the eugenics movement, de-institutionalization, and legal and social change, readers may refer to works such as Carey, 2009; Degler, 1991; Ferguson, 1994; Gallagher, 1999; Kevles, 1985; Largent, 2008; Ludmerer, 1972; Minow, 1990; Noll, 1995; Pickens, 1968; Reilly, 1991; Scheerenberger, 1981; Trent, 1994; Wolfensberger, 1975.

Voices of Pineland: Eugenics, Social Reform, and the Legacy of "Feeblemindedness" in Maine, pp. 9–46

IDENTIFYING A "SOCIAL MENACE"

Feeblemindedness was not fully acknowledged as a serious, genetically transmitted societal threat requiring public attention, restrictive legislation, and punitive action until early in the twentieth century. Advocates and supporting rationales for the "menace" conception of mental deficiency emerged decades before, however, emanating largely from the mid-nineteenth century social philosophies of Herbert Spencer and Francis Galton and the re-interpretation of the scientific discoveries of Charles Darwin, Gregor Mendel, and August Weismann. Even before the work of these important figures gained prominence, a handful of American physicians proposed sterilizing persons they considered sexual deviants and social "degenerates," leading Largent (2008, p. 12) to conclude that Darwin's evolutionary theory served nicely to support the social arrangements some had already envisioned.

In the last decades of the nineteenth century, physicians asserted their control of the "feebleminded," or "degeneracy," problem, promoting the condition as the cause of defectiveness, dependency, and deviance that was transmitted from parent to child through some combination of biological and environmental factors. Within this medical framework, defect and deviance rested squarely inside the individual, pointing logically to person-change solutions geared toward control—social segregation sterilization, and marriage restrictions (Carey, 2003, p. 413). Acknowledged but minimized were environmental elements such as poverty and inequality. Not coincidently, the role physicians carved out for themselves placed them in the enviable position of beneficent enforcer, offering care and treatment to diseased individuals and protecting and improving society.

In the early 1850s, Englishman Herbert Spencer coined the phrase "survival of the fittest," becoming a visible proponent of evolution even before Darwin's 1859 classic, *Origin of Species*, linking social status with biology, and arguing that science, not God, determined human destiny (Degler, 1991, p. 11). Demonstrating the potency of biological determinism as a social weapon, Spencer argued in 1874 that schools, asylums, charities, and medical hospitals that undertake "in a wholesale way to foster 'good-for-nothings,' commit an unquestionable injury, since they obstruct the 'natural process of elimination' by which society continually purifies itself" (as cited in Degler, p. 11). Spencer recommended that governments do nothing to assist their least powerful members in order to allow deficiency to dissipate naturally and avoid perpetuating inferiority.

The heredity agenda was propelled by the so-called "pedigree studies." The earliest of these was published 1877 as *The Jukes: A Study in Crime,*

Pauperism, Disease and Heredity by Richard Dugdale, a New York sculptor, dilettante, social reformer, and a member of the New York Prison Association. Despite his lack of scientific education and experience, Dugdale was asked to complete a study on "criminal heredity" initiated by the registrar of the city's Board of Health (Bruinius, 2006, p. 145). While interviewing prisoners in an upstate New York jail, he discovered that many were related to each other, leading him to trace their lineage back to one family and estimate the economic cost of multiple generations of crime, dependency, disease, and immorality. Replete with figures and charts, Dugdale's study impressed social reformers, politicians, and professionals who were not only dazzled by its detailed cost estimates of one family's cumulative degeneracy, but also convinced that it confirmed the inheritability of social deviance (Degler, 1991, p. 37). Although he had little praise for poor families, Dugdale was more cautious in his interpretation than many of his readers, pointing to the influence of the family's long standing social deprivation on their circumstances (p. 37).

Dugdale's work spawned a series of similar studies where the authors' conclusions were more definitive. One of these, the "Tribe of Ishmael," was presented in 1888 by Indiana minister, Oscar McCullouch, who argued at the National Conference of Charities and Corrections that this clan was characterized by generations of incompetence, poverty and crime, all of which he attributed to the "hereditary scourge blocking American progress" (as cited in Black, 2003, p. 25). In 1897, the Kansas's "mixed-breed and tramp family—the *Smokey Pilgrims*—was described, followed by the *Hill Folk* of Massachusetts, and the in-bred, *Nam* family of upstate New York. Perhaps the most notorious pedigree study of them all was that conducted by eugenic psychologist, Henry Goddard, on a New jersey family he called the *Kallikaks*.

As a more aggressive eugenics perspective emerged, apparently Dugdale's original, more equivocal, findings were too ambiguous for some. In 1915, Arthur Estabrook, a field surveyor for the Eugenic Records Office in New York, and author of the *Nam Family: A Study in Cacogentics*, re-analyzed and re-interpreted the *Jukes* results, concluding definitively that heredity was the cause of the family's history of poverty and "degeneracy" (Scheerenberger, 1981, p. 152). The overall intent and effects of such research was to illuminate the genetic nature of not only physical characteristics but also temperament and behavior, tying together the beliefs of social Darwinists and the work of Italian criminologist Cesar Lombroso who argued for the biology and inheritability of criminality (Kevles, 1985, p. 71). Surrounding such findings with the aura of science, pedigree studies linked proliferating poor families with spreading social pathology, ranging from crime and drunkenness to prostitution and illegitimacy (Trent, 1994, p. 178).

Following up on Spencer's and Darwin's theories, Sir Francis Galton, an Englishman and cousin of Charles Darwin, coined the term "eugenics" in 1883 from the Greek phrase "well born." Galton became the movement's leading spokesman and as early as 1865 was proposing that improvement of the human race could be achieved by the same methods used in the selective breeding of horses and cattle (Ludmerer, 1972, p. 10).

Galton was an intellectual innovator, "a rough-cut genius" who, according to Kevles (1985), "moved from one new field to another, applying methods developed in one to problems in another, often without rigor, but usually with remarkable effectiveness" (p. 10). Some of his more notable accomplishments included devising the first weather maps and discovering human fingerprinting. In 1865, Galton first published his research on "natural ability," (later expanded and published in the book, *Hereditary Genius),* where he described the biographies of citizens whom he selected (from existing biological dictionaries of the day) as the most eminent citizens spanning two centuries (Kevles, 1985, pp. 3-4). Galton determined that many of those he selected were related, pointing to a biological link between genius and ancestry, and advancing the startling proposition that attributes like talent and character were genetically determined (p. 4). While acknowledging his eugenic equations were speculative, Galton did not shrink from recommending them as the basis for strong social policy, such as strict marriage regulation that prohibited "eugenically flawed unions" and endorsed "well-born partnerships" (Black, 2003, p. 18).

Following publication of *Origin of Species,* Galton was elated that his cousins had moved the question of "the nature of man" from the realm of religious superstition to that of scientific doctrine (Kevles, 1985, p. 12), a compliment that may have also been applied to Galton, himself. Incorporating decades of his heredity studies with his innovative statistical work on regression and correlation, Galton published an influential book, *Natural Inheritance,* in 1889 in which he went beyond the ambiguous analyses of his predecessors applying to heredity the sharp scientific focus it lacked: "the quantitative, hence measurable, relationship between generations for given characteristics" (p. 18).

Both Spencer's social Darwinists and Galton's eugenicists claimed a close affiliation with Darwin's evolutionary theories, dividing the world into the fit and unfit and linking social status and biology (Pickens, 1968). They were split, however, on how best to achieve human perfection. For eugenicists, the social Darwinists' laissez faire solution of natural human selection was too passive, slow, and inefficient. Eugenicists favored active intervention that emphasized "doing something," whatever that might be, to control heredity (Degler, 1991, p. 44). According to Galton, "what Nature does blindly, slowly, and ruthlessly, Man can do providently, quickly, and kindly" (as cited in Black, 2003, p. 18). Such activism eventually encouraged Alexander Johnson, President of the National Conference on Charities and Correction, to remark in 1901: "I do not think that to prevent the propagation of this class it is necessary to kill them off or resort to the knife; but if it is necessary, it should be done" (as cited in Wolfensberger, 1975, p. 37).

Although, Galton's own research led him initially to be more cautious and skeptical than his followers toward methods of social intervention, he remained intrepid and optimistic in his newly discovered "secular faith" (Kevles, 1985, p. 12). He argued that eugenic improvement could be achieved indirectly, guiding human evolution whenever possible by acting on opportunities to intervene, checking "the bad and giving free play to the good" (p. 19).

While most reformers had not yet fully endorsed the dramatic measures suggested by Johnson and others, they began segregating identified groups in greater numbers by the end of the nineteenth century. Between 1890 and 1903, the population of institutionalized people more than doubled. In 1890, 14 states had public and private institutions for approximately 5,250 people called feebleminded. By 1903 the number of institutionalized people totaled 14,300, held in 44 facilities (Trent, 1994, p. 166). Despite such expanded incarcerations, public officials and superintendents insisted that only 10% of the total feebleminded population had been properly segregated, with as many as 150,000 people remaining undetected (p. 167). Citing the 1904 census, reformers claimed that the nation's almshouses alone accounted for 16,551 feebleminded, more than all of those housed in large institutions (p. 166).

The successful scientific indictment of "unfit" groups was finally achieved early in the twentieth century when biologists connected Galton's eugenic views with the rediscovered genetic research of Gregor Mendel (1868) and linked them to August Weismann's (1889) theory of *germ plasm* (Ludmerer, 1972, p. 14). Weismann's work supported Galton's position that "race improvement could occur only when nature provided a distinct and heritable change … upon which selection, natural or eugenic, could act" (Kevles, 1985, p. 19). Weismann discredited the prevailing neo-Lemarckian theory (named after French naturalist Jean Baptiste de Lamarck) of "acquired characteristics" which posited that inherited and transmitted human characteristics included those affected positively and negatively by one's environment (Degler, 1991, p. 42). The Lamarkian view of natural selection allowed social reformers to argue that successful environmental improvements like sanitation, educational, and family reforms could produce more "fit" human beings and improve the "human stock" (Stern, 2005, p. 14). As a cytologist, Weismann contended, however, that human *germ plasm* was the major source of human variation, pointing out that the human body contained two types of cells—germ and somatic—and that the former constituted the seat of hereditary material producing sperm and eggs that affected the expression and arrangement of somatic cells but remained reciprocally unaffected by them (pp. 14–15).

Cross fertilizing pea plants, Gregor Mendel identified governing inheritable traits, termed dominant and recessive, that he could mathematically represent and predict (Black, 2003, p. 26). Rediscovered and reinterpreted in light of Weismann's work and applied to humans, Mendel's laws were heralded in 1900 as confirmation of the inheritability of human traits according to predictable patterns that could only be altered by selective breeding and control of procreation. Protecting and cultivating "good" germ plasm and neutralizing or eliminating "bad" material became the driving determinants of racial and national fitness (Gallagher, 1999, p. 2).

By 1905, eugenicists had articulated a two-part strategy for upgrading the hereditary character of America through: (1) *negative eugenics*: eliminating undesirable traits by discouraging unworthy parenthood in those considered mentally defective, criminal, epileptic, alcoholic, feebleminded, insane, prostitutes, and others having hereditary defects; using methods such as compulsory marriage restrictions, sterilization, and segregation; and (2) *positive eugenics:* increasing desired traits in the population by encouraging "worthy" parenthood by the educated, established, upper classes who, by producing too few children contributed to a dearth of desirable germ plasma and committed what Theodore Roosevelt called "race suicide" (Gallagher, 1999, p. 3; Trent, 1994, pp. 137–138).

Galton as been referred to as a conservative eugenicist, emphasizing positive, voluntary methods like education and contraception (Kevles, 1985, pp. 85, 90), rejecting the pro-Mendelian notion of breeding men and women like "cocks and hens," and terming control of marriage as "unrealistic in democratic societies" (Black, 2003, pp. 27–28). Early in the twentieth century, however, Galton revised his outlook downward, suggesting that the problem of degeneracy had become "so clear-cut and dire" as to require "state intervention of a coercive nature in human reproduction" (as cited in Kevles, 1985, p. 91). Unlike many British colleagues, Galton argued that sterilization seemed the only way of "checking the produce of the unfit who are allowed their liberty and are below the reach of moral control (as cited in Kevles, p. 94).

Galton's closest eugenic collaborator and leadership successor in Britain was Karl Pearson, a brilliant socialist statistician who, along with zoologist

Walter Weldon, invented the discipline of biometry—"the statistical study of evolution and heredity" (Kevles, 1985 p. 34). Together, the three founded the scholarly journal *Biometrika* from which emanated much of the supporting literature for the new "science" of eugenics (pp. 34–35).

Pearson reworked Galton's theory of ancestral heredity not only adding scientific legitimacy to the idea that humans could be permanently improved by biological manipulation but also the important notion that heredity was such a powerful force in determining attributes that selective breeding was the only approach that assured heightened societal improvement (Kevles, 1985, pp. 33–34). Pearson was also among the first and most widely cited sources for the alarmist warning of differential birthrates for "a proliferating menace," claiming in 1903 that Britain was in "a state of national deterioration" because half of every generation was produced by no more than a quarter of its married predecessors and the prolific quarter was disproportionately represented by the most unfit, for example "the habitual criminal, the professional tramp, the tuberculoses, the insane, the mental defectives, the alcoholics, and the diseased" (as cited in Kevles, p. 33).

As Galton, Pearson and their biometric colleagues infused the subject with heightened scientific legitimacy, American eugenicists were developing momentum of their own as more biologists joined physicians and other professionals in endorsing the idea that complex social conditions and behaviors were innate, unchangeable, and transmittable (Largent, 2008, pp. 2–3). In addition, eugenic proponents were becoming more organized, lending the movement leadership and clout and beginning to attract generous support from the nation's financial, intellectual, and political elites (pp. 6–7).

MAINSTREAMING AND EXPANDING EUGENICS THEORY AND PRACTICE

Emerging as a social force to be reckoned with, the eugenics movement was aided by the U.S. progressive movement, an influential, loosely defined and amorphous coalition of intellectuals, scientists, politicians, social reformers and philanthropists who sought political and social reforms at the end of the nineteenth and early twentieth century. An important part of the progressive group were large numbers of middle and upper class women who spearheaded many of the philanthropic and reformist campaigns aimed at assisting society's vulnerable populations such as poor children and adults, orphans, widows, immigrants, and persons with disabilities (Minow, 1990, p. 243).

Eugenics and Progressivism are terms that elude simple definition and are increasingly considered broad and changing entities that are often inconsistent in their claims and activities (Gallagher, 1999, p 2). Progressives criticized the abuses they felt were caused by unfettered capitalism, defining their mission as "caring for those in need," and proposing concrete solutions for individual and societal betterment, ranging from settlement houses and juvenile courts to compulsory education and protective labor laws (Minow, 1990, pp. 245–267). This movement stood for benevolent and responsive action based on enlightened thought, offered by educated, established citizens to less fortunate members of society. Progressives developed new social science disciplines to explain economic, political, sociocultural, and psychological phenomena and advocated for specialized services and professionals, such as social workers, public health nurses, labor statisticians, and probation officers (p. 245). Their ranks included such American icons as Teddy Roosevelt, Margaret Sanger, John Dewey, Jane Addams, Alexander Graham Bell, Woodrow Wilson, and Oliver Wendell Holmes and for several decades they attracted the major political parties to their causes.

Progressives were attracted to the eugenics movement because it appealed widely to their faith in science, trust in specialized experts, and infatuation with the prevention of human social and health problems. Eugenicists provided "a unifying paradigm, common themes and a new language of biological determinism," offering a more scientific approach to ensuring national fitness, preventing crime and poverty, and preserving the national's moral character (Gallagher, 1999, pp. 2–3). They also provided progressive intellectuals from different fields with an interdisciplinary forum to obtain financial resources for their research, apply their findings to the common goal of human betterment, and generate an influential literature that would be of interest to politicians, policy makers and philanthropists (Largent, 2008, p. 53).

The seeds of widespread support for an organized, scientifically-based, eugenics movement in America were sown with the emergence of Charles Davenport, a young and promising Harvard zoology instructor (later a University of Chicago professor) who was heavily influenced by the biometrics of Karl Pearson and Francis Galton (Kevles, 1985, p. 45). Acting as the summer director of the Brooklyn Institute's biological laboratory, Davenport wrote a proposal in 1902 to the Carnegie Institute to establish a biological experiment station at Cold Springs Harbor, New York. The proposal was accepted, and in 1904 the newly funded facility was formally inaugurated as The Station for Experimental Evolution of the Carnegie Institution (Pickens, 1968, p. 51). This was one of three important biological research organizations with which Davenport was closely involved, the other two being the American Breeders Association (ABA) and the Eugenic Records Office (Largent, 2008 p. 39). Considered as perhaps "the most influential American biologist of the twentieth century," Davenport profoundly enhanced the prestige and visibility of American biologists by forming alliances and attracting huge sums of money to fund research facilities and initiatives that demonstrated to policy makers and prominent philanthropists how evolutionary and heredity research and its applications could improve the nation (pp. 39-40).

In order to broaden scientific support for evolutionary research, biologists formed an alliance with the American Breeders Association (ABA), a newly formed group comprised largely of animal breeders and plant experts. In 1906, the ABA formally established a Committee on Eugenics, a step that was followed in 1910 (at Davenport's urging) by a full-fledged Eugenics Section. The latter became the precursor to the Eugenics Record Office (ERO) and the American Eugenics Society (Stern, 2005, p. 22). By 1913, the ABA had changed its name to the American Genetic Association and renamed its journal, formerly the *American Breeders Magazine*, to the *Journal of Heredity* (Pickens, 1968, p. 52).

In 1910, Davenport secured substantial funding from the widow of railroad tycoon, E. H. Harriman, to create the Eugenics Record Office with the expressed goal of gathering and documenting the genetic backgrounds of the American citizenry, separating "defective strains" from "desired lineages" (Black, 2003, p. 45). To direct this massive undertaking, Davenport selected Missouri biology teacher, Henry Hamilton Laughlin, an energetic and passionate eugenicist who would devote his life to promoting eugenic laws, research, and education. Under Davenport and Laughlin, the ERO would prove to be a key factor in the expansion of the eugenics movement throughout the United States, particularly in attracting funding, publicizing the cause, and passing legislation (Largent, 2008, p. 56). In 1913, Laughlin described the specific functions of the ERO as providing: a repository for eugenic records, a source of information about human heredity, a service to advise the public on the subject of "fit marriages," a place of employment and training for field workers collecting eugenic data, and a resource for the dissemination of eugenic research and conclusions (pp. 56–57).

Over the years, until his death in 1938 (ironically from complications surrounding epilepsy) Laughlin served as the "expert eugenical agent" for the U.S. House of Representatives; helped to draft and pass state sterilization laws and federal immigration restrictions. In 1922, he wrote the book, *Eugenical Sterilization in the United States*, "an encyclopedic collection of documents and commentary on the surgery that also contained a 'Model Eugenical Sterilization Law' " upon which many state statutes were based (Largent, 2008, pp. 56–57). Using this law, Laughlin sought to sterilize the "socially inadequate," referring to "anyone who by his or her own effort, regardless of etiology or prognosis, fails chronically in comparison to normal persons, to maintain himself or herself as a useful member of the organized social life of the state" (as cited in Largent, pp. 57–58). On the list of those considered socially inadequate were: "feebleminded, insane, criminalistic, epileptic, inebriate, diseased, blind, deaf, deformed, and dependent" (p. 57). By 1920, the ERO had secured millions of dollars from America's wealthiest citizens, including the Carnegie, Harriman, Eastman, and Rockefeller families (Black, 2003, pp. 93-95)

Despite Laughlin's best legal efforts and to the dismay of eugenic reformers, the courts were not as cooperative as anticipated, especially when dealing with the "moral imbecile," the most maligned of those considered feebleminded and a precursor to Henry Goddard's "moron." Moral imbeciles were the menacing culprits who possessed numerous traits of social inadequacy, none more threatening than their innate and incurable criminality. In 1909, Walter Fernald had no problem indicting and incarcerating this group early and permanently although they had committed no crimes:

> Cases of imbecility with criminal propensities—"criminals who have committed no crime"—will be recognized at an early age before they have acquired facility in crime, and permanently taken out of the community and given life-long care and supervision in special institutions.... Every imbecile, especially the higher grade imbecile, is a potential criminal, needing only the proper environment and opportunity for the development and expression of criminal tendencies.... From a biological standpoint the imbecile is an inferior human being. (as cited in Trent, 1994, pp. 160–161)

The term "moral imbecile" not only combined biological deficiency, economic dependency, and incurable criminality but also posed a particular threat due to its frequent invisibility. In 1912, Walter Fernald described the problem as "stealth" imbecility, arguing that "the unrecognized imbecile is a most dangerous element in the community" (as cited in Wolfensberger, 1975, p. 35). Despite the urgings of Fernald and other reformers, judges sometimes could not distinguish those identified as feebleminded from average citizens, questioning the diagnosis of moral imbecile, especially when applied to those accused of crimes, and resisting indefinite institutionalization in favor of finite prison terms. Apparently, eugenicists needed more convincing evidence to persuade their legal and political colleagues of the deviance-feebleminded link, to address lingering judicial resistance to full eugenic reform, and to expand the restrictions imposed on targeted groups (Trent, 1994, p. 161). Enter Henry Goddard.

A well-educated psychologist, Goddard was referred to as perhaps "the most unsubtle hereditarian of all" (Gould, 1996, p. 190). As much as any social scientist, he fueled eugenic fires across the country by developing and promoting a scientifically-based picture of a social villain that combined all the fearsome ingredients of the period: foreign birth, innate feeblemindedness, criminality, and invisibility. Goddard was a champion of the Binet intelligence test in America and, along with fellow psychologists, L. M. Terman and R. M. Yerkes, was an early and prominent promoter of the genetic IQ (p. 29). Although Goddard would perform some of the most controversial and ultimately discredited research in the history of intellectual/developmental disabilities, he was an influential force in constructing and promoting a new and more formidable conception of mental deficiency and devising and disseminating methods for its widespread identification.

A native of Vassalboro, Maine, Goddard gained prominence as research director at the Vineland (NJ) Training School for Feebleminded Boys and Girls (Scheerenberger, 1981, pp. 143–44). Traveling in Europe in 1908, he became aware of an intelligence test developed by Alfred Binet and Theodore Simon to assist "slow learners" in the school system (Trent, 1994, p. 157). Soon after, he began administering the test to Vineland residents and reporting success in identifying higher functioning, feebleminded students. His work caused what Trent (1994) terms "frenetic praise," inspiring numerous variations of the test and launching the intelligence test movement and the efficient sorting of people on the basis of innate functioning (p. 159).

Goddard concluded that perhaps 2% of all school children suffered from inherited, permanent, and low intelligence but were not sufficiently impaired to be classified as feebleminded. Beginning in 1909, he redefined "backward" children from intellectually slow to mentally deficient; from educationally improvable to permanently abnormal; and from special education students to institutional candidates (Trent, 1994, pp. 159–160). In 1910, he proposed that because of the prevalence, distinctiveness, and permanence of their condition, these children required a new label: "moron," derived from the Greek word, "foolish" (Gould, 1996, p. 189).

Goddard proposed to the classification committee of the American Association for the Study of Feeble-Mindedness (AASFM) that a new diagnostic schema be implemented, using Binet's concept of mental age as its centerpiece (Gould. 1996, p. 189). Following his recommendations, AASFM adopted an intelligence system in 1910 consisting of three levels based on the Binet-Simon test scores. The association applied the term "idiot" to individuals with a measured mental age of less than 2 years; "imbecile" to people with scores of 3–7 years; and "moron" to those who measured between 8 and 12 (Trent, 1994, p. 162). Adding the moron to the revised classification system expanded the incidence of mental deficiency by a full percent, wrapped the idea of an insidious menace in respectable scientific garb, and quantified the condition, transforming it from ambiguous to specific, invisible to detectable (pp. 160–62).

While Goddard appropriated Binet's instrument, he distorted his ideas and intentions. Binet had resisted a hereditarian interpretation of intelligence, insisting that his test was a guide to learning assistance, not simply a classification tool, and arguing that using his scales as hereditary measures would serve only to stigmatize children as uneducable, producing a result opposite to the test's intent (Trent, 1994, p. 29). Goddard (1919), however, considered an individual's measured intelligence as "by far the most important fact about him" (as cited in Gould, 1996 p. 191). Considering Binet's scales as valid measures of innate, immutable intelligence, he advocated the test's widespread application "to identify in order to recognize limits, segregate, and curtail breeding to prevent further deterioration of an endangered American stock, threatened by immigration from without and by the prolific reproduction of its feeble-minded from within" (p. 189).

Goddard went further than most of his professional colleagues in proposing that feeblemindedness was not just associated with social pathologies through some murky human trait-environment interactions, but was the primary genetic cause of societal disorder through what he termed the "cancerous growth of bad protoplasm" (cited in Trent, 1994, p. 162). According to Gould (1996):

> Goddard worked in the first flourish of excitement that greeted the rediscovery of Mendel's work and ... joined the transient bandwagon with a hypothesis that must represent the ultimate reification of intelligence ... and concluded that "feeblemindedness" obeyed the Mendelian rules of inheritance. Mental deficiency must therefore be a definite thing, and it must governed by a single gene undoubtedly recessive to normal intelligence. (p. 192)

To verify his view of feeblemindedness as a transmissible genetic flaw Goddard pointed to the Kallikak clan, a family that clearly illustrated the effects of Mendelian heredity, intergenerational breeding, and the proliferating birthrates of feeble minds (Trent, 1994, pp. 163–164). Goddard invented the term "Kallikak," combining the Greek words, "kallos" (beauty) and "kakos"(bad) (Gould, 1996, p. 198). Using the memories of older family members as primary sources, Goddard traced the family lineage of a Vineland School resident he named Deborah Kallikak back to the time of the American Revolution. Goddard's research was the most famous and influential of the pedigree studies because he claimed to have isolated two parallel family lines, emanating from the same father, Martin Kallikak, but involving different mothers, one a feebleminded prostitute, the other a respectable, Quaker woman. Goddard asserted that by successfully isolating two parallel family lines of descendants differing only in maternal roots, he had isolated and proven that generations of inherited traits, as opposed to environmental influences, led to a family history of feeblemindedness, criminality, and debauchery on one side, and of intelligence, morality and lawfulness on the other (Gould, 1996, pp. 198–201; Trent, 1994, pp. 163–165).

Describing the implications of his research for understanding social pathology and deviance, Goddard concluded in 1912:

> No matter where we traced them whether in the prosperous rural district, the city slums to which some had drifted, or in the more remote mountain regions ... an appalling amount of defectiveness was everywhere found.... If all of the slum districts of our cities were removed tomorrow, and model tenements were built in their places, we would still have slums in a week's time because we have these mentally defective people who can never be taught to live otherwise.
>
> There are Kallikak families all around us. They are multiplying at twice the rate of the general population, and not until we recognize this fact, and work on this basis, will we solve our social problems. (as cited in Trent, 1994, pp. 164–165)

Confidently identifying deviants by their unconventional behavior, Goddard cast a wide net that could include the indictment of almost anyone defined as troublesome, unsuccessful, or unconventional: "We know what feeblemindedness is, and we have come to suspect all persons who are incapable of adapting themselves to their environment and living up to the conventions of society, or acting sensibly, of being feebleminded" (as cited in Gould, 1996, p. 191).

The alarm was sounded around a proliferating, stealth, scientifically-verified, moron class, leading state officials across the country to propose larger facilities and separate institutions for men and women as the best way to ensure proper sexual quarantine, giving institutional expansion added urgency and momentum. Goddard preferred large scale segregation to compulsory sterilization as the best defense against the growing threat, arguing that humanely run colonies where people were treated as children and made content were not as fiscally hopeless as many believed (as cited in Largent, 2008, p. 61).

Despite Goddard's reassurances, institutional expansion involved such escalating numbers and costs that even the most ardent reformers began to worry that there were far too many morons breeding at prodigious rates to institutionalize them all (Trent, 1994, p. 192). Superintendents assured legislators, however, that institutions with 1,000 or more residents were both "economically and therapeutically ideal" (Wolfensberger, 1975, p. 49). Some urged that new facilities be built to hold as many as 2,000–3,000 people. One proposal called for the construction of national reservations similar to the government's approach to Native Americans (p. 43). As ever-larger institutions were built, admissions continued to exceed capacity, long waiting lists persisted, and new or expanded facilities were contemplated.

Overcrowding worsened as more states began restricting the use of almshouses, adding increasing numbers to the roles of feebleminded, committing more children and adults to specialized institutions, and failing to sufficiently underwrite the heightened costs (Wolfensberger, 1975, p. 44). In Pennsylvania, a facility built in 1906 to relieve the overcrowding at a nearby institution, was designed for 1,200 residents, but housed 2,300 in 1928 with a 500 person waiting list (p. 49). In Rome, New York, a state institution designed for 1,200 actually held 1,554 people in 1916 (p. 49). The Lincoln (Illinois) State School had an enrollment of 1,888, and a capacity of 1,700, and in 1918 Lincoln's superintendent resigned, complaining that in some quarters residents were sharing beds (Trent, 1994, pp. 188–191). Following World War I institutions across the country continued to expand dramatically. Between 1923 and 1936, the number of people institutionalized as feebleminded nearly doubled, from 43,000 to 81,000 (pp. 188, 199). By 1923, 90% of the states had at least one public institution specializing in persons considered mentally deficient. Some had more. Massachusetts, New Jersey, and Pennsylvania, for example, had three and New York had six (p. 185).

WORLD WAR I, IMMIGRATION AND IQ

Kevles (1985, p. 72) points out that neither the burgeoning eugenics literature nor the "pre-existing intellectual climate of social Darwinism" were sufficient to create the ensuing and widespread movement. Additional societal changes were needed, such as "industrialization, the growth of big business, the sprawl of cities and slums, and the massive migrations from the countryside and abroad. Gould (1996, p. 29) refers to this period as the age of restricted immigration, the spread of Jewish quotas, Sacco and Venzetti, and the peak period for Southern lynchings. Moreover, while urban problems such as alcoholism, crime, prostitution, and disease were very familiar, their magnitude and costs were being revealed through the new and increasing use of statistics, imbued with an aura of mathematical certainty and detailing to an increasingly fearful public the extent of the worsening social threats of mental defectives and social deviants (Kevles, 1985, p. 72).

In the last decades of the nineteenth century, the U.S. experienced a large influx of immigrants from Southern and Eastern Europe, inducing public fear and suspicion, associating foreigners with crime, disorder, deficiency, and worst of all, attributing to them proliferating birthrates that far exceeded those of native born citizens. In 1904, census data estimated that 33% of institutional residents had at least one foreign-born parent and by 1910 these facilities were characterized as repositories for the nation's poor and immigrant populations, due to deficiency not disadvantage. (Kevles, 1985, p. 185). Building on public anxieties, eugenicists campaigned vigorously for immigration restrictions following World War I. Initially they emphasized the economic threat, warning that unconstrained immigration would overrun urban centers and overwhelm an already glutted labor market (Ludmerer, 1972, p. 96). Soon they shifted their focus to racial fears. Adding to the pervasive bigotry regarding African Americans, eugenic reformers used the debates surrounding the 1924 Immigration Restriction Act to issue dire warnings regarding the dangers of replacing Anglo-Saxon, or "Nordic" type citizens with biologically inferior Southern and Eastern Europeans who were also characterized as racially inferior (p. 96). Lobbying for immigration restrictions, proponents linked immigrants with feeblemindedness, a connection to which eugenic researchers lent considerable scientific legitimacy, influencing national immigration policy for decades. Again, Goddard emerged as a leading figure.

Perhaps Goddard's most outlandish claims emerged from his research at Ellis Island where, in 1912–13, he began using the Binet Intelligence Test to evaluate newly arriving immigrants. He tested four groups he classified as Italian, Russian, Hungarian, and Jewish and generated such astounding data that even he questioned its validity (Gould, 1996, p. 196). In 1917, Goddard concluded that 79% of the Italians, 80% of the Hungarians, 87% of the Russians, and 83% of the Jews he tested were feebleminded (p. 196). Although he later adjusted his calculations down to 40-50 %, he defended his results as reflecting a newer wave of poorer, intellectually inferior immigrants and remained staunchly supportive of restrictive immigration policies (p. 196).

Another notable scientific project that fueled immigration fears was one directed by Harvard psychologist, Robert Yerkes, and his team of prominent psychologists, notably Goddard and Louis Terman, a Stanford University psychology professor who specialized in psychometrics and was a "pivotal figure to the national eugenics movement: (Stern, 2005, p. 18). Terman's 1916 book, *Measurement of Intelligence,* was an instrumental force in championing the passage of the 1924 immigration restrictions and molding thinking about IQ distinctions between people of different races and levels of mental abilities (p. 19). From 1917–1919, the group administered the Army Alpha and Beta Mental Tests to 1.7 million World War I recruits, publishing their findings in 1921 that "reverberated through the 1920s with a hard hereditarian ring" (Gould, 1996, p. 226). The data revealed that 37% of White males and 89% of African Americans had mental ages under 13 years, causing Yerkes to proclaim that "we are a nation of nearly half-morons," and point to foreigners as a leading cause, particularly those from Southern and Eastern Europe (as cited in Gould, 1996, p. 227).

Yerkes's World War I Army tests that initially spurred eugenic fervor also served to allay some of the worst public fears, since no calamitous intellectual or social deterioration ensued and an increasing skepticism about the inheritability issue was creeping beyond just the scientific community. As early as 1913, two respected researchers, Edith Spaulding and William Healy, challenged the degenerate family myth in a presentation to the American Academy of Medicine (Reilly, 1991, p. 55). After studying 1,000 young criminal recidivists, the researchers concluded that there was no proof that criminality was inherited. According to Rafter (1997, pp. 173, 176), after 1915 those writing about "defective delinquents" referred to them as "psychopaths" and attributed the condition less to hereditary feeblemindedness than to mental disturbance. In a widely read 1922 series published in the *New Republic* by nonscientist, Walter Lippmann, referred to the Army Test data as beyond "inaccurate" and "incorrect;" calling the results "nonsense," having "no more scientific foundation than a hundred other fads, vitamins, and glands, and amateur ... courses in will power (Kevles, 1985, p. 129). Such criticism aside, the "hereditarian interpretation of IQ" in the U.S. arose in no small measure from the combined work of Goddard, Terman and Yerkes in importing and popularizing standardized intelligence testing (Gould, 1996, p. 29).

A schism between mainstream eugenicists and the emerging community of genetic scientists became visible around World War I, as the latter group came to view the former as a kind of "pop science," that to some was "morally and scientifically offensive," and most importantly was seen as "slipshod in method, evidence and reasoning" (Kevles, 1985, pp. 121–122). A biometry proponent from the Galton Lab referred to the interpretations of Davenport and his colleagues as "Mendelism run mad." (p. 149).

Despite the fledgling skepticism, eugenic advocates were about to record impressive policy triumphs. In 1921, Congress passed immigration legislation that created a quota on immigration keyed to the national census of 1910. Three years later, legislators made the restrictions even harsher, pushing back immigration quotas to 1890 census figures, promoting the superiority of Nordic and Teutonic races, and excluding groups who were considered racially "inadequate," such as Italians, Greeks and Poles whose immigration rates were reduced by 80% (Reilly, 1991, p. 65). Gould (1996, pp. 261–262) argues that although immigration restrictions would most likely have occurred without scientific legitimacy, the 1924 Immigration Restriction Act went far beyond previous legislation and was likely harsher and more extreme than might have been the case without scientific support (p. 262). Ludmerer (1972, pp. 89–90) argues that eugenicists scored their greatest national victories in restricting immigration quotas and rekindling public support for stringent sterilization laws, both of which depended on scientific-biological arguments.

MARRIAGE RESTRICTIONS AND THE SURGICAL SOLUTION

While banishing increasing numbers of allegedly defective and deviant persons to a rapidly expanding number of large residential facilities proved publically popular, the practice always attracted its share of critics who characterized it as physically impractical and economically unsustainable. As identified menaces multiplied, institutions grew in size and number, waiting lists persisted, and overcrowding worsened, the chorus grew louder for other methods of control.

At the end of the nineteenth century, states began imposing marriage prohibitions, beginning in Connecticut in 1895 (Pfieffer, 1994, p. 485). That state passed a statute that prevented men who were "epileptic, imbecile, or feebleminded" from marrying any woman under child bearing age (45 years old). Women under 45 and classified as mentally deficient were prohibited from marrying any man, regardless of age (p. 485). Thus, began a national movement to bar people considered feebleminded or insane from marrying (Wolfensberger, 1975, p. 40). By 1913, over half the states had enacted marriage restriction laws (Trent, 1994, p. 165), although by then even eugenic icon, Sir Francis Galton, considered the measure ineffective and unenforceable (Black, 2003, p. 28). That same year, Murdock warned in the *Journal of Psycho-Asthenics* that although marriage restriction was "no doubt advisable" it was futile since "'the unfit reproduce their kind regardless of marriage laws" (as cited in Wolfensberger, 1975, p. 40). Despite such early disenchantment, laws banning or restricting marriage for those with intellectual disabilities persisted through the 1980s in over 30 states (Pfieffer, 1994, p. 486).

A surgical solution to an increasingly medically defined problem would gain momentum as logical, viable, and cost efficient, but prove to be controversial. Eugenic sterilization was initially referred to as "asexualization" germinating in mid-nineteenth century America as a way to "cure" people of everything from idiocy, insanity, and epilepsy to masturbation, promiscuity, and criminality (Lombardo, 2008, pp. 20-23). In 1849, Gideon Lincecum, a Texas physician, introduced a bill to castrate people convicted of certain crimes (Largent, 2008, p. 11). Between 1860 and the end of the nineteenth century, persons found guilty of sexual and violent assaults, nearly all African American, were reportedly castrated, while prison inmates and mental patients in Kansas, Oregon, Indiana, Illinois and Pennnsylvania were involuntarily sterilized before any laws permitting the surgery were passed (p. 11). The superintendent of the Winfield Kansas State Home for the Feebleminded, Dr F. Hoyt Pilcher, began castrating older boys and men in 1893 to curb masturbation (Trent, 1994, p. 193). Replaced after a public outcry, Pilcher was reinstated and soon resumed his surgical activities, eventually sterilizing a total of 44 boys and 14 girls (Pfieffer, 1992, p. 482). Between 1899 and 1912, a physician at an Indiana mental institution performed 236 vasectomies, most of them illegally, until legislative authorization was enacted in 1907 (Pickens, 1968, p. 87).

An early leader in advocating sterilization was physician Orpheus Everts, head of the Cincinnati Sanitarium (Largent, 2008, pp. 12–13). He argued that the operation was an appropriate way to deal with convicted criminals who reflected "constitutional depravities that are recognized as transmittable by heredity." Such an approach, he predicted, would "eventuate in an effectual diminution of crime and the reformation of criminals" (as cited in Largent, p. 13).

Women were targeted for sexual surgery to treat "hysteria" and other types of "nervous" disorders, "sapphism" (homosexuality), "masturbation" and "promiscuity" (Largent, 2008, pp. 18–19; Pickens, 1968, pp. 90–91). In 1866, a Swiss psychiatrist sterilized a woman he claimed suffered a "sexual neurosis" (Degler, 1991, p. 87). In the Unied States, a young woman at the Pennsylvania Training School was given a hysterectomy in 1892, reportedly to reduce her sexual desires (Trent, 1994, p. 193).

Advocates of sterilization defended the practice as not only scientifically valid and fiscally wise but also universally beneficial to all, including its victims. The surgery's popularity among superintendents was boosted when feeblemindedness was scientifically verified to be primarily hereditary in nature and the operation was presented as a cost-effective way to discharge more residents without fear of procreation, reducing the spiraling expense of institutional enlargement (Noll, 1995, pp. 41–42). Further propelling involuntary sterilization were new surgical methods (tubal ligation and vasectomy) that proponents touted as less dangerous and severe than castration and even claimed to be "liberating" to its victims. While some feared that such "liberation" would result in accelerating licentiousness (Reilly, 1991, p. 44), others like Pennsylvania superintendent Kerlin cited sterilization's effect on one woman as her "salvation from vice and degradation," enabling her to enjoy a more "tranquil well ordered life," and demonstrate heightened "industry and usefulness" (as cited in Trent, 1994, p. 193).

By the end of the nineteenth century, a large and expanding group of U.S. physicians were transforming their campaign for compulsory sterilization as an antidote for sexual deviance into a wider movement, promoting the surgery as the most effective "treatment" for criminal behavior and preventing the "defective" classes that caused it (Largent, 2008, p. 17). It would not be long before physicians would be joined by a broad array of other professionals, scientists, philanthropists, and social activists.

Initial efforts to legalize eugenic sterilization stalled. A Michigan proposal to sterilize certain classes of criminals and feebleminded was defeated in 1897. In 1905, the Pennsylvania legislature passed the first sterilization law in the country, only to have it vetoed by the governor (Macklin & Gaylin, 1981, p. 65). Finally, in 1907, the governor of Indiana signed the first compulsory sterilization law targeting state institutional residents who were classified as insane, feebleminded, convicted rapists or other criminals who were designated by a board of experts (Ludmerer, 1972, p. 93). By 1915, thirteen states had eugenic sterilization laws (Pickens, 1968, p. 90).

Even as compulsory sterilization was growing more popular, it attracted an array of critics, none more persistent and vocal than the Roman Catholic Church. In 1930, Pope Pius XI issued a marriage encyclical, referring to eugenics as "that pernicious practice" (as cited in Black, 2003, p. 232) and condemning "divorce, birth control, and companionate marriage" (as cited in Kevles, 1985, p. 168). Some judges and politicians were also skeptical, as legal challenges to compulsory sterilization persisted. By 1913, laws were struck down in seven states (Reilly, 1991, p. 50). In 1915, Cornell could confidently assert that at the National Conference of Charities and Correction, sterilization as a viable way to control reproduction was dead:

> The sterilization of feebleminded is now universally acknowledged to be impractical, principally because the hereditary influence in this field has not been quantitatively determined, because the operation is dangerous, the idea more or less revolting, and possibly because it is not in consonance with the religious thought of a certain proportion of the community. Sterilization, therefore, need not be further discussed at this time. (as cited in Wolfensberger, 1975, p. 41)

Between 1918 and 1921, no new sterilization statutes were passed due to flagging scientific and legal support (Reilly, 1991, p. 71). The surgery was rejuvenated several years later, however, due to post-World War I anti-immigrant sentiments; the increasingly prominent role played by biologists who added scientific authenticity to the eugenic claims that some socially and physically undesirable human traits were inherited (Largent, 2008, p. 39); and the indefatigable activism and lobbying of ardent eugenicists, Charles Davenport and Harry Laughlin.

In 1922, Laughlin amended the language for a national sterilization law that addressed the constitutional questions that had clouded its more widespread acceptance. In earlier statutes, some states had declared the operation to be cruel and unusual punishment despite the inclusion of a therapeutic rationale, claiming physical and mental benefits to the individual (Davies, 1959, p. 56). Changing to an entirely eugenic focus, Laughlin clarified that the sole purpose of the law was "to prevent the procreation of persons socially inadequate from defective inheritance" (p. 56). He also expanded the list of targeted groups to virtually anyone who could be considered by authorities as troublesome. Propelled by continuing public fear and the increasing support of a growing number of professional supporters and social groups, as well as Laughlin's work, legislators began to revise their opinions in favor of sterilization, starting gradually in 1922 when the state of Washington passed its bill. Five more states passed legislation between 1923–24. In 1925, nine states passed eugenic sterilization laws (Reilly, 1991, pp. 83–84).

Although eugenic sterilizations were again on the rise, touted as an explicitly medical treatment—a vaccine against inherited human pathology that would prevent the infection of society—it was not so compelling to several prominent eugenic icons like Walter Fernald, Henry Goddard, and even Charles Davenport. While still seeing social menaces as the pre-eminent sources of society's problems, these individuals counseled against applying sterilization as the primary solution (Largent, 2008, pp. 60–61). Not only questioning whether there was sufficient scientific evidence to justify its widespread application, they also thought that sterilizing such large numbers, estimated by Davenport to be 38% of all children, was impractical and possibly unjust since many would likely be high functioning and some would not constitute a threat (p. 60). Fernald argued that debauchery and disease would inevitably result when already morally deficient people were "set free" by sterilization "to gratify their instincts without fear of consequences in the form of children" (as cited in Largent p. 61). These eugenic proponents preferred large-scale institutionalization, acknowledging that it was more immediately expensive, but more just, because people could be released if a mistake was discovered. Davenport also estimated that since segregation would reduce the incidence of mental deficiency in 15–20 years, large-scale institutionalization would eventually pay for itself (Largent, pp. 60–61). Despite such views, apparently Davenport did little to rein in his assistant, Henry Laughlin, from pursuing strident pro-sterilization activities.

As for Goddard, he did not reject sterilization entirely or recant his views on inherited intelligence, but he favored large scale institutionalization as the treatment of choice. By 1928, however, he had recanted as much of his early views as any of his eugenic colleagues. Goddard acknowledged that few people with a measured mental age of 12 were feebleminded and unable to manage their affairs; that proper education could greatly reduce the incidence of mental deficiency; and that the danger of "moron parents having imbecile or idiot children" was probably neglible" (as cited in Gould, 1996, p. 202).

Medical superintendents generally supported sterilization, but did so as much for practical and professional reasons as scientific ones. As larger facilities became harder to defend politically and fiscally, superintendents embraced sterilization as a persuasive economical strategy to increase "safe and well-supervised" discharges, and expand their professional influence and authority beyond the walls of the institution (Trent, 1994, p. 200).

At the beginning of twentieth century, medical superintendents were experiencing a kind of professional malaise and increasing lack of respect. Presiding over large institutions increasingly viewed as custodial and ineffective in treating patients who were considered chronic and incurable, medical superintendents faced the very pessimistic prospect of being considered irrelevant, treated as institutional managers and out-of-touch administrators rather than dynamic medical practitioners and researchers (Rafter, 1997, p.169). To extract themselves from the professional doldrums, many looked beyond the institution for new career opportunities, treatment tools and prospective clientele, reinventing themselves in the progressive reform image of the day: "optimistic and activist, introducing scientific reforms, stressing the need for prevention and intent on creating a new, manageable and efficient society" (Rafter, 1997, p. 170; Scull, 2005, p. 59).

Emerging from the effort to reinvent themselves was the National Committee of Mental Hygiene (NCMH), a group of reform-minded, "progressive alienists" who eventually began referring to themselves as more modern-sounding "psychiatrists" (Rafter, 1997, p. 170; Scull, 2005, p. 59). The NCMH was a fascinating organization that was founded in 1909 by Clifford Beers, a Yale educated, former resident of the Connecticut Hospital for the Insane. As a patient there, he experienced harsh, abusive treatment that he described vividly in a remarkable and compelling book titled, *A Mind That Found Itself*. Published in 1908, his book attracted a wide audience and led Beers to begin a national campaign to reform the nation's asylums and treatment of the mentally ill (Grob, 1983, pp. 147–149). Although the NCMH began as the first, ex-patient reform organization, it was quickly diluted and diverted by medical professionals who persuaded Beers to change direction. Forming an unlikely alliance with Dr. Alfred Meyer, superintendent of the Worcester (Massachusetts) State Hospital, Beers was persuaded by Meyers to adopt a less critical posture toward psychiatry. Comprised mostly of medical superintendents, the committee's stated mission became: "protect the public's mental health; promote research into and dissemination of material pertaining to the etiology, treatment, and prevention of mental disease; enlist the aid of the federal government; and establish state societies for mental hygiene" (p. 153). Beers intention to stop the abuse of mental patients and improve their treatment was redirected to the more amorphous goal of preventing mental illness and eventually to preventing all forms of social dependency, including feeblemindedness (Grob, 1983, pp. 162–164; Scull, 2005, p. 58).

Meyer, one of the most eminent psychiatrists of that period, attempted to present a gentler image of psychiatry through the NCMH, focusing on research and prevention of mental disease, and avoiding close alignment with what he considered "eugenic excesses" (Scull, 2005, pp. 14, 59). The new lexicon of progressive psychiatry included terms like community adjustment, supervision, and services and emphasized the professional (psychiatric) treatment of the potentially large "extra-institutional" populations of people considered feebleminded, e.g. those located physically outside the facility (Trent, 1994, p. 181). The NCMH was eventually funded by powerful and wealthy foundations established by John D. Rockefeller, Andrew Carnegie, and E. J. Harriman, and supported emerging community social work settings and practices such as child guidance clinics, in-school interventions, and mental and psychological testing (Gallagher, 1999, p. 74).

The NCMH took no official position on eugenic sterilization (Grob, 1983, p. 173), although its membership consisted of many eugenicists who easily mixed the language of menace and mental hygiene (Gallagher, 1999, p. 74; Rafter, 1997, p. 176). As Beers's influence waned, and despite the growing costs of large scale institutionalization and an emerging caution among some scientists concerning the "menace of feeblemindedness," medical superintendents retained a vested interest in institutional growth (Trent, 1994, pp 179–183). It is not surprising that after 1912, the NCMH provided the professional rationale, leadership, and support for promoting and constructing institutions across the country, particularly in the Southeast (Dowbiggin, 1997, p. 127; Noll, 1995, p. 16). NCMH members were particularly distressed about losing influence to psychology rivals within The Committee on Provision for the Feeble-Minded and were at least as interested in using their own organization to further their professional ends as they were in reforming or reducing the nation's institutions (p. 178).

THE *BUCK V. BELL* DECISION: THE SUPREME ENDORSEMENT OF EUGENIC STERILIZATION

In 1927, the U.S. Supreme Court trumped emerging scientific skepticism and religious objections, endorsing eugenic sterilization of institutionalized residents considered to have inherited feeblemindedness. In its notorious *Buck v. Bell* decision the Court upheld the right of the State of Virginia to involuntary sterilize a 17-year old, pregnant Caucasian woman named Carrie Buck who, like her mother, was admitted to the Virginia Colony of Epileptics and the Feebleminded and gave birth to an allegedly mentally deficient daughter, Vivian. Both Henry Laughlin and Arthur Estabrook of the Eugenics Records Office certified Ms. Buck and her daughter as having "inherited feeblemindedness," and in need of the surgery (Kevles, 1985, pp. 110–111).

The Court that included such notable Justices as Oliver Wendell Holmes, Louis D. Brandeis and former President, William Howard Taft, voted eight to one, the lone dissenter being Pierce Butler, a Catholic who issued no dissenting opinion. The decision was announced by Chief Justice Oliver Wendell Holmes in what Gould (1996) referred to as "one of the most famous and chilling statements of our century" (p. 365):

> We have seen more than once that the public welfare may call upon the best citizens for their lives. It would be strange if it could not call upon those who sap the strength of the state for these lesser sacrifices ... in order to avoid our being swamped by incompetence. It is better for all the world, if instead of waiting to execute degenerate offspring for crime, or let them starve to death for their imbecility, society can prevent those who are manifestly unfit from continuing their kind. The principle that sustains compulsory vaccination is broad enough to cover cutting the Fallopian tubes.... Three generations of imbeciles are enough. (as cited in Lombardo, 2008, p. 287)

Supporting the constitutionality of compulsory sterilization for all people deemed mentally deficient, institutionalized or not, the Court bolstered not only the flagging inheritability and menace myths, but also the need to extend the surgery beyond the institution in order to control an ever expanding menace. In a less quoted section of his statement Holmes explains that:

> But, it is said, however it might be if this reasoning were applied generally, it fails when it is confined to the small numbers who are in the institutions named and is not applied to the multitude.... Of course so far as the operations enable those who otherwise must be kept confined to be returned to the world, and thus open the asylum to others, the equality (between institutionalized and non-institutionalized defectives) aimed at will more nearly be reached. (as cited in Lombardo, 2008, p. 287)

Overall, the Great Depression should have had a mixed effect on the eugenics movement. Not sparing the upper classes, it debunked the Social Darwinist claim that wealth and social standing reflected genetic superiority and weakened arguments for large-scale sterilization and incarceration of the poor (Ludmerer, 1972, p.127). On the other hand, blame for the economic disaster could be more easily attributed to societal deterioration due to the differential birthrates among the unfit (Kevles, 1985, p. 114). In addition, the spreading financial calamity led to increasing pressure from town officials and some families for institutional relief from rising poverty (Trent, 1994, p. 218). Large state institutions also provided well-established economic benefits, functioning like sizable local businesses, employing numerous workers and requiring a variety of goods and services, all of which offered fiscal and employment stability to the surrounding area.

Following *Buck v. Bell*, sterilizations increased dramatically from 1932 to the beginning of World War II and were being performed in more states than ever (Kevles, 1985, p. 116). Before that decision, less than 6,000 people had been sterilized across the country, mostly in California. After the Court's ruling, the total of those castrated or sterilized soared to almost 36,000 by the end of 1940 (Black, 2003, p. 123). Endorsed as constitutional, the surgery could be extolled on virtually all fronts, claiming to benefit all parties including its victims. Harvey Watkins, superintendent of the Polk (Pennsylvania) School and future president of the American Association on Mental Deficiency (AAMD), proclaimed in 1930 that after 10,000 reported surgeries, it was clear that sterilization "saved thousands of taxpayer dollars," was a "blessing" to the community "freed from worries about future defectives," and but also benefitted "mental defectives, who could now be paroled, freed from the constraints of parenthood" (as cited in Trent, 1994, pp. 200–201).

Watkins titled his paper "Selective Sterilization," reflecting the emerging trend of using the term "selective" to denote a more limited policy that targeted those certified by physicians as "clearly" having a hereditary form of mental deficiency" (Paul, 1965, pp. 171–172). A 1933 White House Conference on Child Heath and Protection also used the term "selective sterilization," although it is difficult to discern what specific limitations were being proposed:

> There are at present no legal, surgical, or humanitarian obstacles to the extensive practice of selective sterilization of the adult feebleminded; these facts should be impressed upon the consciousness of every responsible citizen.... When adequately safeguarded, little individual or social danger attends sterilization ... and ... selective sterilization may be regarded as a highly desirable, although perhaps not indispensable, adjunct to any program of prevention. (as cited in Paul, 1965, p. 71)

Carrie Buck's daughter, Vivian, died in 1932 at age 8. Her teachers reported that while in elementary school, she was considered "very bright" (Kevles, 1985, p. 112).

Despite the continuing endorsement of the surgery by the Court and medical community, times were dramatically changing economically and scientifically. As Gould (1996, p. 29) observed, "most of the men who built biodeterminism in the 1920s recanted their own conclusions during the liberal swing of the 1930s when Ph.D.'s walked depression breadlines and poverty could no longer be explained by innate stupidity" (Kevles, 1985, p. 148). As importantly, a group of outspoken, highly respected, and well published British biologists, J. B. S. Haldane, Lancelot Hogben, and Julian Huxley, and their American colleague, Herbert S. Jennings, began arguing that mainline eugenics reflected racial and class prejudice more than proven scientific fact (pp. 122–128). A widely circulated book, *Human Sterilization*, written in 1932 by lawyer, Jacob H. Landman, coupled with a 1934 report from England's Department Committee on Sterilization, seriously challenged the evidence behind widespread sterilization, terming compulsory sterilization unscientific and speculative (Paul, 1965, pp 73–77). Around the same time, the American Neurological Association (ANA), "the only scientific organization to make a systematic study of state eugenic sterilization in America (p. 77), formed a committee titled the Committee for the Investigation of Sterilization. Under the leadership of Tufts University professor and sterilization critic, Abraham Myerson, the group issued a widely regarded and read report in 1935–36 that slowed the national momentum of the harshest eugenics practices across the country and signaled the beginning of the end of involuntary sterilization in the United States (Sofair & Kaldjiian, 2000, pp. 316–317). The Committee dismissed the ideas that: (1) "feeblemindedness and other forms of social deviancy" were rapidly increasing; (2) "defectives" were reproducing at higher rates than those considered "fit;" (3) the societal threat posed by those considered unfit was sufficiently great to warrant their sterilization; and (4) most mental diseases were "clearly or solely hereditary in origin" (Largent, 2008, p. 122; Paul, 1965, pp. 77–78; Sofair & Kaldijian, 2000, p. 316).

In the early 1930s, the boards of both the *New England Journal of Medicine* and the *Journal of the American Medical Association* began to retreat slowly from their pro-sterilization views, particularly surgeries considered "mandatory" (Sofair & Kaldjiian, 2000, pp. 316–317). Referring to the ANA report, the *New England Journal of Medicine* wrote that "until a deeper scientific understanding of mental disorders was achieved, laws to prevent propagation by sterilization are unwise, and sterilization should certainly not be mandatory" (p. 317). The *Journal of the American Medical Association* (*JAMA*) had endorsed the surgery as a solution to the "economic and criminal problems associated with mental illness," but narrowed its endorsement to persons whose "mental diseases were clearly heritable," and warned that "the established genetic foundation must not be exceeded" (p. 317). The journals' editors did not explicitly reject the idea of sterilization, per se, only indirectly criticizing involuntary surgeries, and supporting the operation as a "rational procedure" in "voluntary" form and when applied "selectively" (p. 317). Neither organization addressed the coercive nature of many "voluntary" operations.

WORLD WAR II, NAZI ATROCITIES, AND THE DEMISE OF MAINSTREAM EUGENICS

In 1933, Germany's Nazi government passed a "mass, compulsory sterilization law," targeting "defectives," including those classified with "feeblemindedness, schizophrenia, manic depression, Huntington's chorea, epilepsy, hereditary body deformities, deafness, hereditary blindness, and, selectively alcoholism" (Black, 2003, p. 299). Legally redefining religion as race, the Germans passed what became known as the Nuremberg Laws in 1935. The laws effectively transformed religious prejudice into eugenics science, legally defining Jews as a separate race, stripping them of their citizenship, restricting their marriages, and disenfranchising those determined to be "half or quarter Jews" as well as practicing Christians suspected of having Jewish ancestry (Black, 2003, p. 311).

In the United States, despite heightened criticism of the underlying science and growing international outrage at German social policy, eugenic advocates applauded the new German laws, touted their American origins, and emphasized their own influence on German policy makers (Black, 2003, pp. 299-300). In 1936, editorials in the *New England Journal of Medicine* referred to Germany as "the most progressive nation in restricting fecundity among the unfit" (Lombardo, 2008, p. 203). While *Buck v. Bell* continued to offer legal cover for U. S. sterilization laws, criticisms and legal challenges continued (Lombardo, 2008, p. 219). Eugenic surgeries receded during World War II largely due to an absence of available physicians, coupled with the 1942 *Skinner v. Oklahoma* Supreme Court decision that prohibited the use of compulsory sterilization as punishment for criminal acts (Nourse, 2008; Paul, 1965, pp. 86–87).

Following the war, and despite the revelations of Nazi atrocities, the number of eugenic sterilizations in the U.S. again rose. Although more scientists were critical of eugenic practices and the fledgling community of geneticists were trying to separate themselves from mainline eugenic activities and organizations, they had less impact than might have been expected, underscoring the extent to which eugenic ideology had become more ingrained in the national psyche than is generally acknowledged (Black, 2003, p. 7; Largent, 2008, p. 7). In fact, eugenics proved to be a prominent American export to Germany and elsewhere. The U.S. sterilization campaign of the 1920s and 1930s influenced Canada, Sweden, Norway, Finland, France, and Japan to enact similar laws (Barondess, 1998, p. 892). Moreover, while the histories of the U.S. and German eugenic movements contain some important differences, they include "many similarities of motivation, intent, and strategy" (Sofair & Kaldjiian, 2000, pp. 312–314). The passage of Germany's first eugenic sterilization law was based directly on U.S. statutes, while Germany's euthanasia practices toward disabled children during the 1930s was based on eugenic science emanating from the United States and the United Kingdom (Mitchell & Snyder, 2003, p. 857). German officials acknowledged the important role that California's "successful" compulsory sterilization campaign played in their policy decisions, and bestowed on the tireless American eugenic advocate, Henry Laughlin, an honorary doctor of medicine which he accepted in New York in 1939 (Kevles, 1985, p. 118).

Following World War II, eugenic ideas, increasingly associated with Nazi horrors, were widely discredited but not entirely discarded. In fact, for decades afterwards, eugenic sterilization, rights restrictions, and social segregation were promoted by "progressive" physical and social scientists, lawyers, judges, politicians, philanthropists, educators, as well as a collection of "do-gooders, racists and utopians" (Largent, 2008, pp. 6–7). Institutionalization continued to rise throughout the United States until 1968 for persons with intellectual disabilities, and like other rights restrictions, continued into the new millennium in some states. Decades after the war, eugenic advocates continued to emphasize contraception, referring to "population control" at home and abroad, the latter focusing on circumstances in the "developing world" while the former attending to birthrates at the low end of the social stratum which in the U.S. increasingly meant African Americans (as cited in Kevles, 1985, pp. 258–259). Legal scholars and social scientists in the U.S. did not begin shifting their positions completely on sterilization until the late 1950s and early 1960s, while the American Medical Association did not end its support of involuntary sterilizations until after its legal and socioeconomic committee issued its report critical of the practice in 1960 (Largent, 2008, pp. 8, 124–125).

In 1954, biologists, James Neel and William Schull condemned the eugenics of the past in their widely circulated text, *Human Heredity*, but carefully endorsed "a reform version" with the stated intent of "advancing the science of human genetics" (Kevles, 1985, p. 251). As a group, biologists, perhaps the most authoritative body on the topic, did not explicitly connect the eugenics movement with the Nazi holocaust and treat the term "eugenics" as an epithet until the late 1970s and early 1980s (Largent, 2008, pp. 8–9). More broadly, popular recognition of the link between the American eugenics movement and the Holocaust did not occur in the U.S. for decades after the war (p. 117). It might still be argued that this association has not yet been fully acknowledged.

The decade of the 1960s saw the rise of a reconfigured eugenics movement, propelled by a group of American intellectuals whose views became well publicized within both the scientific community and the general public, causing intense and widespread controversy and debate (Kevles, 1985, p. 267). By the late 1960s, based on new and revolutionary discoveries in the field of human genetics and biochemistry, biologists could uncover and diagnose a rapidly growing list of chromosomal and genetic disorders. By the next decade, "carriers of at least 50 different genetic disorders could be identified; virtually all 100 chromosomal disorders could be detected in uterus, as well as 23 inborn errors of metabolism, … and 40 more seemed potentially detectable" (p. 267). Such remarkable progress led Robert Sinsheimer, a well respected California Institute of Technology molecular biologist, to announce the arrival of a "new eugenics" that would permit in principle the conversion of all of the unfit "to the highest genetic level with the potential to create new genes and new qualities yet undreamed" (as cited in Kevles, pp. 267–268). In the mid-1970s, Harvard zoologist, Edmund Wilson introduced the idea of "sociobiology" and appeared to revive Herbert Spencer's doctrine of social Darwinism by endorsing the biological social status quo, and arguing that human social behavior should be more carefully controlled by "precise steering based on biological knowledge" (pp. 272–275).

Berkeley professor, Arthur Jensen, sparked a national debate in 1969 when he reported that his research on human intelligence revealed racial differences that were largely biological and inherited. At the same time Nobel laureate William Shockley, a physicist, proposed paying voluntarily sterilized individuals according to how many IQ points they scored below 100 (Gould, 1996, p. 24). He also endorsed the idea of collecting and making available to "healthy and intelligent females" the sperm of prominent intellectuals like himself (Kevles, 1985, p. 263). Summing up the decades following World War II, Kevles (1985, p. 276), concludes that

> in renewed claims of a dependence of intelligence upon race or class, the popularity of sociobiology, the revived apprehensions about a differential birthrate, the fresh resorts to sterilizations, there is a good deal that would have warmed the heart of an early-twentieth-century mainline eugenicist. (p. 276)

THE EMERGENCE OF FAMILY-LED ADVOCACY AND ORGANIZATIONS

After the war, an ebullient and optimistic America was bombarded with images of domestic tranquility, security, materialism and fulfillment. Social life was idyllically portrayed in advertisements for a dizzying array of new household products, later presented in television sitcoms like *Father Knows Best* and *Leave It To Beaver*, and increasingly lived in freshly excavated housing tracts on the outskirts of America's cities. Family togetherness was the main message and having children was considered the key ingredient to family bliss. As Jones (2004) remarked, however, "No where in this picture of familial bliss was there space for a child who failed to measure up, who was not 'perfect,' or in the 1950s discourse on mental retardation, 'normal' " (p. 324). Such idealized images of "normal" American family life, so integrally linked with trouble-free fulfillment, exacerbated a family's sense of difference, adding new rationales for the removal of a child with disability. Difference, conflict, and pathology were also reinforced in professional writings and advice that urged removing children with disabilities, claiming their inclusion in the family would adversely affect its cohesion, mental health, and stability, psychologically damaging nondisabled siblings (Castles, 2004, p. 361). Institutional officials would often discourage parents, from frequent visits and ongoing contacts with their child following placement, purportedly for their own emotional well being and that of their child's (Carey, 2009, p. 106).

Despite the existing professional wisdom, many parents who placed their child in an state facility remained actively involved, taking them home, visiting frequently, and participating as volunteers and donors. Moreover, most families did not institutionalize their children, sometimes due to long waiting lists and/or concerns about the existing institutional conditions, but most frequently because of their desire to apply what they considered typical child rearing practices to their child with a disability (Carey, 2009, pp. 106–107).

Many young, middle class, mostly suburban women, often separated from extended family, discovered that raising a child with a disability was often atypical and began reaching out to each other in increasing numbers to form social networks and join local civic and community groups (Metzel, 2004, p. 433). The ensuing parental activism, initially stimulated by mutual support, was further fueled by a lack of noninstitutional options and services, and the exclusion of large numbers of their children with disabilities from public school (p. 433). Parent-led groups also benefitted from well publicized disclosures in the early 1950s by celebrities, like author Pearl Buck and actors Roy and Dale Rogers, who publically revealed having children with disabilities (Trent, 1994, p. 234). In an another widely read book, John Frank, a noncelebrity, law professor, described in detail the experiences he and his wife had after learning they had a child with a disability. As he related their personal dilemmas and financial struggles in seeking the best quality care for their young son, Frank's experiences resonated with many other families in similar circumstances (Carey, 2009, p. 111). Years later, the family of Massachusetts Senator and Democratic Party presidential nominee, John F. Kennedy, revealed that one of their members, Rosemary, had a disability, virtually eliminating the family stigma associated with such circumstances and opening the door to national reform.

In 1946, a New Jersey housewife named Laura Blossfeld who had a 9-year old son identified as mentally retarded published a plea in her local newspaper for other parents to join her in forming an organization to help their children with disabilities. This action led to the formation of the first New Jersey Parents Group for Retarded Children in 1947 (Jones, 2004, p. 328). Two years later a similar ad in a New York City paper started the Association for the Help of Retarded Children (Castles, 2004, p. 351). Such groups were not entirely new, dating back to the 1930s in New York, Ohio, and Washington State, and were initially started by parents of institutionalized children who saw themselves as supplementing and supporting the facility's programs (Carey, 2009, pp. 105–106; Jones, 2004, p. 328). As associations expanded in the late 1940s to many states, parental membership became more varied and included those who institutionalized their children and those who did not; those who favored large state facilities and those who did not. By1950, 88 parent groups existed in 19 states with over 19,000 members. (Castles, 2004, p. 351; Jacobs, Weingold, & Dubrow, 1965, p. ix). That same year, chapters from 14 states joined together to form the National Association of Parents and Friends of Mentally Retarded Children, a group that in 1952 became the National Association for Retarded Children (NARC)

(Jones, 2004, p. 328). By 1960, the NARC had 681 local affiliates and a membership of 62,000 (Castles, 2004, p. 351).

What was particularly notable about the parent-led movement was how effectively families supported each other in breaking from the social isolation and stigma that marked the experiences of prewar families; declaring their normality and that of their families; openly questioning expert theories and advice that encouraged quick and permanent institutionalization of their children; and publically calling for more community connectedness, support, and organization (Farber, 1968, p. 147). As Jones (2004) points out:

> The claims of domesticity brought these particular families together and structured the activities of the NARC units.... [T]he units pressed the traditional goals of mother's groups-mutual support and public awareness. In addition, the groups voiced a spirit of entitlement that was decidedly new and grounded in the family ideology of togetherness. Their children were part of the family and deserved the same degree of care, concerns, and ultimately services that the family (and the community) offered "normal children. Their definition of family and children also went beyond the biological boundaries. (p. 329)

The NARC emerged not only as a large, interconnected parental support network, but also as a national political advocacy force that changed forever the way in which people with mental retardation and their families were defined and treated. The movement effectively wrestled with mental retardation professionals for control and change, started their own schools and day programs, called for expanded educational opportunities for children who were considered lower functioning, and proposed legal reforms and institutional service alternatives.

Since membership in NARC chapters now included parents with diverse views about state institutions, the relationship between factions who favored such facilities and those who did not became increasingly strained. Each group reflected different perspectives on family life and what constituted proper treatment of children, whether disabled or typical, within the family. To avoid a schism, NARC chapters attempted to navigate a middle course, supporting institutional reforms while advocating for more community options. NARC executive director from 1957–63, Gunnar Dybwad, criticized the role, conditions, and centrality of large-scale state institutions and called for smaller, home-like residences, but also acknowledged that large facilities would be needed for the foreseeable future (Carey, 2009, p. 123).

Ongoing differences between parent groups within the NARC led to divergent and often conflicting priorities and proposals. Eventually, proponents of state institutions began forming their own chapters and organizations (Castles, 2004, p. 353). As both sides began to compete for political allies, the rift caused considerable political and public confusion over who truly represented the "parent" perspective.

Although parental supporters of state institutions were a minority, they lobbied hard and effectively for continued state and federal support, vigorously opposing institutional reductions and de-institutionalization legislation. Like the NARC, proinstitutional families allied with some union groups and professionals to form a national alliance called the "Congress for Advocates of the Retarded, Inc." (Landesman & Butterfield, 1987, p. 811). The perspective of this group is illustrated by their "friend of the court" petition to the Supreme Court during its review of *Haldeman v. Pennhurst State School and Hospital* (1977), the landmark "anti-institutional" case:

> The degree of disabilities suffered by the mentally retarded residents of public institutions is far more severe than the court believed. The reality of mental retardation is inconsistent with a presumption in favor of deinstitutionalization. It cannot be assumed that a CLA (community living arrangement) will be "less restrictive" or "more normalizing" than an institution; for many retarded people, only an institution can provide adequate services and programs. A system relying more heavily on CLAs would be unstable and inadequately monitored and would not assure quality of care. (Gottesman, Weinberg, & Collins, 1980, as cited in Landesman & Butterfield, 1987, pp. 6–7)

Despite the best efforts of some parental groups to portray institutions and their staff positively, they were dealt a severe setback in the mid-1960s when vivid accounts and lurid photographs publically revealed unimaginably dehumanizing conditions within state institutions in the Northeast United States. In 1965, New York Senator Robert Kennedy visited the Willowbrook State School on Staten Island where he expressed outrage at the squalid conditions he found. The following year a university professor, Burton Blatt, and a photographer, Fred Kaplan, published graphic images of institutional life they took surreptitiously during the Christmas holidays inside several state institutions for persons with intellectual disabilities. Calling their collection *Christmas in Purgatory* (Blatt & Kaplan, 1966), they revealed shocking photos that appeared in 1967 in *Look* magazine, dramatically revealing to a wide public audience living conditions that legal advocates, families, media, and politicians immediately declared a national disgrace. Soon local media were examining conditions within their state's facilities, exposing conditions similar to those revealed in *Look*. Largely hidden from public view, grossly overcrowded, underfunded, and deteriorating, state facilities quickly became the object of public and legal outrage, debate and reform.

Even before the shocking series of institutional revelations, deinstitutional activities had begun quietly across the country. The discovery and widespread application of tranquilizing medications dramatically altered the treatment of all institutionalized persons, beginning with those in psychiatric hospitals where enrollments went from a peak of 559,000 in 1955 to 475,000 in 1965, and to less than 200,000 twenty years later, a drop of 65% (Bassuck & Gerson, 1978; National Institute on Mental Health, 1979, as cited in Lakin & Bruinicks, 1985a, p. 13). Following John F. Kennedy's election to the presidency in the early 1960s and the elevation of mental health and mental retardation to more visible national priorities, heightened research and practice funding was offered in order to expand existing programs, offer community alternatives, and reduce the enrollments of large state facilities.

From the mid-1960s through the mid-1970s, the country became deeply and bitterly divided along political, racial, and generational lines, buffeted by spreading civil rights confrontations, escalating Vietnam War protests, and growing government scandals. Taking a cue from the civil rights struggles of African Americans, disability activists began defining disability as a legal issue and institutionalization as a form of discrimination. According to Minow (1990, p. 109), a rights analysis begins with the view that legal rights apply to everyone and is skeptical about the accuracy of particular assumptions and classifications of abnormality or mental incompetence when applied to those who have endured a history of unjust and/or cruel treatment.

The fledgling disability rights movement arose in Berkeley, California in the late 1960, through the efforts of a small group of University of California students, the most prominent of whom was a young man named Ed Roberts. Roberts and his colleagues called themselves the Rolling Quads and rebelled against the physical, social and professional restrictiveness they experienced as students that isolated them from typical campus and community life and minimized their personal choices and control (Shapiro, 1993, pp 49–51). Eventually, they developed the first "Center for Independent Living" (CIL) in the country, establishing a setting from which to conduct social and political advocacy, and offer peer services and supports to assist people with disabilities lead more self-directed lives (pp. 41–55). From the groundbreaking work of Roberts and his colleagues sprung an alternative, activist definition of disability and model of services that contrasted sharply with the predominantly medical approach that treated people with disabilities as primarily patients and was dominated by nondisabled professionals. As disability was seen primarily through the lens of civil rights rather than medicine and the problem was seen as more societal than individual, the solution became focused on social change more than person change.

The concept of "independent living" became widely popular. The language was included in the landmark 1973 Rehabilitation Act, and expanded into to an accepted rehabilitation service in the 1978 Rehabilitation Act Amendments. By the late 1980s, there existed more than 300 federally funded CIL's nationwide (Carey, 2009, p. 137).

Across the country, disability activism was increasing and gaining widespread visibility. In 1970, Judy Heumann, was denied a teaching certificate by New York City's Board of Education despite having competed all the requirements (Shapiro, 1993, pp. 55–58). Heumann who would eventually join Roberts in Berkeley and become an internationally known disability rights advocate in her own right, sued the board and formed a political coalition, called Disabled in Action that drew wide media and public attention for its disability rights and antiwar protests (pp. 57–58).

Due largely to the political activities and public protests of disability activists and returning Vietnam wounded and disabled veterans who were protesting their treatment, the 1970s yielded unprecedented disability rights and educational legislation that included pioneering federal laws such as the 1973 Rehabilitation Act, the 1975 Developmental Disabilities Act, and the Education for All Handicapped Children Act of 1975 were passed. Fashioned on the Civil Rights Act of 1964, the 1973 Rehabilitation Act was the first civil rights bill for persons with disabilities, and the precursor to the broader 1990 Americans With Disabilities Act.

Using this landmark legislation, and newly enacted state statutes, the National Association of Retarded Children (NARC) became a primary plaintiff in numerous state class action lawsuits advocating for services that would be offered to persons with disabilities in the "least restricted environment." This phrase was interpreted in varied ways, illustrated by phrases like, "as normal a way as possible," "maximum reasonable level of [community] integration" and/or "settings that enhance societal participation" (Lakin & Bruinicks, 1985a, p. 16). While the term, "least restricted environment" would serve as the legal antidote for institutionalization, an emerging concept called the "Principle of Normalization" would form the conceptual and practical framework for the de-institutionalization movement that was about to dominate the field of mental retardation.

The normalization idea originated in Denmark, by the head of the Danish Mental Retardation Services, Niels Erik Bank-Mikkelsen, as "letting the mentally retarded obtain an existence as close to the normal as possible" (Wolfensberger, 1972, p. 27). Subsequently, Bank-Mikkelsen was instrumental in having that principle written into Danish law in 1959. The term "normalization" was virtually unknown in the

U.S. until 1969 when the Swedish director of that country's Association for Retarded Children, Bengt Nirje, wrote a chapter in the widely-read federal publication, *Changing Patterns in Residential Services of the Mentally Retarded* (Carey, 2009, p, 141). Nirje (1969) defined normalization as "making available to the mentally retarded, patterns and conditions of everyday life that are close as possible to the norms and patterns of the mainstream of the society" (p. 181). Later, Wolf Wolfensberger, a Syracuse University professor, operationalized the concept, adding specific rules for its implementation, offering training to those who wished to apply it in their organizations and practices, and later renaming the concept *Social Role Valorization* in 1980. Through his training materials and activities, coupled with his book, *The Principle of Normalization in Human Services,* Wolfensberger, was instrumental in disseminating the idea throughout the United States.

Although Normalization would serve as a framework for the de-institutionalization movement, it would prove to be controversial. As a powerful critique and a practical alternative to traditional rehabilitative practices, it challenged societal attitudes and policies, parental domains, and entrenched professional interests. Dramatic social reforms were looming, however, and while advocates of Normalization were premature in the 1970s, they would prove to be prescient in a few short years.

Nowhere was change more evident than in the legal arena. The first important "right to education" litigation occurred when Pennsylvania's Association for Retarded Citizens (PARC) challenged the exclusion of their children from community public schools, only to be the institutionalized in deplorable state facilities As Laski (1985) describes the situation:

> Throughout the country, state laws, excluding children from public schools codified and legitimized the practice of institutionalization of young children and continued to encourage institutional admissions of school-age children even during the late 1960s when the institutional census began to decrease.
>
> Given this background, it was no accident that early litigation efforts were the result of parents who began to organize out of concern for inhumane conditions in institutions and their frustration with traditional political solutions to chronic neglect, abuse, and maltreatment.
>
> The 1972 federal court decision in the *PARC* case marked the beginning of the end of school exclusion for severely handicapped children and, if not the beginning of the closing of state institutions, at least stemming the tide of admissions to institutions by securing needed alternative services

> and by establishing the importance of habilitation in programs for severely handicapped persons. (p. 69)

The 1970s also saw a series of "right to treatment" court cases that focused on the living conditions in state institutions and represented the first significant attempts to use constitutional arguments to improve the living arrangements within these settings, thereby enhancing the lives of those considered to be mentally disabled (Bradley, 1985, p. 83; Laski, 1985, p. 70). The first of these cases, *Wyatt v. Stickney*, 1972, was directed at the mental health system of Alabama, and was followed by rulings in Nebraska, New York, and Minnesota (see *Horacek v. Exon*, 1973; *New York State Association for Retarded Citizens v. Rockefeller*, 1973; *Welsch v. Likins*, 1974) in which the courts ruled that residents of state institutions had a constitutional right to habilitation or at least a right to protection from harm (Laski, 1985, p. 70)

Up to this point, both the right to education and habilitation cases focused primarily on institutional improvement, allowing for the continuing segregation of certain individuals, such as those considered severely impaired. Shortly, however, this perspective would dramatically change. As Laski (1985, p. 71) points out, advocates would apply the *PARC and Wyatt* rulings, with their underpinnings of equal protection and due process, coupled with newly enacted state and federal laws, to *replace,* not merely *improve,* state facilities. This "anti-institutionalization" focus emerged unexpectedly in another Pennsylvania case, *Haldeman v. Pennhurst State School and Hospital,* in which a class action was filed on behalf of Terri Lee Haldeman and her fellow residents of the notorious Pennhurst facility. Initially arguing for institutional reform and minimum standards of care, the lawyers for the plaintiffs successfully argued that Pennhurst, due to its segregated character and deplorably overcrowded and neglectful conditions, was by its very nature incapable of offering adequate care (Bradley, 1985, p. 84). In this way, the argument "moved beyond institutional improvement to a community imperative based on constitutional and statutory bases" (p. 84).

Another, less publicized, court decision also contributed to the de-institutionalization cause by both illuminating and prohibiting the long standing and exploitive practice of using institutional residents as unpaid or underpaid workers. In 1972, a federal class action suit in Maine, *Jorthberg, et al v. U.S. Department of Labor and Augusta State Hospital*, was filed seeking an end to an institutional labor practice that originated with the first institutions built in the United States and was legitimated as both justifiable resident payment to the state and as an effective rehabilitation tool. While *Jorthberg* specifically addressed unjust employment practices within the Maine psychiatric facility, its ensuing consent decree effectively required residents of any institution to be paid at least minimum wage for their work. Eliminating the blatantly exploitive policy of retaining residents in state institutions because of their value as workers, the decision served as an incentive for facility officials to discharge more individuals in order to reduce their enrollment costs. Unfortunately, it did not lead to great increases in employment among skilled residents. Too often, institutional officials simply terminated workers from doing the jobs many had been performing competently for years.

Releasing institutional residents into community living and working situations was not a revolutionary idea. Dating as far back as 1916, Charles Bernstein demonstrated in upstate New York that residents could be successfully employed outside of a state institution, while many subsequent studies documented that released residents could adjust and function successfully within the community, if adequately supported (Lakin, Bruinicks, & Sigford, 1981, as cited in Lakin & Bruinicks, 1985a, p. 10). The most widely publicized study of this kind was one conducted in the early 1960s by a California anthropologist, Robert Edgerton, who described the lives of 48 former residents following their release from Pacific State Hospital in California. Edgerton's work was widely interpreted as showing the resiliency and adaptive capacities of formerly institutionalized people despite years of incarceration and a lack of preparation. According to Edgerton (1967), ex-residents could "achieve some notable successes in the community despite the fact that they received inadequate preparation from the institution" (p. 211). Often overlooked in his research, however, is the caveat that not all who were discharged blended seamlessly and successfully into community life after years of societal separation:

> These former patients do some things quite adequately, but ... usually fail in their attempts to cope with the exigencies of everyday life; it would appear that, with a few exceptions, they would not be able to maintain themselves in the outside community without the assistance of normal benefactors. They usually fail to pass as well. They are often surprisingly clever in their techniques of passing and they are always dogged in their efforts. Nonetheless, they are successful in deceiving relatively few people. (Edgerton, 1967, p. 217)

Despite Edgerton's warnings, facilities across the country released people with little or no planning and support, resulting in many inappropriate, unsuccessful and tragic placements and leading to public reservations, even resistance, to de-institutionalization slowing its acceptance and progress nationwide.

Interestingly, the resistance of local communities to the release of institutional residents often provided individuals with disabilities a forum to tell their own stories about institutional life, opening the door to developing a collective voice. And in speaking out against institutionalization, they were not alone. Despite well documented problems and setbacks, deinstitutionalization was actively promoted by disability rights organizations, becoming an integral part of their legal offensive that eventually culminated in the passage of the 1990 Americans with Disabilities Act. People with intellectual disabilities were not, however, considered integral players in the first wave of disability rights and independent living efforts by those in or outside the movement (Gilson, 1998, p. 6). In order for people with intellectual disability to gain more recognition and control, they needed to find a collective voice and learn how to effectively express it.

The parallel cry for equal rights and self-determination by persons with intellectual and developmental disabilities has been termed the "self-advocacy" movement (Shapiro, 1993, p. 185). Like normalization, the movement started in Sweden and migrated to Canada several years later (Williams & Shoultz, 1982). The first human rights-focused coalition that was organized and run by persons with intellectual disabilities in the U.S. was reportedly formed in Oregon by a small group of individuals who were inspired by a conference they attended in Vancouver, British Columbia (Cone, 1998, p. 36). Naming their organization "People First of Oregon," the group held a conference the following year that surprisingly drew over 500 attendees (Shapiro, 1993, p. 1997). By 1990, there were 374 such chapters, consisting of approximately 10,000 members (p. 186). The following year, self-advocates held their second national conference and named themselves "Self-Advocates Becoming Empowered" (SABE). Positioning themselves as a disability rights organization, SABE has developed a collective and independent voice, actively supporting institutional closure and community inclusion, criticizing proinstitutional parent groups such as "Voices of the Retarded," both for their name (which SABE found offensive) and their continuing support for state institutions (Carey, 2009, p. 188). SABE also opposes segregated vocational programs, like sheltered workshops, placing the group at odds with old allies such as Arc, the new name for the NARC—the National Association for Retarded Children (later Citizens) (p. 188). Other issues taken on by SABE have included reform of Medicaid and the criminal justice system, the former for its funding of segregated placements like nursing homes and large group residences, and the latter for what they consider its unjust treatment of persons with intellectual disabilities (pp. 185–186). According to Carey (2009, p. 187) by the end of the twentieth century, SABE had become a respected and influential part of the disability rights community and the developmental disabilities field. Clearly, much had changed.

CHAPTER 3

OPENING THE INSTITUTIONAL DOORS

In the winter of 1903, the fledging campaign to build Maine's institution for people considered feebleminded made its way to the state legislature. Predictably, lawmakers appointed a committee to look into "the advisability of establishing a Home for the Feeble-Minded of the State" (S. Rep. No 6, 1905, p. 1). The effort to approve the facility would take 4 more years to become law and entail considerable debate and the intervention of influential individuals from within and outside the state. There seemed little doubt, however, that the newly formed "Committee on the Home for Feeble Minded" would strongly recommend a new institution.

The original idea for the facility emanated from a handful of determined reform-minded women from Portland. As Mosher (1991) notes, progressive social reform efforts led by women of the upper and middle classes were common during this period, propelled by moral principles of charity and societal improvement and directed toward improving the plight of the poor (p. 2). The women's delegation reportedly impressed lawmakers, canvassing the state and producing statistics and "startling and convincing statements" regarding the deplorable living and working conditions facing the feebleminded of Maine, and successfully "arousing public sentiment in favor of starting a home for the unfortunate feeble-

Voices of Pineland: Eugenics, Social Reform, and the Legacy of "Feeblemindedness" in Maine, pp. 47–71

minded of our state"("Maine Home For Feeble Minded At West Pownal, ME," n.d., in *Clippings Pownal State School, 1909–1946,* 1989, p. 7).

It is not surprising that Maine reformers would propose a new facility at this time. Specialized institutions for persons with disabilities were well established regionally, most closely in New Hampshire and Massachusetts where there were designated facilities and schools for those with psychiatric, visual, hearing, and intellectual disabilities. Next door, New Hampshire also had separate institutions for individuals considered insane and mentally defective. Over the years, Maine had built numerous facilities to segregate troublesome men and women, ranging from "insane hospitals" to reformatories and prisons. In 1840, the state built its first asylum, the Maine Insane Hospital, in Augusta. After a hiatus of more than 50 years, during which time state officials sent many of those considered, "feebleminded, blind, deaf and dumb" to facilities in Massachusetts, they embarked on a building spree of sorts. In 1897 they opened a residential school for the deaf, followed in 1901 by a second "insane asylum" in Bangor. In 1908 the Maine School for Feebleminded was constructed, around the same time that Helen Keller helped the Maine Institution for the Blind raise money for a building and property that the state later funded.

In 1904, Bigelow T. Sanborn, superintendent of the Maine Insane Hospital in Augusta from 1883–1914, added his support for a new institution, indicating that the state's two psychiatric facilities were now overcrowded and the state should "extend its protection" to Maine's idiots who were "deprived of all higher mental power"; imbeciles "hedged in by "quite serious limitations"; and feebleminded whose judgment was "defective" by the "same degenerative processes" as the idiot and imbecile (Sanborn, 1904, p. 49). Sanborn's arguments for the new facility reflected both the paternalistic sentiments of Maine's women reformers who emphasized "care for the unfortunate," as well as "the burden of feeblemindedness" perspective that he characterized as plaguing families and reducing their economic productivity.

> The one dependent member often commands the physical resources of the entire family. Production is at a standstill, ... not only from the family but the community as well.... [E]liminate this class from undesirable home care and almshouses and place them under institutional treatment where proper environments can be afforded and opportunities for improvement and in some cases recovery ... [and perhaps] "a return to a life of usefulness and productiveness." (Sanborn, n.d., p. 49)

Also reflected in Sanborn's arguments were the emerging fear of a proliferating defective and immigrant class that 3 years later was further fueled by the largest influx of foreigners in history. By 1910, the poor, working class and immigrant classes largely filled the nation's specialized institutions (Trent, 1994, p. 185). According to Sanborn:

> If ... we are to attain to even higher standards of moral and intellectual prosperity, we should see to it that such measures are inaugurated as shall make it impossible for the propagation of this weakened and degenerative humanity which if allowed to continue will dwarf manhood, and physical and moral decline will inevitably result.... The families throughout the State who are so seriously handicapped and burdened by such objectionable and dangerous members of the household should be relieved.
>
> In the end the establishment of a home or school for the feeble-minded will contribute to the material welfare of the State, especially when we take into consideration the large influx of laborers from Canada and foreigners from continental Europe. (Sanborn, n.d. pp. 48, 51–52)

At the turn of the twentieth century, Maine had a population of around 750,000 and was a growing but volatile place socially, economically and politically. Babcock, Frenette, Scontras, and Eagan (1995, p. 452) termed the period between 1880–1910 as the "apex of competitive capitalism in Maine," as the number of wage earners doubled and industries like cotton goods, lumber, boots and shoes, pulp and paper, and woolens added 28,000 new jobs, accounting for two thirds of the state's wage earners. New or expanding industries such as tourism, shore fishing, paper and hydro power accelerated into the twentieth century, replacing declining industries such as banks fishing, timber and canning as the linchpins of Maine's economy (pp. 420–441).

During this period, there was considerable rural migration to the state's industrial centers of Portland and Lewiston, accompanied by uncertainty and instability (Babcock et al., 1995, p. 448). In 1890, 26% of Mainers lived in urban areas, but by 1930 that figure had reached 40% (p. 452). Many rural migrants came from foreign countries, the most important of which were the people from French Canada. By 1900, French Canadians comprised 12% of Maine's population, many of whom lived in Aroostook County and the textile producing areas of central and southern Maine (p. 453). In the 1890s, the cotton mills employed 70% of Lewiston's labor force, 80% of whom were from Quebec (pp. 457–459).

Ethnic conflict was part of the social landscape in the early twentieth century. Initially, protestant Mainers resigned themselves to incoming French-Canadians as necessary laborers in industrial cities, but as the numbers grew and foreign groups became more politically active, tensions increased. Anti-Catholicism expanded, often playing out dramatically in neighboring towns. In the white collar city of Saco, for example, officials tried to restrict French Canadians from residence and allowed the Ku

Klux Klan to operate openly (Babcock et al., 1995, p. 469), infuriating citizens of neighboring Biddeford, a city with many French-speaking Catholics from Canada.

Despite the state's aggregate growth, the economy's changing nature created an often unpredictable and unsettling local employment climate for working people. Pockets of poverty and unemployment were evident, living and employment conditions were often deplorable, and working people moved frequently disrupting family life and transforming some towns into transient communities (p. 449). In Biddeford, for example, the turnover of French Canadians was 50% every 3 years, making it one of the most transient cities in New England (Babcock et al. 1995, p. 466).

In order to survive economically, poor families required multiple working members, including children, and often lived with extended members (Babcock et al. 1995, p. 465). The percentage of women in the work force increased from 14% to 22% between 1880 and 1930, 30% of whom worked in domestic and personal service jobs (p. 453). Most women worked between ages 10–29, before they married and had children, although many took in boarders and worked within the household (p. 460). Until 1907, child labor was permitted in Maine and even after it was outlawed, the practice continued for years as enforcement lagged (p. 465)

MAINE SCHOOL'S EARLY DEVELOPMENT, 1908–1919

Walter Fernald's Massachusetts School for Feeble-Minded in Waverley, Massachusetts served as the model for Maine's proposed institution. After visiting the facility, the Home Committee issued a report in 1905, describing it as one of the oldest, largest, and best managed institution in the country (S. Rep. No. 6, 1905, p. 3). In 1904, Walter Fernald attended the National Conference of Charities and Corrections Convention in Portland and advocated strenuously for expanded colonization and reported on the great progress achieved at his facility in turning "hopeless cases" into workers who "progressed sufficiently to be useful about the farm ("Maine Home For Feeble Minded At West Pownal, ME," n.d., in *Clippings, Pownal State School, 1909–1946*, 1989, p. 7). At the time, about 10% of Waverley's residents were Maine citizens, admitted at a total annual cost of $3,000 (p. 3).

Maine already had built specialized institutions for those considered insane and deaf and would soon add a facility for those who were blind or visually impaired. In light of the growing trend toward such specialized facilities, Bigelow Sanborn, superintendent of Maine's asylum, argued that congregating people considered feebleminded with those classified as insane was not only becoming physically impossible, but also scientifically outmoded and therapeutically unsound:

> The institutions at Augusta and Bangor which have already practically reached their maximum capacity should be left to devote its *[sic]* institutional energies to care for the absolutely insane and not be expected to extend aid to the idiot, imbecile, or feebleminded.... The progressive and indefatigable investigations ... during the past quarter of a century have demonstrated beyond a doubt the necessity of widely different methods of treatment.... The domiciling of the two classes is incompatible and one is frequently a menace to the other. (Sanborn, 1904, in S. Rep. No 6, 1905, p. 11)

With the continued assistance and support of the women's council, Sanborn, and other progressive reformers, the Committee on the Home for Feebleminded recommended construction of the proposed facility (S. Rep. No 6, 1905, p. 3). State Senator L. M. Staples of Knox County, one of the committee members, sponsored the first formal bill to establish the institution. Other reformist women's civic organizations and prominent professionals soon joined the ranks of supporters, emphasizing humanitarian goals, societal benefits, and family relief.

In 1905, reformers brought the bill to the full legislature, but it was referred to the Committee on Appropriations and Financial Affairs for consideration in the next legislative session (*First Report of the Maine School for Feeble-Minded*, 1911, p. 3). Concerns about the cost were cited as the reasons for the bill's deferral (Kleinberg, 1974, p. 17).

In the years leading up to final approval, supporters offered diverse rationales ranging from charity to custody, citing, on one hand, the need to humanely protect pitiful, helpless victims and unburden their families, and on the other, the importance of protecting society from a rapidly proliferating and genetically inferior menace. Although most acknowledged that not everyone was equally dangerous, by this time most reformers subscribed to a increasingly menacing definition for those considered higher functioning and of "deviant character," but often softening their eugenic rhetoric behind the language of care (Lazerson, 1975, p. 37).

The Home Committee's report illustrates the emerging public hysteria that would eventually engulf the feeblemindedness issue, warning of unfettered genetic transmission of mental deficiency, and "the great benefit to be derived ... by an institution of this kind [for] ... this class of feebleminded so that there will be no fear of reproduction (S. Rep. No 6, 1905, p. 3). According to the report, about 2,000 people, including 300 children under age 21, could be classified as "incapables" in Maine and were reproducing at an alarming rate. While young men posed a serious threat, the greatest need was to exert reproductive control over young women of child bearing age (p. 6):

> The adult males become the town loafers and incapables; the irresponsible pests of the neighborhood; petty thieves, purposeless destroyers property, incendiaries, and very frequently violators of women and little girls.
>
> It is well known that feebleminded women and girls are very liable to become sources of debauchery and licentiousness which pollute the whole life of the young boys and youth of the community. Almost every town has one or more of these defective women, each having one to four or more illegitimate children, everyone of whom is predestined to be defective mentally, criminal, or an outcast of some sort. There is widespread and insistent demand that these women be put under control. (p. 5)

Reformers also characterized feeblemindedness as a serious threat to family stability, defining afflicted children as "unbearable burdens," for family members and declaring institutionalization a "public duty'" essential for the community's welfare and the family's emotional, social, and economic survival (S. Rep. No 6, 1905, p. 5). Quoting Walter Fernald, the report calls the feebleminded child "a foreign body in a family or a modern American community, an emotional and financial burden, the source of grief, shame and humiliation, a detriment to siblings, and a reason for poverty due to loss of wage earner energy and vitality" (pp. 4–5). The committee warned that the genetic threat could be latent, residing deeply within a family's history undetected until it was too late:

> The terrible misfortune of having a feebleminded child ... does occur in families without a mental, moral, or physical taint for generations back, and where no cause can be assigned. The rich and poor, the great and the humble are alike liable to this dreaded visitation.
>
> Only small premiums ... insure training and life care to any member of the family who may need it in the future. No family is absolutely secure. (pp. 6–7)

The committee took pains to reassure families and the public that the facility would offer even better care than residents would receive in their own homes. After visiting institutions in New Hampshire and Massachusetts, committee members held the facilities up as ideal settings, describing the Waverly (Massachusetts) institution as directed by "Dr. W. E. Fernald, a Maine man by birth and education [who] is doing wonderful work" (S. Rep. no 6, 1905, p. 3), and claiming that residents were happy, contented, and improved as a result of the "faithful and competent teachers in the school, on the farm, and in the workshops." Moreover, "no parent, however kind, can possibly give to a feeble-minded child, the care and attention as can be done by facilities such as [Waverly and Laconia]." (S. Rep. No 6 1905, p. 4).

Reformers rebutted the reservations expressed by some legislators regarding the proposed cost of building, maintaining, and perhaps expanding a new institution by arguing that failing to construct such a facility would be even more expensive, both fiscally and socially. They added that using prudent management and resident labor would also minimize costs. The Home Committee pointed out, for example, that it already cost Maine about $30,000 per year, to care for all its feebleminded citizens. That includes paying local towns and cities and reimbursing Fernald for admitting people to Waverly (S. Rep. No. 6, 1905, p. 6).

Home Committee members presented resident labor as legitimate care, pointing out how much of it was occurring at other institutions. At Waverly, they observed "good workers who are nearly made self-supported" doing all the laundry work and making all the resident clothing. At Laconia, "inmates under supervision raise all the vegetables, beef, and pork consumed" (S. Rep. No 6, 1905, p. 6).

Deflecting narrow concerns about financial costs, State Senator Staples, the original sponsor of the bill, used both societal interest and humanitarian rhetoric to support his case, deflecting cost concerns and warning about the proliferating danger of doing nothing:

> You know … there are 2,800 [feebleminded] in the State of Maine today. It has cost the state year in and year out $27,000 … for the support of the feebleminded by the different towns of the State.
>
> Besides that, we have been paying Massachusetts some $3,000 every year. It is not a question of money. If you will go to this institution and see how … hundreds of them come to the Waverley hospital almost every year, and how their minds are strengthened, you would confess that it is not a matter of money. It will purify our towns in Maine.
>
> Let us … stop the propagation of idiots in the different towns of the state. If you do, the people will not find fault with you for this appropriation, because it goes right home to the essence of economy and justice." ("Maine Home For Feeble Minded At West Pownal, ME," n.d., in *Clippings Pownal State School, 1909–1946*, 1989, p. 7)

The final argument justifying the institution's costs was the availability of cheap land. Following Fernald's model, the committee envisioned a farm colony where residents would be "educated" in how to perform farming and domestic chores, helping to support their institutionalization. The facility would be located far from large villages or cities on a large enough tract of land and away from the eyes of the curious and families, ensuring privacy and minimizing interference and publicity (Rep. No. 6, 1905, p. 7).

Locating institutions in remote, rural locations may have met the state's fiscal and segregation needs, but it presented some rehabilitation and personnel problems. Edward Seguin, the nineteenth century authority on institutional education, stressed the importance of community proximity for maximum learning of practical skills of living. This was much less of a concern for institutional officials of this era who did not aspire to prepare people for community living, but for indefinite institutional life. A geographically isolated setting would, however, present staffing difficulties especially as the facility expanded.

On March 6, 1907, the legislature voted to establish Maine's first specialized institution for persons with "feeble minds." According to the legislation:

> The state shall establish and maintain a school for the care and education of the idiotic and feeble minded six years of age and upward and shall be known as the Maine School for Feeble Minded. All such feeble minded persons supported by towns in the state, who, in the judgment of the municipal officers of towns or state board of charities are capable of being benefitted by school instruction, shall be committed to this institution. (S. Rep. No 44, 1907, pp. 336–337)

The legislature allocated $60,000 for the facility's first 2 years of operation, primarily for the purchase of land. The project had the full endorsement of Governor William T. Cobb, who emphasized that "one of the most important duties of the State at this time is to provide a suitable establishment where these unfortunate people might receive proper care, and such employment as their clouded brains might be able to accomplish" ("Much Being Accomplished" 1909, p. A15).

A five-person board of trustees, appointed by the governor and consisting of only Maine residents, would oversee the new facility. One trustee was a woman, in deference to the legislative and reform efforts of the various women's groups. The trustees were given authority to "make all necessary rules and regulations as to admissions" and do all that was required to "properly care for and educate the feeble minded of the state" (S. Rep. No 44, 1907, p. 336).

Those deemed to be "indigent and destitute," having "no parents, kinsmen or guardian able to provide for them," and considered to be "proper subjects" for admission, could be admitted as state charges without cost. Others, considered to have the means for payment would be charged "for their care, education, and maintenance in the amount determined by the trustees." Out-of-state residents without access to such a facility were admissible "when there is room for them without excluding state charges, at a cost ... of not less than $3.25 per week"(S. Rep. No 44, 1907, p. 336).

Legal commitment of individuals "not already in any almshouse, the instructional school, or hospital in Maine, or supported by any town," and considered appropriate, could be conducted by a judge using an order "directed to the trustees of said school by a certificate of two physicians who are graduates of some legally organized medical college and have practiced three years in this state," verifying at a formal hearing that such a person was a proper subject for the institution. Commitments could be appealed "in the same manner by the same persons and to the same extent that [is used to appeal] decrees of the judge of probate appointing guardians over persons alleged to be insane or incompetent or spendthrift" (S. Rep. No 44, 1907, p. 336).

Discharge of residents was possible if ordered "by any three of the trustees or by a justice of the supreme or superior court of the state" whenever they believed that further detention was unnecessary (S. Rep. No 44, 1907, p. 336). After discharge, any residents with unexpired prison sentences would be transferred to prison to complete their full sentence.

Admission priorities were also established. First in line were

> feeble minded persons who are now in public institutions supported entirely at public expense; second, feeble minded persons in public institutions not supported as aforesaid; third, feeble minded persons who are not at any institution of the state, have no parents, kinsman, or guardian able to provide for them, or who are committed by a judge of probate; fourth those residing with the state whose parents kinsman or guardian by law to support such persons are able to pay; fifth persons of other states whose parents, kinsmen, or guardians are willing to pay. (S. Rep. No 44, 1907, p. 336)

Although the new facility was called a "school," it adhered to general and ambiguous admissions criteria that could apply to virtually anyone older than 6 years and include many not found in a typical school. Lawmakers made little effort to define what they meant by education and targeted poor people who were given priority for admission and were most easily committed as they were considered troublesome and expensive by town and municipal officials. In fact, the admission criteria was defined as much in terms of one's socioeconomic status as one's intellectual functioning.

Maine's institution was one of those considered "voluntary" since formal commitments could only be conducted in court and with the concurrence of two properly credentialed physicians. Commitment appeals were permitted, although being deemed a "proper subject of the institution" was an amorphous criterion, subjectively determined and applied, and difficult to contest, especially by individuals or families with little education, few resources, and no knowledge of legal procedures.

Following passage of the 1907 bill, a group led by then former Governor William T. Cobb was appointed to a Governor's Council by newly elected Governor Bert Fernald to find a proper location for the facility. The governor charged the council with securing a large tract of land "which should be removed from any large town or city, but at the same time easy of access by rail" ("Much Being Accomplished," 1909, p. A15). The committee finally decided on property that was situated across the four towns of Pownal, New Gloucester, Gray, and North Yarmouth. Equally distant from the state's largest cities, Portland and Lewiston, its location was considered "most excellent," and its campus idyllic:

> It is on the high ground and commands a magnificent view. Casco Bay is on one side and the White Mountain on the other being plainly visible which means an overlook of wide range of country. It further means pure air and plenty of sunshine. The tract includes 1,500 acres of land. Part of this is good woodland and there are many fine springs of water on the premises. The open land is fair farming land and the hay cut is excellent. (p. A15)

As more information about the land emerged, however, descriptions of it became less flattering. Moreover, the circumstances surrounding the purchase of the land became the institution's first major scandal, centering on how the land was selected and secured. The Governor's Council secured the services of Charles Dow and Albert Larabee of West Pownal to purchase the property (Bateman, 1912, p. 8). Soon after, but before other farmers learned of the state's interest in the land, Dow convinced the council to accept his proposal to buy not only his large farm, but also 10 surrounding properties for which he had secured purchase options (p. 8). Without informing his neighbors of the state's intentions, Dow bought the surrounding farms, then promptly sold them to the state, making a hefty profit. Some newspaper accounts described the deal as astute and economical. Presumably Dow's neighbors were not as generous in their praise.

News stories did not describe how Dow convinced the council why his property was superior to the more than 60 other possible sites, or explain what the price difference was between what he paid his neighbors for their farms and what he received for selling the properties to the state. Apparently the deal festered with some legislators who years later protested a new funding request for the Maine School, citing the expense, political favoritism, and possible fraud surrounding Dow's land brokering

("On the Grill," 1912, p. A1). Lawmakers were further incensed by the emerging reality that the land was far less fertile than advertised (p. A1).

No one was formally charged with illegal actions in the land purchasing deal, although the episode illustrates the myriad of conflicting professional, financial, political, legal, and social interests that surrounded the institution from its earliest days. This would not be the last time that institutional officials would exaggerate their successes, or that people external to the institution would profit from its existence.

Despite the controversy, advocates of the facility rallied to its defense, citing Walter Fernald's endorsement of the property and the similarity of Maine's site to that in Waverly ("Friends of Home for Feeble-Minded Ready to Aid," 1913, p. A11). Also, reflected in the land controversy were the mix of expectations that various parties held for the facility, ranging from punitive to humanitarian.

Acknowledging that the tract is a "a rocky, rough farm" LeRoy Pike, a member of the original site selection committee, argued that the land was perfect for emulating Waverly's focus on hard labor that was needed for such a troublesome population of residents ("Friends of Home for Feeble-Minded Ready to Aid," 1913, p. A11). At Waverley, Pike recalled seeing "inmates at work … all day lugging rock from one pile and piling them up at another point, only to return them the next day. They had to be given that sort of hard work. It was necessary for them" (p. A11). The chair of the trustees, Dr. Seth Gordon, reminded legislators that the institution was not purchased to become "a money making farming enterprise," but a school with loftier humanitarian and therapeutic goals. According to Gordon, "It is acreage we want. We are not farming, not calculating how much we are going to make. We want something to keep these poor unfortunates employed and do them good" (p. A11).

Despite the differences in tone between those advocating punitive work versus therapeutic activity for human betterment, the focus remained on resident labor as an integral and vital part of indefinite segregation. Resident work was not considered training for community re-entry, but for permanent custody and it was not coincidental that it reduced the state's associated costs. Unpaid resident labor would continue for decades, even after one superintendent in the 1960s criticized the practice as "indentured servitude."

The Maine School for Feeble-Minded officially opened in the fall of 1908 with a few male residents. They lived in the existing farm buildings until a new building could be completed in February, 1909 for 50 boys (Hedin, 1914, p. 1894). Dr. George Bliss was the institution's first superintendent and he appeared to be the ideal candidate. A New Hampshire native, graduate of Dartmouth College Medical School and a former official of the Waverly School, he was not only an experienced institutional physician from Northern New England, but also a disciple of the renowned Walter Fernald ("Remarkable Progress Made," 1909, p. A11; Report of the Trustees of the Maine School for Feeble-Minded, 1911). Bliss was the first of five physician-superintendents who would direct the Maine School for the first 64 years of its 88 year existence. While these men did not exclusively determine the institution's shape and functions, they operated nearly autonomously and were visible, powerful and influential figures.

Bliss began the tradition of visible physician—superintendents by effectively constructing and projecting a strong public definition and image of feeblemindedness as a primarily medical problem requiring proper therapeutic care. As the state's anointed expert on feeblemindedness, Bliss became a noted public figure who attracted legislative attention, media coverage, and public curiosity and effectively used the media and public presentations to disseminate his views.

It was incumbent on the new superintendent to educate and assure the public of the institution's value and present a clear, positive image of the facility as well-run, cost effective, and humane. In this regard, Bliss effectively juggled numerous, complex roles, including public spokesman, professional reformer, political operative, institutional administrator, and state bureaucrat. Through public speeches, carefully staged media visits, and favorable news stories, Bliss crafted a positive public image of the Maine School that would serve as a useful model for his successors and prove particularly helpful when conditions within the facility were found wanting. In his first report, dated 1909, (inserted in the school's first annual report dated September, 30, 1911), Bliss described a farm colony for 50 boys and a domestic service for 12 girls. (*First Report of the Maine School for Feeble-Minded*, 1911, p. 5). All 62 residents lived on the Hill Farm, situated at the southern end of the property, where they performed gender-differentiated work assignments that included familiar farm chores for the boys and sewing and washing for the girls-all carried out in what Bliss presented as an idyllic rural setting that would be familiar and comfortable for most Maine citizens. A second farm-the Valley Farm—was planned for the northern end of the property (pp. 3–4). According to the superintendent:

> Here we have a farm colony ... where the boys live the simple outdoor life of a farmer's boy, caring for the farm stock and crops, improve the fields by clearing out stones, bushes, and stumps, getting up their own wood for heating and working up the same. The last has been done by the very lowest grade boys we have, the boys so defective mentally as to be of very little use in the garden and other farm work. We have had seven acres under cultivation at this place under cultivation cared for by these boys and one attendant. We have raised all the green vegetables we could use this summer.... The boys

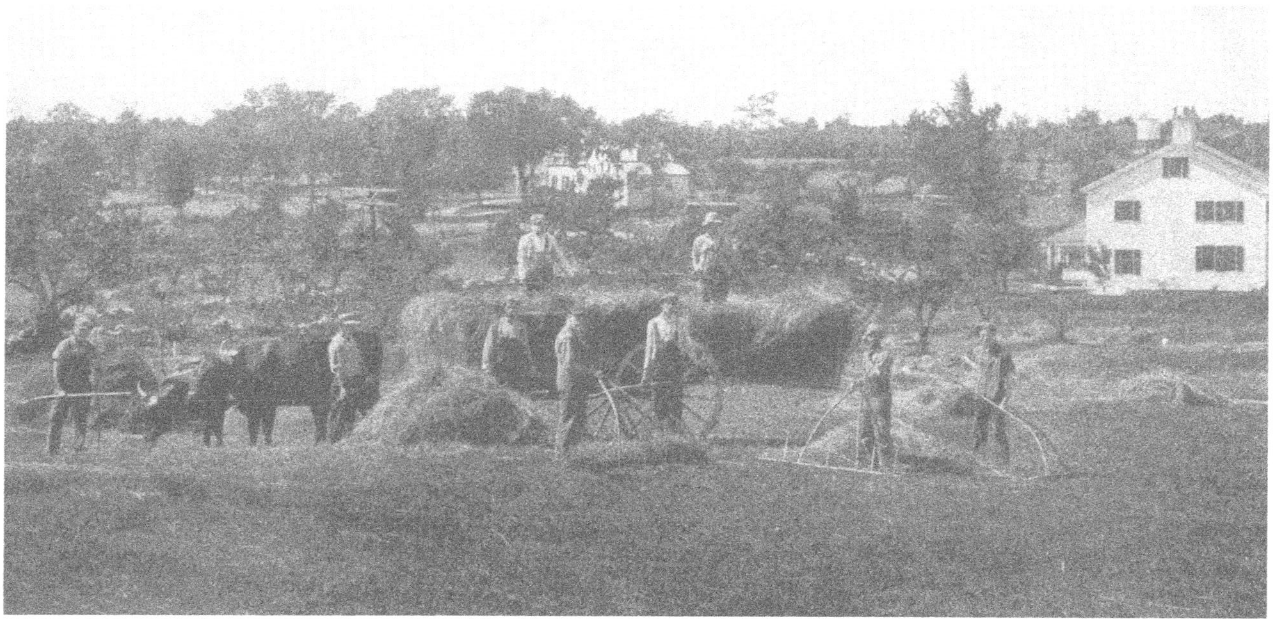

Figure 3.1 Resident Farm Workers. From the Sixth Annual Report of the Maine School for Feeble-Minded at West Pownal. 1914. From the collection of Debra and William Barry

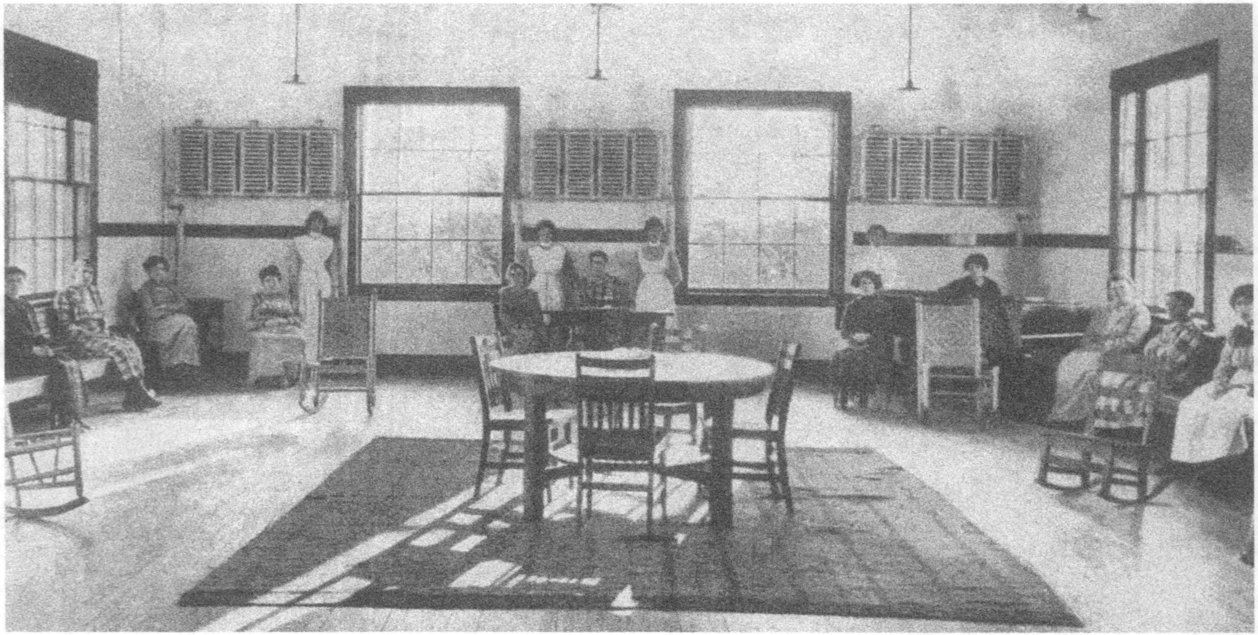

Figure 3.2 Womens' Dormitory. Sixth Annual Report of the Maine School for Feeble-Minded at West Pownal. 1914. From the collection of Debra and William Barry

> have cleared about one half mile of road of bushes besides a large filed ... and we expect by winter to plow and completely clear and seed down this land. (p. 5)

Bliss characterized the women as equally productive and contented as they performed their work: "The girls do the sewing for the school, the washing for themselves and the women employees. . . They are of all grades, four of them almost helpless from their defect. They seem very happy and contended [*sic*] in their new home" (*First Report of the Maine School for Feeble-Minded*, 1911, p. 6). Extolling the merits of hard work for all, Bliss argued for its character building virtues and benefits for both resident and institution:

> Occupation with some definite thing to do is the activation of the defective as well as of the normal being. Hence, I believe thoroughly in giving every inmate of the institution a task or tasks adapted to his physical and mental capacity, and insist that he do that work as well as it lies in him to do it, repeating it if necessary until he has done the best he can..., Give him some occupation and intelligent supervision and such a case, even though of very low grade, will become a useful and helpful inmate. ("School at Pownal," 1910, in *Clippings Pownal State School, 1909-1946*, 1989, p. 22)

The superintendent also constructed an image of the institution's environment as pastoral and promoting self-support reflecting Yankee independence:

> This dairy farm ... is one of the prettiest on the State's land here. It lies in a fertile valley at the base of the hill.... Here a herd of 18 Holsteins browse contentedly on the green slopes and furnish all the cream and milk for the employees and inmates of the Home. Here also are a score of fat porkers ... which will furnish meat for the State's tables throughout the year. Timber is plentiful over the 1300 acres, and judicious and scientific cutting will enable ... the two colonies ... [to] supply their own wood. Already the gardens ... are furnishing wholesome green stuff. ("Remarkable Progress Made," 1909, p. A11)

Within the facility, the importance of healthy, humane and safe living circumstances are emphasized as Bliss related that proper care "is best accomplished by placing [residents] in groups of not more than fifty or sixty in a building.... It requires sunny, well ventilated, well warmed buildings, with abundant toilet facilities" ("Remarkable Progress Made," 1909, p. A11). The superintendent added that institutional life must include a rigorous, plentiful schedule of "outdoor exercise with proper food, regular occupation, and suitable amusements ... [that] makes the feebleminded boy or girl, or man or woman, a happy human being" (p. A11).

Initially, Bliss defined feeblemindedness as an incurable, irreversible, and only superficially improvable disorder, accompanied by discernible physical pathology:

> a permanent thing that once established does not grow better or worse if left alone. It is always established in very early life, either before birth, during birth, or in small children by something occurring that destroys a portion of the brain. This destroyed portion of the brain cannot be restored by any means within our power, all we can do is to take what is left and train it until the defect is less noticeable. ("Had Varied Program," 1910, p. A11)

The superintendent classified residents as one of three types, each corresponding to assigned levels of cognitive impairment, learning prognosis, and personality characteristics. The three levels were "idiot, low grade imbecile, and high grade imbecile" ("Had Varied Program," 1910, p. A11). Idiot was the designation for the lowest functioning group, described by Bliss as "noisy, excitable, dull, and apathetic," performing destructive behaviors such as destroying their clothing, eating plaster, and breaking windows; and exhibiting functional deficits such as inability to eat properly, dress themselves, and/or use the toilet (p. A11).

Bliss considered those with low cognitive ability to have very limited potential but not innately dangerous or deviant:

> They [residents] are not degenerates.... I mean they are more unfortunate than vicious. They are simpleminded, incapable of doing independent work in which initiative or any great skill is required. They are, as a rule, kindly in disposition, tractable and obedient. ("Remarkable Progress Made" 1910, p. A11)

Referring to "idiots" as acutely impaired, Bliss related that most were marginally improvable within the institution but only if admitted early, though not too early:

> Of the real idiots there are only a few, nearly every case is susceptible of [*sic*] a certain degree of improvement.... If a low grade child ... can be taught to acquire reasonably tidy habits, and to dress himself, the burden of his care is lessened immensely. To make such work successful, the child must come under careful training early in life, from 7 to 12 years. During these formative years, habits may be modified, and correct ones established which, if taken later in life, could not be accomplished. Below 7 the child is much better off

at home under the care of his mother or friends than in an institution. ("Had Varied Program," 1910, p. A11)

In defining the highest functioning group, "the high grade imbecile," Bliss dramatically changed his paternalistic tone, dredging up the older image of "moral imbecile" and soberly warning of individuals who are "quite a different proposition," requiring tight control:

> He is probably already tidy in his personal habits. He can be taught to read and write, perhaps to figure a little; he often has considerable musical ability and can be taught to do many kinds of work well. His defect shows most in his relations with his fellow men. He is always improvident, always a liar, a petty thief, perhaps cruel to animals and children, and he may be so strongly inclined to set fires that he finds the impulse impossible to resist. Because of his weak will and deficient judgement, he is likely influenced for evil, and is likely to become a drunkard, a vagrant, or if a woman, a prostitute. ("Remarkable Progress Made" 1910, p. A11)

However threatening people were characterized when allowed to roam freely in their communities, Bliss assured Maine citizens that once behind institutional walls, they were harmless and malleable children. In fact, perhaps the most prevalent image the superintendent projected of his charges was that of a physically damaged, perpetual child, a description that he applied regardless of age. One visiting reporter, observing physically mature adults, remarked that even though some residents were "over 30 years old," they were referred to as "boys and girls" ("Remarkable Progress Being Made," 1909, p. A11).

Child-oriented pursuits dominated Bliss' review of resident activities, interests, and opportunities:

> For amusements, the out of door sports such as baseball and football in summer by boys, and crochet for the girls, and sliding and skating in winter are always good.
>
> Indoors, childish games like "drop the handkerchief," "roll the platter," and "Jerusalem" are very popular even with grown men and women. Dolls and toys of all descriptions are cherished as by any children. The brighter ones love to sing. Some of them dance very nicely, and they enjoy popcorn, apples and fudge as much as children can. ("School at Pownal,"undated, in *Clippings Pownal State School, 1909–1946*, 1989, p. 22)

Questioned about the need for discipline, the superintendent responded:

> Discipline? Why, we need very little of it here. The boys and girls are very good. Now and then it is necessary to send one early to bed or to deprive him or her temporarily of some amusement. This is all the

> discipline needed to secure obedience. ("Remarkable Progress Made," 1909, p. A11)

Bliss's description of institutional routines was based on the training regimen of French reformer, Eduard Seguin and an idealized middle class life of reformers' imaginations. Seguin argued that "idiocy" represented a lack of personal will, self-control, and motivation requiring institutional observation and technical instruction in the everyday skills designed to combat innate, perpetual childishness. As Mitchell and Snyder (2003, p. 853) note:

> It should not be surprising that the origins of restrictive disability regimens such as eugenic science come out of professedly humanitarian efforts.... Training in separate institutional/educational sites recognized "idiocy" as a state of infantilism ... that could be overcome by modern disciplinary techniques.
>
> The bulk of this disciplinary regime at Seguin's institutional training sites sought to correct "behavioral aberrancy" by providing his subjects with a fully regimented daily routine; one that was orchestrated from dawn to dusk with tasks of self-care.

Reflecting an increasing medical portrayal of feeblemindedness, Bliss emphasized residents as having broken and inferior bodies:

> The feebleminded have many congenital as well as physical defects. That is, they are poorly made human beings. Very few of them have symmetrical heads, ears or limbs; cleft and narrow palates and poor teeth are very common. Along with this the organs of digestion and assimilation of food are often defective.
>
> The feebleminded child needs more food than the normal child, and it must be in easily digestible form, such cereals, bread and milk, meat in soups and stew, and fish in chowders ,and plenty of fresh vegetables. ("School at Pownal," n.d., *Clippings Pownal State School*, 1909–1946, 1989, p. 22)

By 1912, Bliss had downgraded residents' medical condition further:

> The average age of the feebleminded is not great, as that class die comparatively young. They have but little control of the vital organs and are naturally weak and can stand but little strain. A small sickness that an ordinary person would survive will often prove fatal with them. (Bateman, 1912, p. 8)

It was apparently not sufficient to limit the concept of feeblemindedness to a cognitive disorder if it was to fall fully under the domain of medicine and be applied as widely as possible. Medical superintendents led the way in pairing "feeble minds" with "feeble bodies" not only to devise a "discernible map" for identifying an otherwise invisible, internal defect, but also to use the identification of "intellectual shortcomings" to search the body for "the inevitable signs of inferiority" (Mitchell & Snyder, 2003, p. 855). Tying "feeblemindedness" to such multidimensional dysfunction permitted eugenicists to use one term only to discredit people in every conceivable way and more easily justify increasingly punitive and restrictive actions (p. 855). Practices such as permanent incarceration, marriage prohibition, coerced sterilization, and ultimately extermination, were considered initially by even their supporters as "whispered," extreme, and/or unlikely possibilities, but in a relatively short time were described overtly and widely accepted as beneficial, necessary, and humane (p. 856).

Resident labor was critical to the institution's economy and efficiency, although Bliss downplayed its institutional benefits and rejected the idea that the facility could be completely self-supporting. Instead, he focused on the health and rehabilitative merits of work for males, and on its protective qualities for women:

> Those inmates able to do so, are required to assist in the work, but there is no intent to work them with the idea of making the institution pay its way-the object is to instruct and to furnish healthful exercise for they are boys and men committed to the care of the State—for no fault of their own. The girls are kept busy with sewing and doing washing and are kept under closer observation than the boys. The object of this is to protect the girls who, as is well known, are almost certain to come to grief at the hands of men. ("An Institution of Great Value, n.d., in *Clippings Pownal State School, 1909–1946*, 1989, p. 12)

Bowing to both cost-conscious legislators and earnest social reformers, Bliss couched his description of resident labor as both a humanitarian and fiscally responsible way of combating crime, salvaging damaged lives, saving money, and doing social good:

> The modern scientific study of the deficient and delinquent class ... has shown that a large proportion of the inmates of our almshouses, reform schools, jails, and prisons are mentally defective. This class are always cared and maintained at public expense, and when they have become criminals, as they are almost sure to become, involving repeated and expensive trials ... or support in prisons, jails or public institutions, the burden becomes greatly multiplied. How much better then to send them to an institution where they can be employed and their own work turned to good account in caring for

> themselves and other less bright feebleminded persons. ("An Institution of Great Value," n.d., in *Clippings Pownal State School, 1909–1946*, 1989, p. 12)

As he highlighted the importance of resident labor, Bliss manipulated his description of residents' health, contradicting his previous image of them as medically vulnerable and physically fragile, in favor of a robust image more consistent with that of able laborer:

> They [residents] are of New England country stock, for the most part, sturdy of body and possessed of rugged physical health. We have little illness so far ... and this is where Maine has a different class from that found in other states who draw their feebleminded in no small degree from the large cities and slum element. ("Remarkable Progress Made," 1909, p. A11)

Alongside Bliss's emphasis on humane treatment is the emerging eugenic message of preemptive control, e.g. "to prevent these people from becoming fathers and mothers" ("Remarkable Progress Made," 1909, p. 8). Asserting that "every feebleminded girl and woman is the prospective mother of defectives ... [and] every feebleminded man may be the father of foolish children" ("School At Pownal," undated, *Clippings Pownal State School, 1909–1946*, 1989, p. 22), Bliss contended that the primary institutional mission is the "entire and absolute separation of the sexes in their dormitories, in their work, and in their play" ("Had Varied Program," 1910, p. A11). He expressed full confidence that, if effectively implemented, large-scale segregation would reduce society's social ills in short order:

> Many troubles like crime and intemperance and disease can be controlled but not often stamped out; but in this affliction segregation, living the community life in a school where the inmate is sheltered, the men on one farm, the women on another, can so change conditions in a single generation that the pity of it is that there cannot be such complete foster care held over all cases in the State today as to insure safety to the community and to futurity. ("At Pownal," n.d., *Clippings Pownal State School, 1909–1946*, p. 22)

Although young men were portrayed as problematic, reformers considered women of "child bearing age" particularly troublesome. Using the language of care and control interchangeably, Bliss pointed out the threat this group represented and the tragedies that surrounded a lack of timely and widespread prevention:

> I believe that the custodial care of feebleminded women of child bearing age is going to mean a very material reduction in the number of paupers in the next twenty years. The absolute segregation of the sexes necessary to

> accomplish this cannot be brought about in our poor farms and only in a few homes.
>
> A feeble-minded girl of the higher grade was accepted as a pupil at Massachusetts School for the Feeble-Minded when she was fifteen years old. At the last moment the mother refused to send her ... as she could not bear the disgrace of publically admitting she had a feebleminded child. Ten years later the girl was admitted to the public institution by the court after she had given birth to six illegitimate children, four of whom were still living, and all feeble-minded.
>
> Care in an institution stops this but only the greatest care can do so. Some of the girls and women who come to us have already lived the life of the street walker and prostitute and only extreme care and incessant supervision can protect such girls. ("School at Pownal," n.d., in *Clippings Pownal State School, 1909–1946*, 1989, p. 22)

Properly executed, segregation and training required removing children from their family at an early age since they created a heavy burden on their families and the earlier the intervention the easier was the instruction. Initially, Bliss claimed that families concurred, acknowledging the burdens and becoming major sources of referrals:

> It is a striking fact that the reason for the great majority of the applications for admission to our institutions is based upon the relief needed for the mother, the family, or the neighborhood..., Hundreds of mothers and fathers, friends and guardians of these people in the State are asking that a burden too great for them to bear be taken from their shoulders. ("Had Varied Program," 1910, p. A11)

A few years later, however, he characterized families as more troublesome since "few parents or relatives will acknowledge that a member of their family is feebleminded" (*Report of the Maine School For Feeble-Minded*, 1912, p. 15). Combating family resistance was becoming a higher priority for eugenic reformers who began indicting the family as integral to the problem of feeblemindedness—a condition eugenicists were increasingly portraying as genetic in nature and exacerbated by family incompetence and shame. Indeed family "resistance" to institutionalization would prove nettlesome to reformers of any era, since it proved to be the rule rather than the exception. Despite the campaign that began in the mid-nineteenth century to portray disabled children as family and community burdens and the subsequent efforts to characterize the family itself as a primary obstacle to successful reform, pre-empting familial authority in this regard proved insurmountable. Historically, the great majority of families have successfully raised their children with intellectual disabilities at home, despite little or no government support and often against the strong advice of family physicians and other professionals.

In an attempt to maximize family cooperation, Bliss took great pains to present institutional segregation in the most positive light, labeling it an unqualified success, emphasizing its caring staff, technical instruction, and professional supervision and describing it as the best hope for achieving maximum individual potential and the only legitimate source of family relief:

> All of our boys and girls have shown marked improvement physically and mentally. The regular hours, steady occupation under careful, intelligent supervision, and encouragement to do their best have worked wonders with some of these unfortunates. (*First Report of the Maine School for Feeble Minded*, 1910, p. 5)
>
> We expect, by and by, to be able to take others from families who may wish to put their children where they may have expert care, careful supervision, and such training mentally and morally as the children can make the most of. ("Remarkable Progress Made," 1909, p. A11)

During the institution's first 2 years, enrollments doubled from 62 to 135, its waiting list reached 300, and Bliss pronounced the Maine School an unqualified success. This, however was not the view of a politically-appointed Standing Committee assembled by newly elected Governor Frederick Plaisted in 1911. The committee's report was highly critical and reflected a wide discrepancy between official reports and observed conditions, illustrating dilemmas, conflicts, and contradictions that would plague the facility for decades.

The committee's report refutes many of the claims made by the superintendent, and illustrates how quickly the facility was used as a repository for those considered community liabilities, discarded as too old, sick, unproductive and expensive. The report also reflected the tension that existed between those advocating segregation primarily for care of those who could assist in their own (and the institution's) support versus those who saw the facility as a mechanism for controlling a wide variety of troublesome people; although each camp supported aspects of both objectives.

Visiting the school for the first time in February, 1911, the committee found a population of 135 residents whom they termed entirely inappropriate for admission, given the institution's stated purpose. According to the committee, "the legislature of 1907 passed an Act with the following title: 'An Act to Establish a *School* for the Feeble-Minded,' and 'the chief purpose' of the institution was clearly designed for 'Feeble-Minded persons over six years of age, and capable of being *benefitted* by School Instruction.' " The committee argued that the facility was regarded as a *Home* rather than a *School* (Standing Committee Report, *Report of the Maine School for Feeble-Minded*, 1912, p. 19):

> The prime object for which the Institution was founded ... was being ignored, as the population consisted, to quite an extent, of aged imbeciles, many over forty, and some as high as seventy-five and eighty years of age-a class of people totally deficient mentally, wholly unimpressionable, and incapable of mental improvement. (pp. 19–20)

The Standing Committee also criticized the Maine School for having no designated school or manual training department and spending far more per resident—seven dollars per week—than was spent for "this elderly class" in their own towns where they were "given good homes and were well cared for ... at a cost not exceeding $2.50 to $3.00 per week" (Standing Committee Report, *Report of the Maine School for Feeble-Minded*, 1912, p. 20). The institution was also blamed for accepting too many residents from some regions of the state and not others.

To address the identified problems, the committee recommended that institutional officials: (1) return to their home communities "all the aged ones who were incapable of mental improvement" and replace them with younger feeble-minded "who were capable of being benefitted by school instruction;" (2) establish a "school of learning" and manual training department; (3) apportion admissions of residents among the various counties within the state "in proportion to the number of feeble-minded who live there; (4) reduce per resident cost and focus as much as possible on admitting wards of the state and girls, the latter in order that "communities would be better safeguarded, by lessening the liklihood [sic] of a new generation of imbeciles" (Standing Committee Report, *Report of the Maine School for Feeble-Minded*, 1912, p. 20).

Perhaps the committee's most ominous recommendation was to more aggressively identify and segregate Maine citizens and combat family resistance. Tackling the murky statewide incidence figures on feeblemindedness, committee members argued that the 1910 census total of 722 was too low, estimating the real statewide figure as closer to 1,500. Members proposed to legally require municipal assessors to annually compile and submit to the state an accurate list of the names, ages, and sex of all residents suspected of being feebleminded (Standing Committee Report, *Report of the Maine School for Feeble-Minded*, 1912, p. 22). Following up on such a list, the committee proposed a law that would compel municipal authorities to commit "feeble-minded persons 12 years old or over, girls preferably, who have become dangerous sexually or otherwise and are not properly cared for at their homes" (p. 22). As the committee put it:

> We fully realize the difficulty in obtaining a correct list, as people are very loath to give up, as defective, any of their children. But only in this way does the State know with whom they will have to deal, and this knowledge would add very largely to the efficiency of the Institution. (p. 22)

On July 11, 1911, the governor appointed an entirely new board of trustees. Praising Bliss and his wife for "doing most excellent work under somewhat embarrassing conditions," the new board contradicted Bliss' idyllic descriptions of the facility's condition, the farm's success, and the healthy surroundings. In addition, they contested his enrollment figures and reversed his admission practices (*Report of the Maine School for Feeble-Minded*, 1911, pp. 3–4). The trustees called for improving the physical plant, the poor crop yields, and, most importantly, the lack of "a constant, unfailing supply of good water" (p. 3). They also estimated that the facility could hold 75 more residents, and that every effort should be made to admit more residents "to the full capacity of the buildings" (p. 4).

The new board praised the school's reliance on "labor ... done almost exclusively by the inmates" (*Report of the Maine School for Feeble-Minded*, 1911, p. 3), and reiterated the committee's criticism of school officials for admitting too many "old and feeble men and women who are unable to do any work" (p. 4). The board announced that they were discharging many of these residents and sending them back to their local communities, arguing that room must be made for "a number of State paupers, of the feebleminded class, [who] have been discovered [and] who will be properly cared for in this institution, there being abundant room" (p. 4). Those having been "discovered" likely refer to targeted inhabitants of Malaga Island, a colony of poor people, some of whom were sent to the Maine School following their eviction from the island in what was certainly one of the most shameful chapters in Maine's history.

Near the end of 1912, the board of trustees accepted "with regret" the resignation of George Bliss, who reportedly received "a very flattering offer" from the Indiana School for the Feebleminded" (*Report of the Maine School for Feeble Minded*, 1912, p. 6). As the first superintendent, Bliss became a lightening rod for much of the controversy that quickly surrounded the facility. He left under a cloud of political drama that surrounded the new facility over admissions criteria and numbers, shady land deals, and facility size and costs. As noted earlier, the Board refuted Bliss' claims of overcrowding, and perhaps pushed harder for more admissions and resident self-support than Bliss could accept. Trustees and committee members wanted younger, more capable people admitted, especially women. These were the individuals they considered the most menacing as the eugenic rhetoric escalated, and more essential to the institution as capable, inexpensive labor was needed in an underfunded, understaffed, and overcrowded facility.

Like his medical colleagues, Bliss was a strong eugenicist, supportive of institutional segregation and expansion. He discharged relatively few residents, reporting a discharge/attrition rate of about 10% per year, a bloated figure that included not only community and family parole, but also inter-institutional transfers, deaths, and escapes. The superintendent's rate of discharge was not close to matching the facility's ever-growing waiting list, something Bliss acknowledged and defended vigorously. He emphasized the need for institutional enlargement and indefinite incarceration, despite higher costs, and rejected the idea that residents could be self-supporting outside the facility:

> The feebleminded should never be placed in poor houses. The proper place is on a farm where every movement can be guarded. A poorhouse provides no school and limited guardianship. This place has both.... [W]e are protecting society by preventing propagation of their species. They might be cared for cheaper at poor houses, or at their homes, but ... we are training them here, and to a great extent making them useful. (Bateman, 1912, p. 8)
>
> A very few of the higher grade cases are able to go out from the institution, provided they have relatives or friends to care for them, and do very well, but they are never fitted to assume the responsibilities of citizenship to marry and to produce their kind. ("School at Pownal," n.d., *Clippings Pownal State School, 1909–1946*, 1989, p. 22)

Bliss's views may have made cost-conscience state officials and lawmakers cringe, although institutional expansion would continue for almost 50 years despite legislators' objections and criticisms. While overall discharged rates remained consistently low after Bliss departed, what did change was *who* was discharged. Before 1912, enrollments within the Maine School slightly favored males, but after that, female residents outnumbered males and generally were discharged at a lower rate until the middle 1920s. Only after 1925 did officials reverse this trend, although the rates of release would be consistently low for decades despite what superintendents might claim.

CHAPTER 4

EUGENICS, RACISM, AND STERILIZATION

STATE SPONSORED EVICTION ON MALAGA ISLAND

The national persecution of people considered feebleminded intensified between 1908 and 1920 (Trent, 1994, p. 141), coinciding both with the formative years of the Maine School and the saga which unfolded on Malaga Island, an incident that vividly illustrated how the effects of the eugenic indictment could combine with local economic interests, political forces, and social fears to oppress a vulnerable group of people under the guise of "progressive" social reform.

Richard Dugdale's publication of the Jukes family in 1877, replete with carefully constructed charts and startling numbers, lent an air of scientific legitimacy to eugenic claims about the menace of proliferating, inbreeding rural clans living in huts and hovels and characterized by crime, dependency, and illicit sex (Rafter, 1997, pp. 37–38). The *Jukes* research was followed by numerous other accounts of "defective families" and "intergenerational deviance" that had a profound and longstanding effect on social reformers, legislators, and state officials. They remained impressed for decades with the detailed accounting of how much one degenerate family could cost the tax-paying public and used this research to ratio-

Voices of Pineland: Eugenics, Social Reform, and the Legacy of "Feeblemindedness" in Maine, pp. 73–101

nalize building and/or expanding new institutions, unearth "unfit populations" and document the proliferating problem of "criminal families" (Bruinius, 2006, p 146).

As these studies were "scientifically" verifying the inherited, inter-generational character of feeblemindedness and degeneracy, highlighting rural areas, and advocating for aggressive measures, the drumbeat for action was growing in Maine where state authorities had identified a "retrograde settlement" living on coastal Malaga Island. Many of the islanders were multi-racial, referred to as "degenerates" and "sub-normals," particularly dangerous labels to be assigned to anyone since they represented human inferiority and primary sources of genetic infection. They were also amorphous descriptions, largely invisible, easily applied, and readily inferred from "deviant" values and behavior. In the case of the Malaga Islanders, identification was greatly simplified by the presence of racial differences and the community's isolation. Mosher (1991) described the Malaga eviction:

> By July 1, 1912 the last of the residents of a poor fishing village located on Malaga Island ... had taken heed of the eviction notice issued by the Cumberland County sheriff. At the order of Governor Frederick Plaisted, houses which were not taken down by their owners were torn down and destroyed.... A small cemetery containing the remains of several generations of islanders was exhumed, and the bodies sent to the Home for the Feebleminded (now Pineland Center) in New Gloucester, Maine. Former residents were left to find communities willing to accept them. Some were able to float their homes to the mainland with little incident. Others were met by angry residents intent on sending the newcomers packing. And one family was institutionalized at the New Gloucester facility to which the Malaga Island cemetery had been re-interred. (p. 1)

The 10-acre island was inhabited by 45 people, many reportedly descendants of former slave Benjamin Darling, and some of whom descended from the area's first settlers with familial origins dating back to at least 1794 (Mosher, 1991, p. 39). Settled as a community around the middle of the nineteenth century, the island consisted of mostly poor residents who eked out a living fishing and working seasonal jobs and was largely ignored until the end of the nineteenth century. Malaga, like other island communities, became a casualty in the economic battle with an increasingly important coastal tourist industry (Barry, 1980, p. 55).

Near the end of the nineteenth century, Maine was becoming an increasingly popular resort area for upper—and middle-class people from New England and other eastern states. As land values increased, many poor families who had settled on property they had never officially purchased became increasingly unwelcome since they required local financial assistance, and reportedly despoiled the scenery of coastal communities bent on attracting affluent summer tourists and residents (Mosher, 1991, p. 3). As DuBrule (1999) concluded, "by 1900, towns along the Maine coast were fighting for possession of abandoned or un-deeded islands ... so that they could be sold, developed and taxed" (p. 51). According to Mosher (1991), by 1910 there were few, if any, islands along the Maine coast without a resort hotel, and many Malaga Islanders were refugees, "island hopping to keep ahead of the real estate market" (p. 3).

Local and state officials had additional reasons for wanting to rid the area of poor residents. Because of their unsavory reputations and the growing tensions over fishing grounds and local jobs, Malaga residents were increasingly resented by their neighbors and vilified by the local press (Barry, 1981, pp 55–56; Mosher, 1991, p. 46). State officials began referring to poor communities as "pauper colonies" (Mosher, 1991, p. 107), and considered them literal breeding grounds for social pathology and disorder. In the mist of the eugenic persecution and fears of "race suicide" expressed by national leaders and where Anglo-Saxons were seen as experiencing "biological defeat" under the onslaught of fecund, "sub-normals" and immigrant groups (p. 12), such language resonated with many Maine citizens. Between 1900 and 1910, news accounts became more sensational and racist, referring to Malaga as "a curious populace of blacks and whites" where "children have married and intermarried;" a place replete with "sexual and moral depravity [and] shiftlessness," and "peopled by sub-normals in ancestral shacks." (pp. 59, 106–107). State officials sounded the alarm as they characterized Malaga residents as vivid examples of the "retrograde" families and "decaying family stock" that resulted from genetically transmittable feeblemindedness (Barry, 1981, pp. 55–56). This was nearly identical to the language used by the authors of the "pedigree studies" and the rationale authorities used to assign people to the Maine School.

In 1905, the state annexed the island, making its residents wards of the state and promising them care and protection (DuBrule, 1999, pp. 49, 51). For a few years things improved as some resources came to the islanders. Malaga's annexation and the accompanying publicity regarding conditions there attracted the attention of Massachusetts missionaries and local reformers who established an island school, donated supplies and money, and, in the best progressive tradition, began converting Malaga's residents to middle class respectability (Mosher, 1991, p. 2). In 1908, a schoolhouse was built and according to Breed (2006, p. 72), the school did well as children reportedly learned, state funding was obtained, and some mainlanders enrolled due to the school's positive reputation.

Shortly after taking office in 1911, Governor Frederick Plaisted convened a three-person committee to investigate conditions on Malaga Island. It was not coincidental that he appointed as chairman, Dr. Charles Kilgore, head of the Governor's Committee on the Home for the Feebleminded (DuBrule, 1999, p. 91). Mosher (1991) referred to Governor Plaisted as a " 'good barometer' of the middle class values of early-twentieth century Mainers" (p. 110). The governor left little doubt about his intentions for Malaga after a visit to the island in 1911:

> The best plan would be to burn down the shacks with all their filth. Certainly, the conditions are not credible to our state, and we ought not to have such things near our front door, and I do not think that a like condition can be found in Maine, although there are some pretty bad localities elsewhere. (as cited in Mosher, 1991, p. 110)

Beginning legal maneuvers to remove the islanders who were described as "squatters," the state declared that descendants of Eli Perry, an early settler of the nearby mainland town of Phippsburg, were the rightful owners of the island (Breed, 2006, p. 73). The ruling was based on deeds from 1818, although rightful ownership of the island remained obscure. One Malaga resident, claimed to have bought all or part of the island but was unable to provide proper receipt although he was listed on the 1870 census as owning $300 worth of unidentified real estate (p. 73). In addition, no one paid taxes on the land or stepped forward to declare ownership when requested to do so (p. 73). In previous, less compelling instances, the state had awarded property rights to long time settlers and could have done so for Malaga residents (p. 73). In December, 1911, state officials bought the property from the Perrys for $400, paid the islanders a small amount for their homes, and ordered them off the property by July, 1, 1912 (p. 73).

Just before the initial eviction notice was given, state officials committed an older woman and the entire Marks family to the Maine School for the Feebleminded (Barry, 1981, p. 84; Breed, 2006, 73), a clear cue from the state regarding how the islanders should be perceived. Mosher (1991) described the eviction as "a classic case of cultural imperialism" that was publically applauded "in a society that condemned pauperism, feeblemindedness, thriftlessness, and idleness, and that reflected increasingly dissonant community values and socio-economic distinctions within the state" (pp. 1–2).

The Malaga Island saga illustrates how culture, economics, politics and science can be tied together in neat rationale of racial and ethnic persecution, portraying targeted individuals as serious and escalating threats to the state's prosperity, order, and stability and legitimating their exclusion and control. Those determined to be unattractive, incompetent and unproductive were merely displaying their biological destiny and it was left to the "socially fit" to dispose of them and the problems they posed.

The Malaga incident also reveals how the indictment of persons considered feebleminded involved a widening net of citizens. Initially, the move to segregate persons at the Maine School was led by social reformers and medical professionals who convinced local and state politicians to support them. The activities at Malaga included these parties while adding some new adherents such as legal professionals, local citizens and business people. Widely portrayed as a racist act, the Malaga eviction was more easily conducted and supported because the islanders were described as "degenerates," "deviants," and/or "defectives," all synonymous with "feeblemindedness" and because it was endorsed by an increasingly receptive and varied group of citizens. Carey (2003, pp. 420–421) points out that people considered feebleminded were by far, the most vulnerable of any in society during the eugenic period. Once assigned, the feebleminded label was emphasized above all others; vigorously defended by powerful interests; and nearly impossible to reverse, despite the intervention of community allies

Five years after the Malaga eviction, the governor appointed the Maine Commission for the Study of the Feebleminded that in turn requested the National Committee for Mental Hygiene to conduct a "thorough investigation of the whole problem of feeblemindedness" throughout the state (*Report of the Maine Commission for the Feebleminded and the Survey of the National Commission for Mental Hygiene*, 1918, p. 3). In the final report, the Malaga community was described as:

> One of the largest of the State's degenerate communities ... has been ingeniously dispersed.... Three consignments of feebleminded children were sent to the State School for Feebleminded and the squatters notified to remove their shacks. In the course of time this was done and little hardship resulted. Before this step was taken, however, dwellers of the nearby main land were often startled by night by the weird shouts, howls, profanity, obscenity, and reports of firearms from the island This colony contained many with mixed African blood. (p. 42)

In 1927, 15 years after Malaga and the same year the Supreme Court declared the constitutionality of eugenic sterilization in *Buck v. Bell,* the *Portland Sunday Gazette and Sunday Press Herald* ran a front page story revisiting the Malaga incident. In it, the reporters again juxtaposed race and feeblemindedness, portraying a community bereft of moral standards, genetically depleted by generations of inter-racial and intra-family breeding, and intellectually incapable of benefitting from the best re-socialization efforts of dedicated reformers. The message to Mainers seemed unmistakable: these were precisely the kind of people to whom

Justice Oliver Wendell Holmes was referring in *Buck v. Bell* when he declared the constitutionality of eugenic sterilization, noting society's responsibility to "prevent those who are manifestly unfit from continuing their own kind. . . Three generations of imbeciles are enough" (*Buck v. Bell*, 274, U.S. 200).

One photo showed two men standing in a row boat with the caption: "Harmless simple-minded folk, were the Malagaites" ("A Few Interesting Tales of Lower Casco Bay," 1927, p. A1). Another depicted an African American woman sitting outside a dwelling with three White children around her, and the caption: "Malaga. A black mother with straight hair and three white children" (p. A1). According to the article:

> True it is that marriages were practically unknown. Men and women lived together and children grew up. Sometimes a Malagaite would trade his "woman" for a boat! Things became pretty badly mixed. White mothers – black fathers—and vice versa. Some children light, others dark.... Deplorable indeed!
>
> It is easy to understand how, with the ever-growing number of vacation folk along the beautiful Maine coast, No Man's Land [the new name for Malaga] became impossible. It was a great problem, to be sure. The people were harmless, but such inter-living had resulted in such intolerable conditions – feeblemindedness, disease, illiterateness.
>
> [Following the eviction, the island] was swept clean of all squatters, and ... beautiful Malaga is at last peacefully primitive again in its undisturbed grandeur. (p. A1)

The article described a local justice of the peace, whose own moral code apparently went unquestioned, attempted to impose "correct" moral standards on the islanders by bringing a "packet full of marriage licenses and a gun to straighten things out" ("A Few Interesting Tales of Lower Casco Bay," 1927, p. A1). Reportedly, he shot several dogs and forcibly married two or three couples, but ultimately failed in his broader mission to impose marital uniformity on the island. Portrayed in the article as ignorant beyond redemption, the islanders were said to have "tacked the [marriage] licenses to the walls of their hovels, and exhibited them to strangers as curiosities" (p. A1).

While the media and the state characterized the Malaga eviction as causing little harm or hardship, the consequences for the evicted and relocated were traumatic, even tragic. The institutional records of those removed to the Maine School indicate that of the seven members of the Marks family—Jake and Abbie, children James, Lizzie, Lottie, and Etta, and grandchild, William (son of Lizzie), only Abigal and Lottie survived their commitment and were eventually released. The others died in the institution.

One newspaper account revealed that the Marks family had some community supporters although the story also illustrated that they had little recourse in the face of public fear and professional authority. The article, unsympathetic to the plight of the family, told of a former Maine School employee who questioned the incarceration of Abbie, and her daughters, Lottie and Etta:

> In her efforts to secure the discharge of these two, the former employee has not only argued with Dr. Hedin [Pownal's superintendent] but has consulted a member of the Governor's Council, a member of the State Board of Charities and Corrections and others and has published letters in the Portland newspapers. Her claim is that this mother and her daughters are normal and should be given their liberty. She sincerely believes that they would be competent help and could easily be self-supporting. Dr. Hedin and the State officials to whom she has told her story have listened courteously. In the first place, considering there are 160 feebleminded on the waiting list, it can readily be realized that, if the authorities deemed it wise, they would be only too glad to discharge these two for the sake of others who are desperately in need of care.
>
> The superintendent and others have attempted to explain why it would be altogether unsafe to allow them to leave. At West Pownal, under supervision and where they have no responsibility, they are apparently normal, but left to their own devices, there is reason to believe they would be harmful to society. Those who know the ins and outs of the situation say they do not doubt the wisdom of the State authorities in keeping them under surveillance. ("Care of Feeble-Minded Big Problem for Maine," 1914, p. A2)

Abbie Marks was released five years after her admission, while Lottie was discharged after 13 years in 1925, the same year as her sister, Etta, died in the institution (DuBrule, 1999, p. 91).

The Malaga incident remains an open wound for Mainers. Gerald Talbot, former state legislator, local historian, and past president of the state's chapter of the NAACP, remarked that for many of Maine's African Americans, "hearing the word Malaga, ... is like hearing the word 'Dachau' " (DuBrule, 1999, p. 49). Maine never acknowledged its role in the eviction (p. 91), although Talbot and others have called for a thorough investigation of the Malaga incident and an official apology to the descendants of the island families (Turkel, 2001, p. B8). Following a series of well publicized accounts of the Malaga incident, the Maine legislature passed what Woodard (2010) termed a "bungled act of contrition" and "strange sort of apology. Woodard (2010) reported that on April 7, 2010, lawmakers passed a unanimous, joint resolution describing the State's numerous injustices toward the islanders, expressing "profound regret," and vowing to "rededicate themselves to the ideals of tolerance, independence, and equality." Unlike other unanimous, joint resolutions, however, this one was never publicized. No notice was sent to island descendents, representatives of the Maine chapter of NAACP, or the news media, so none of these individuals and organizations witnessed or reported the state's only official apology. The legislative action was detected by Rob Rosenthal, the producer of the 2009 radio documentary, *Malaga Island: A Story Best Left Untold,* who posted it on the documentary's Facebook. *Down East Magazine* picked up the story, leading embarrassed state officials to issue a proper apology (Woodard, 2010). In a September 12, 2010 ceremony on Malaga, nearly 100 years after the incident, Governor John Baldacchi stood before Malaga descendents, members of the NAACP, and the media and formally apologized (Fishell, 2010).

Few relics remain of the events on Malaga. The island remains uninhabited. Its schoolhouse was relocated to another community, and the graves of the "uprooted dead," remain in a section of cemetery in

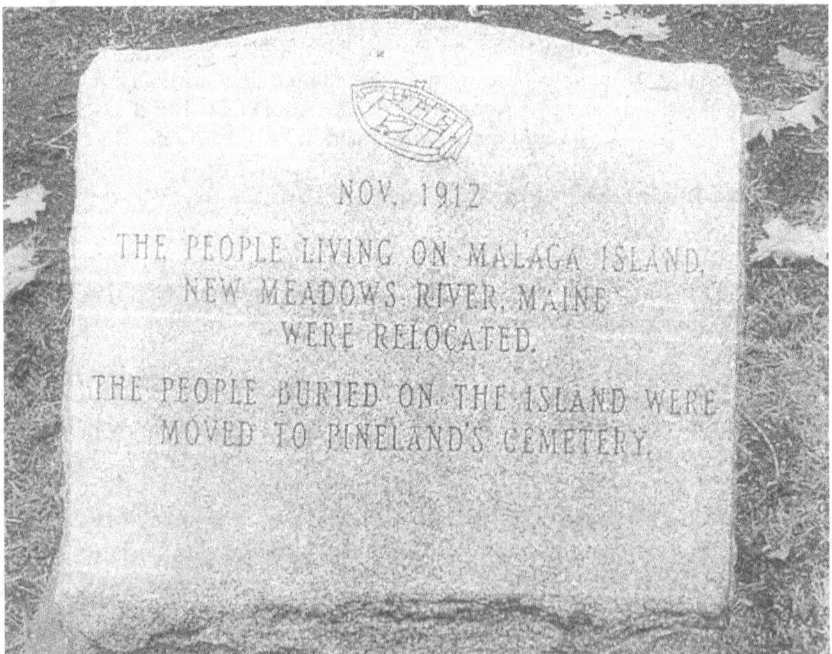

Figure 4.1. Malaga Island Commemoration at Pineland Cemetery (photograph by Stephen Murphy)

New Gloucester reserved for former Pineland residents, attesting to their identity as feebleminded, and far from the island on which they lived. Headstones bear the names of only those whose corpses were easily identified, and the month and year of reburial: Nov. 1912" (p. 91).

Nathan Hamilton, a professor of anthropology, and some of his associates attempted to include Malaga Island on the National Register of Historic Places (Greico, 2004, p. 30). In 1998, Elaine Gallant, a former Pineland employee, "moved by what she saw as a festering injustice" (Turkel, 2001, p. B1), raised $312 for a monument, which she erected at the cemetery where the Malaga re-internment occurred. The monument's simple inscription, however, fails to acknowledge the injustice that characterized this event noting only that: "The people living on Malaga Island, New Meadows River, Maine were relocated. The people buried on the island were moved to Pineland's cemetery" (p. B1).

The construction of the Maine School, and the government-led actions on Malaga Island revealed the mix of factors and parties fueling the eugenic movement in Maine. And there would soon be more to come.

INSTITUTIONAL GROWTH AND EXPANDING LEGAL RESTRICTIONS

In 1913, controversy erupted over escalating costs and squalid living conditions at the Maine School, allegations that contrasted sharply with official accounts and previous media images. Several newspapers began to referring to the facility as a "gold brick," calling conditions "beyond description with no signs of improvement," and predicting that the institution would be condemned and moved elsewhere ("State May Drop Its 'Gold Brick,' " 1913, p. A1). A headline in the *Daily Eastern Argus* blared: "Condemn Home for Feeble Minded;" called legislators "disgusted with conditions at Pownal's institution;" and reported that

> the cottage for boys of feeble minds was located between two barns entirely unsanitary and of foul atmospheric surroundings, that there was no water supply on the place that was at all satisfactory and unless artificial means was employed at considerable expense that there would result great damage to the health of the patients. ("Condemn Home For Feeble Minded," 1913, p. A1)

Faced with a $300,000 budget request, legislators were quoted as believing that the school could never be placed on a sound economical basis in its present location, or be expanded "to the extent that is demanded" (p. A1).

Despite the critical news accounts, Superintendent Carl Hedin defended the institution and raised the eugenic rhetoric, referring to feeblemindedness as the strongest determinant of "crime, pauperism, immorality, and defective, illegitimate children", and calling "morbid heredity" the strongest factor in producing feeblemindedness (*Sixth Annual Report of the Maine School for Feeble Minded*, 1914, p. 15). According to Hedin, segregation of societal menaces was imperative and heightened institutional costs paled in comparison with the price of complacency:

> The public is paying … ever increasing sums and will continue to do so until the feebleminded are properly segregated and prevented from producing their own kind. With this in mind and knowing that there are several hundreds of the feebleminded scattered over the State who are allowed to increase the public burden without restraint, there can be no logical argument against the crying need for enlargement of this institution. It costs money to properly segregate and care for the feebleminded, but it will save money in the end. (*Sixth Annual Report of the Maine School for Feeble Minded*, 1914, p. 15)

Hedin also countered lawmakers' criticisms of the school's location, arguing that the farm would eventually become a model of productivity:

> As a matter of fact, 2/3 of our fields consist of a clay loam which is entirely free from rocks; … By plowing, fertilizing, cultivating and rotating crops, a large portion of the farm has already been brought up to a high state of production. I have no doubt that this farm will be one of the best farms in the State for raising hay, grain and vegetables. (*Sixth Annual Report of the Maine School for Feeble Minded*, 1914, p. 20)

In 1914 enrollment remained steady at 260, although, the waiting list grew to 152. Moreover, the State Board of Charities and Corrections identified four hundred and eighty two additional persons, "the great majority of [whom] ... are in almshouses throughout the State or else are boarded out, as being feebleminded and as receiving public funds" (*Sixth Annual Report of the Maine School for Feeble Minded*, 1914, p. 15). Arguing that almshouses were "disastrous" places for such people, Hedin contended that without specialized facilities, "children receive no training, the men are often allowed to commit arson and other criminal acts, and the feebleminded women are not given proper moral protection which will prevent them from becoming mothers" (p. 15).

Heightening his appeal for institutional expansion, Hedin proposed to not only reduce the waiting list but also to eliminate feeblemindedness across the state by concentrating on the most menacing individuals, precisely those who were avoiding incarceration due to the invisibility of their condition:

> We have now 110 applications for admission.... These figures, however, are no indication of the number of feeble-minded in the State. The people know that the Institution is full, hence many apply only for urgent and troublesome cases. Some have withdrawn their applications and applied to private and state institutions in other states. Then again a large percentage of the high grade imbeciles and morons are not recognized as feeble-minded by relatives and friends, and yet we know only too well that oftentimes these are the most harmful and dangerous to the community, as they are able to reproduce their kind and thus become an important factor in the production of feeblemindedness, insanity, crime, pauperism, intemperance and prostitution.
>
> Since we know that the production of feeblemindedness is largely a question of heredity, and that the only way to reduce the number of defectives is to prevent them from begetting their own kind, why should we not segregate all the feebleminded and thus prevent feeblemindedness? (*Fifth Annual Report of the Maine School for Feeble Minded*, 1913, pp. 11–12)

Two years later, Hedin reversed himself, conceding that perhaps not all feebleminded people required incarceration and that "no serious harm to the community can result" if carefully selected residents are discharged "to suitable homes"(*Seventh Annual Report of the Maine School for Feeble Minded*, 1915, p. 10). During this period, institutional officials were heralding new methods of identifying mental deficiency and screening institutional referrals, replacing Kerlin's classification system and supplementing the interviews, observations and physical exams that staff conducted after people were admitted to the institution. Goddard's invention of the "moron" category and his endorsement of the Binet test and a new classification schema led to diminished use of the generic term, "feeblemindedness" in favor of more specific categories like "idiot" which included those whose mental ages fell below three years; "imbecile "that included people who scored between 3–7 years; and 'moron' that featured individuals with measured intelligence from 8–12 years" (Trent, 1994, p. 162).

During this period, Maine School officials began routinely administering the Binet Test and collecting family histories for each resident. Extolling the intelligence measure, Hedin claimed it "more accurately and scientifically [detected] the exact degree of mental defect present in each child"(*Fifth Annual Report of the Maine School for Feeble Minded*, 1913, p. 12). He also contended that his pedigree screening efforts were highly accurate and improving every year. In 1915, Hedin announced that 39.5% of the facility's admissions showed a family history of feeblemindedness in father or mother, or both, and 44.7% had defective siblings (*Seventh Annual Report of the Maine School for Feeble Minded*, 1914, p. 9). The next year he declared that he found causal heredity links in 76% of new admissions, and, using his family histories, picked up hereditary indicators such as insanity, epilepsy, alcoholism, syphilis, tuberculosis and/or cancer (*Eighth Annual Report of the Maine School for Feeble Minded*, 1916, p. 9).

A SURGICAL SOLUTION FOR THE "UNFIT"

On May 7, 1914, Hedin addressed the Portland Medical Club (remarks later published in the *Journal of the Maine Medical Association*) and presented his standard portrayal of feeblemindedness as the preeminent, inheritable source of social pathology and disorder, with particular warnings about promiscuous women. What made Hedin's speech noteworthy, however, was that he explicitly broached the subject of eugenic sterilization, endorsing the practice, and ushering in the peak period of persecution in Maine. Despite his enthusiasm for the surgery, even Hedin (1914) acknowledged that sterilization was too unpopular in Maine at this time to be considered a realistic possibility:

> Some of you may ask, "Why not sterilize the feebleminded and prevent them from procreating their own kind?" That ... would be a step in the right direction, but public sentiment is so strongly against it that I fear that at best it will be only a partial remedy. (p. 1898)

Hedin also worried that pushing too hard for a sterilization law might create a public backlash toward the institution. As an example, he cited one state where sterilizations were conducted despite public opposition and "people ceased to send their feebleminded to the institution where the officials had the authority to do this operation ... [and] they demanded that those who already were committed there should be released" (Hedin as quoted in Swift, 1914, p. 169).

The sterilization campaign in Maine was led by the medical community and Hedin was not the first physician in the state to mention the surgery. In 1912, Dr. Henry Miller, Superintendent of the Maine Insane Hospital in Augusta gave a presentation to the state's medical association titled "Eugenics," a science he defined as aiming "to produce the best type of men and women, to purify, better, and advance the race" (Miller, 1913, p.1128). Miller's stated the importance of controlling "the production" of all forms of deviance including "the imbeciles, insane, the criminals, inebriate, degenerate, and the other physically and mentally defective members of our community," and he considered it unfortunate that the "science" of eugenics had come to be known only for its "surgical intervention" (pp. 1128–1129). He pointed out that eugenics also emphasized other remedies, such as encouraging fit parents to have more children, and segregating those considered incompetent, deviant, or dangerous. The latter approach he termed "theoretically ideal but practically impossible" (p. 1129).

While describing "asexualization" as permitting the individual "to have the greatest possible liberty but forever preventing him from propagating, Miller, like Hedin, had concerns about adopting the surgical solution. He expressed "certain constitutional concerns," limited applicability to already institutionalized groups, and public wariness (Miller, 1913, p. 1129). Although Miller indicated that Ontario, Canada and 10 states in the U.S. had enacted statutes "inhibiting procreation in habitual criminals, viscous insane, feeble-minded, epileptic, and other defectives," and designated medical boards to oversee the operation, he concluded that "the measure is too radical and is unwarranted in the light of our present knowledge" (pp. 1130–1131).

While Miller and Hedin harbored reservations about the surgery's feasibility in Maine, other state physicians did not. Henry Swift (1914) called the birthrates of feebleminded "alarming," arguing that sterilization would reduce "our dependent classes," and that "a vigorous public education effort would convince the general populace of the surgery's merits" (pp. 161–162). Claiming that the growing numbers of feebleminded were six times larger than current institutional enrollments and that birth rates of this group were twice those of normal people, Swift argued that lifelong incarceration was fiscally unfeasible (p. 164). He recommended that sterilization serve as "the condition for release" of the feebleminded from Maine's prisons, jails and institutions and that space be made for new admissions without the necessity of institutional enlargement (p. 167). In promoting the surgery as the way to facilitate discharge and thereby reduce institutional enlargement, Swift attached to the surgery economic and bureaucratic benefits beyond its medical purpose.

Joining Swift was Dr. Seth Gordon, the president of the Maine School's board of trustees, who emphasized how advantageous wholesale sterilizations would be not only for the state, but for each individual, even those whose only "defect" was his urge to escape:

> If we could absolutely stop the propagation of defectives especially it would be a great thing done for the State.... Anyone who has seen for the last three years as I have seen the defectives at West Pownal, would realize fully that there could be no harm done. It would be no disservice to man or sin against God to sterilize everyone of those men and women who are of child bearing age.
>
> We discharged one boy ... who was absolutely able to take care of himself. He had run away twice and had taken care of himself for several months without any question whatever. He said: "If I am not set free I will run away, and I will go so far that you cannot possibly catch me." He was a bright,

> intelligent man in many ways, but there was a defect about him; and if that man could have been sterilized there is no question that he ought to have been let loose. There are quite a number cases among the women at the institution where the same thing should be done. (Swift, 1914, pp. 168–169)

Gordon went on to suggest that it might be necessary and appropriate to sterilize people without the benefit of law. Citing Indiana, he reported that "they were absolutely sterilizing in the institution for the feebleminded and the state prison without any law at all.... [T]he law was enacted afterwards, and ... public sentiment is absolutely being created in favor of this thing" (Swift, 1914, p. 169).

Gordon's confidence in the public's support of sterilization in Maine was prescient, but a decade premature. Swift (1914, p. 164), on the other hand, wondered why eugenic teachings, marriage restrictions, sterilizations and similar actions had stalled across the country. He could understand the public's reluctance to sterilize the insane where "even in families with bad heredity, some children are normal," and "even genius," but he was mystified as to why anyone could object to sterilizing "defectives"—"idiots, imbeciles, many drunkards and petty criminals," given that they are "unlikely to beget children of even average mental capacity" (p. 165).

Pockets of resistance to the surgery could be found in Maine, none more active or vocal than the Catholic Church. Any obituary for the sterilization movement in Maine or nationally, however, was premature. Though stalled by religious opposition and legal questions, the operation would soon reappear with renewed vigor, even as some scientists were developing doubts about its validity. As it turns out, the sterilization campaign would be reignited as much for fiscal and professional reasons as for biomedical ones.

Most Maine lawmakers continued to strongly support the Maine School, although they often complained bitterly about its escalating costs and perpetual waiting list. In 1915, as state legislators and officials looked for ways to cut costs and address spiraling demand, they resorted to some sleight-of-hand tactics. To reduce demand, they imposed an age limit on admission candidates, eliminating the oldest individuals, a move that immediately reduced the waiting list by one third. Admissions were now specifically limited to males between ages 6 and 40, and females between 6 and 45 (*Seventh Annaul Report of the Maine School for Feeble-Minded,* 1915, p. 11). This opened the door for the release of older residents but even with that action, the institution quickly filled to capacity and the waiting list was soon replenished beyond previous levels.

While enlarging the facility was the overriding priority of institutional officials, controlling the flow of residents was equally essential. Of particular importance was *who* was admitted, especially since all parties had different agendas regarding admissions and discharges. Because the institution required widespread legislative support, admissions decisions were often driven as much by political influence, geographic location and other factors peripherally related to the facility's official admissions criteria. Municipal authorities, law enforcement, social services and judges were anxious to refer troublesome and expensive individuals. Some families, confronted with legal, professional and/or fiscal pressures, were desperate for relief.

On the other side, institutional officials had their own needs to consider. Hedin wanted to decide who entered and exited the facility as the trustees and other outside parties pressured him to accept those he considered unmanageable and/or "worthless." He complained bitterly about turning the Maine School into a custodial setting and not admitting enough younger, higher functioning residents whom he needed to operate the facility efficiently. By selectively admitting and retaining desirable residents, Hedin believe he could show more rehabilitation successes, thereby enhancing the institution's public, political and fiscal support and garnering the professional recognition and legitimacy, and authority to grow and prosper. Clearly, he was frustrated by what he considered his lack of power over such matters:

> Only 21% of the new admissions were of school age and capable of reading and writing.... The great majority were so physically and mentally defective that they were seen as capable of no improvement (p. 9) ... 43.7% of all new admissions were either seen as not improvable at all or only slightly so. Indeed, many were so crippled, paralyzed or helpless that they were hospital cases. There was noted a marked tendency on the part of town and city officials, families and guardians to make the most urgent appeals for the most urgent cases who are not able to benefit from the School's services. (*Seventh Annual Report of the Maine School for Feeble-Minded*, 1915, p. 9)

Hedin added to his complaints, using more vivid language a few years later:

> We have 180 on the waiting list and the school is crowded to the utmost limit. The Trustees give preference in accepting cases to girls of the childbirth period from 15 to 45 who are apt to have children and propagate their kind, and they give preference next to boys who are vicious. We accommodate 282.... Very few are able to go home and support themselves. We have to accept from the different counties in proportion to the population, and we are trying to give each county in the State the same chance.
>
> Of course, we now have a law [giving preference to those] between 6 and 40 [years of age]. After 40, the Trustees ... have the right to discharge them if they are harmless.... [W]hen the school started they dumped into it all the criminals and worthless cases-idiots-that we can do nothing for except to

> keep them in custody and give them care. To be sure, they need a home and proper care but they are taking the place that these younger cases should have for treatment. I have done all I could to change that. You understand the pressure from the people is great to keep the most helpless there, and when you try to return a helpless case, or one that cannot take care of himself, the whole community rises against it, and sends its selectmen and other prominent representatives to oppose it.... Yes, it is now a home for helpless cases. (as cited in Fernald, 1918, pp. 117–118)

Tension over institutional control in general and admissions in particular would continue for decades, reflecting the political character of the facility and the reality that the institution's professional and bureaucratic needs for efficiency and legitimacy were as influential in driving its policies and operations as any medical or scientific factors. With so many people being referred and admitted for so many varied reasons, the Maine School quickly became crowded with a very diverse population of residents, some of whom needed more extensive attention and supervision than existing paid staff could provide. This required that the onus of care for many of the most difficult residents was placed on the shoulders of capable, unpaid resident workers, a group that was also performing much of the farm, maintenance, and domestic labor. Consequently, people with the most obvious impairments for whom the facility might be most persuasively justified were now characterized as the least desirable residents–referred to as chronic, custodial cases, too "worthless" to be of use to the facility. Conversely, those considered the most physically and cognitively skilled were seen as the best candidates, making them more likely to be admitted and less likely to be discharged despite their evident abilities.

Maine School officials discussed as early as 1913 the possibility of discharging selected residents "if they had suitable homes," although worrying that such discharges were risky since "feeble-mindedness is largely hereditary [and] the unfortunate trouble might skip a whole generation without showing up and then when least expected it will crop out" (as cited in "The Home for Feeble-Minded at Pownal," 1913, p. A15). In 1914, Hedin reiterated both his belief that "morbid heredity," caused social ills ranging from crime to illegitimacy, and the urgent need to segregate everyone in Maine determined to be feebleminded (*Sixth Annual Report of the Maine School for Feeble Minded*, 1914, p. 15).

In 1915, however, the superintendent dramatically and suddenly reversed himself, proposing the radical idea of discharging more residents and beginning a community placement, supervision, and education program:

> There are a few of these cases who after certain periods of care become quite industrious, and seem to show no further criminal or immoral tendencies.

> In my opinion no serious harm to the community can result if such boys and girls are given a trial outside the institution, provided that they are sent to suitable homes, preferably in the country, where they will receive proper care and supervision. I further believe that in such cases there should be some provision by which the institution could supervise the treatment of the feeble-minded boy or girl thus sent out with authority to have the case returned to the institution if the best interests of the patient or the community required such action. This, I think, could, be accomplished by an intelligent and trained visitor, who would visit these boys and girls at certain intervals and report to the institution how each case was being treated. These trained visitors would, in addition, be able to acquire information in regard to feeble-minded persons in the surrounding neighborhood and report the same to the institution. They would also be able educate the public and give much intelligent advice in reference to the feeble-minded in the various communities. (*Seventh Annual Report of the Maine School for Feeble-Minded*, 1915, p. 10)

Why did the superintendent so suddenly change his mind? Several reasons may explain his dramatic reversal. Compelling evidence was emerging from Charles Bernstein's practices in upstate New York and Walter Fernald's startling follow-up study of discharged residents in Massachusetts, both of which documented the successful adjustment of released individuals to community life. In addition, respected scientists such as Edith Spaulding and William Healy were raising serious questions about the inheritability of social pathology and the need and practicality of costly and large-scale segregation. Finally, the mental hygiene faction was gaining influence within the psychiatric community, and softening its indictment of feeblemindedness as the sole cause of all social deviance, promoting more institutional discharges with community supervision, and focusing on wholesale prevention (Scull, 2005, p. 59).

Despite his emerging community-oriented rhetoric, however, Hedin continued to build up the institution and retain its residents. From 1913 until 1915, Pownal's discharge rate hovered around 4%, including home visits and escapes. In the years 1916–18, the rate increased modestly to 5.7% but the superintendent carefully characterized his discharges as minimal and benign:

> Only eleven cases were discharged from the institution this year. Four were discharged at the request of relatives; four were discharged because, on account of advanced age, they had become harmless, and therefore did not need further institutional care; one was discharged into a private family where she could support herself; and two high grade boys were discharged because they did not return from elopement. They were both capable of self support. Of the eleven cases discharged 7 were discharges as improved and 4

> as capable of self support. (*Eighth Annual Report of the Maine School for Feeble-Minded*, 1916, p. 10)

During the same period, enrollments increased by 12%. In 1917, the state completed a huge new dormitory for 105 boys and Hedin followed that up by proposing an equally large girls' building. He argued that overall demand was great and that even with the new boys' facility the school would still be able to care for only half of those who were applying for admission (*Ninth and Tenth Annual Report of the Maine School for Feeble-Minded*, 1917–1918, p. 10).

Although Hedin was sympathetic to the recently hatched mental hygiene approach, like many of his colleagues, he continued to espouse a hard eugenic line. Despite the looming war along with accompanying fiscal constraints and personnel shortages, he called for accelerating institutional growth. Referring to segregation as a good investment, he recommended building a new female dormitory "even under present war conditions," "for as surly as the feeble-minded girl is allowed to be at large unprotected, she will increase mental deficiency, immorality, crimes, and other social problems, for which the state must pay" ((*Ninth and Tenth Annual Reports of the Maine School for Feeble-Minded*, 1917–1918, p. 19).

Institutional officials also continued to justify as cost-efficient and rehabilitative the admission and retention of able and competent residents to serve as facility workers. Assistant Superintendent, Dr. Lewis Robinson, pointed out that "the boys and girls do a moderate amount of work which is considered essential to their treatment" (The Home for Feeble-Minded at Pownal," 1913, p. A15), while Hedin termed resident labor as "education," reinforcing the facility's mission and image as a school:

> I believe that the best educational treatment of all mentally defective is to give them an opportunity to do things with their hands. The lower grades in mentality should be taught the simpler things, while the higher grades should be taught more complex work, but all should be taught to do useful and common things.
>
> All of the older boys who are physically able to work take an active part on the farm, and other work about the institution. They have assisted in clearing many acres of land ... in the planting, hoeing, weeding, and harvesting … in excavating the earth and laying the foundations for a day room and a vegetable cellar … [digging] several hundred feet of trenches for steam, water, and sewer pipes … grading and building roads and walks about the buildings and grounds … hauling of wood and dressing … helping the teamsters … assisting the engineers … work[ing] in the horse stables,

> the cow barn, and the piggery.... In the winter, the boys cut wood and help to get the ice. At the farm colonies ... the boys do much of the housework.
>
> The older girls are regularly employed in the various household departments. They assist with various kinds of work in the kitchens, serving in the dining rooms, in the laundry, and in the sewing and mending room.... The girls also take care of the hens and chickens, and care for their own flower beds. (*Sixth Annual Report of the Maine School for Feeble-Minded*, 1914, pp. 16–19)

Admission and discharge figures for 1917-20 revealed that more younger people were admitted, although many candidates older than 20 were also added and overall discharges actually decreased. Moreover, the highest number of new admissions occurred for those between fifteen and twenty years of age, many of whom would be considered older than school age and all of whom were old enough to perform institutional work.

Justifying his need to admit younger, more capable residents and discharge many older ones, Hedin again contradicted himself. In 1914, he proclaimed:

> While it may be possible to support a certain class of feeble-minded in the almshouses, we know only too well the disastrous result of such treatment of the feeble-minded as a class. The children receive no training, the men are often allowed to commit arson and other criminal acts, and the feeble-minded women are not given the proper moral protection which will prevent them from becoming mothers (*Sixth Annual Report of the Maine School for Feeble-Minded*, 1914, p. 15)

One year later, he argued that "older persons, who after they have passed the school age are not capable of being trained to any extent, and are not apt to become a source of future danger to the community and can therefore be cared for in the various almshouses" (*Seventh Annual Report of the Maine School for Feeble-Minded*, 1915, p. 11). Hedin's commitment to "mental hygiene" seemed rather narrowly confined to those he considered too old and incapable of performing institutional work. Apparently, the dreaded almshouses posed no dangers to those considered "untrainable." As importantly, Hedin seemed untroubled by his seemingly contradictory views, underscoring his own self-interests and a willingness to manipulate definitions, policies and practices to suit his own professional needs and the changing economic, political, and/or social priorities around him. As Gallagher (1999, p. 200) demonstrated in Vermont, despite historians' tendency to see the eugenic and mental hygiene movements as "separate and theoretically antagonistic," they could be compatibly maneuvered and dovetailed to meet individual ends.

1917–18 REPORT OF THE MAINE COMMISSION FOR THE STUDY OF THE FEEBLEMINDED

Just before the country's entry into World War I, the cost and control of Maine's feebleminded citizens assumed central importance. In his inaugural address on January 4, 1917, Governor Carl Milliken called "the expansion ... care, segregation, and treatment of the feebleminded one of the State's most urgent needs," but added that the problem was becoming expensive during a period of economic uncertainty (as quoted in *Report of the Maine Commission for the Feebleminded and the Survey by the National Committee for Mental Hygiene*, 1918, p. 5). Before directing further expenditures toward its solution, the governor ordered an investigation that was eventually contracted to the National Committee of Mental Hygiene (NCMH), a group that was started by an ex-patient, turned popular author and institutional critic, Clifford Beers. Unfortunately, Beers soon lost control of his original movement to a new breed of reform-minded medical superintendents who called themselves "psychiatrists" (Rafter, 1997, p. 170) and were able to divert Beer's original purpose away from institutional critique and treatment reform and toward professional expansion and perpetuation (Grob, 1983, pp. 162–164; Scull, 2005, p. 58).

One of the NCMH's primary tactics was the use of statewide surveys to study incidences of feeblemindedness not only in mental hospitals, but also throughout the states' cities and towns in public schools, reformatories, prisons, and facilities for those considered mentally defective (Dowbiggin, 1997, p. 127). Maine's version of the NCMH survey was directed by Dr. Guy Fernald, a physician at the men's reformatory in Concord, Massachusetts. He conducted the survey from 1917–1918 and reported the results to the governor in February, 1919 *(Report of the Maine Commission for the Feebleminded and the Survey by the National Committee for Mental Hygiene*, 1918, p. 3). Fernald also published periodic bulletins in local papers, reporting on selected topics and findings, publicizing the "feebleminded" problem and urging public and political action.

Guy Fernald was a leading proponent of the "defective delinquent" concept. This was a term similar to Goddard's "moron," and its increasing use represented the beginning of a change in the way people, formerly called "feebleminded," were labeled. According to revisionist, or "softening," eugenicists, part of the feebleminded population consisted of relatively harmless defectives while others were considered morally corrupt, "defective delinquents," later referred to as "psychopathic" (Rafter, 1997, p. 190). This newly constructed type of "deviant feebleminded" caused a host of social maladies, was found in nearly all prisons and reformatories, and. like the "moron" was often invisible and therefore particularly threatening:

> Under this generic heading represents the Moron and the Characterologic Deviate as types of mental defectiveness whose behavior and mental eccentricities differentiate them in kind and degree from the low-grade feebleminded on the one hand and from the adult minded and the subnormal on the other.... Many offenders, petty grafters, forgers, panderers, prostitutes, thieves, vagrants, and unskilled laborers are of this grade and mentality.
>
> The cost of supporting this parasitic group, including as it does, many of the court cases of theft, sex offences, arson, vagrancy, assault, gambling, etc is enormous. (*Report of the Maine Commission for the Feebleminded and the Survey by the National Committee for Mental Hygiene*, 1918, p. 16)

The commission warned that, within this collective, no one was more dangerous than women, whether as menacing perpetrators or innocent victims:

> From 50% to 80% of prostitutes are feebleminded.... The unsupervised feebleminded girl is a very grave menace, potential or actual, in any community. She becomes an actual menace of the gravest kind when she becomes infected with either of the two principle venereal diseases, gonorrhea and syphilis. (*Report of the Maine Commission for the Feebleminded and the Survey by the National Committee for Mental Hygiene*, 1918, pp. 34–35)
>
> The victims of infection seek to hide their shame and the boys and girls with poisoned minds and defiled bodies may not be casually distinguished, but as every physician knows, blighted homes are often left along the trails of these often feebleminded females. Any state will do well indeed when it segregates medically, intellectually, and morally these misguided women. (p. 31)
>
> Having the same passions as the well equipped mentally, but lacking, as they do, the inhibitions and higher motives to self-control, the feebleminded women and girls are easily tempted and easily become the victims of the contemptible pimps and panderers who profit by woman's shame.... They must be quarantined and the community safeguarded against their return as prostitutes. p. 34)

The commission cited Maine as a particularly troubled state. It's population of 793,000 included at least 3,000 people considered feebleminded, but likely the number was much higher since the state had approximately 12,000 "dependents" and "the problem of poverty and failure is the problem of dependency, or in popular parlance, the problem of feeblemindedness" (*Report of the Maine Commission for the Feebleminded and the Survey by the National Committee for Mental Hygiene*, 1918, Bulletin 5, pp. 88–89; *Report of the Maine Commission for the Feebleminded and the Survey by the National Committee for Mental Hygiene*, 1918, Bulletin 6, p. 93). In addition, the commission reported that Maine's military-eligible pool of young men rated among the nation's most infected, ranking 43rd out of

48 in the number of recruits rejected for military service because of mental disability. Claiming that the situation in Maine was a long standing problem that caused the state to lose its "best young blood and brains" and its "best human breeding stock to other states since 1850" (*Report of the Maine Commission for the Feebleminded and the Survey by the National Committee for Mental Hygiene*, 1918, Bulletin 3, p. 81), the commission argued that the remaining population consisted of large numbers of "defectives" and "degenerate families" who are following the "usual course of natural race selection," and would soon overwhelm the state "since they tend to perpetuate their own kind and cling to their own communities" (p. 81).

Reflecting the "progressive" mental hygiene side, the commission recommended that Maine should pursue several key actions, such as: professional identification and registration of young, extra-institutional feebleminded; removal of children from their families or institutional training; and selective parole and professional community supervision (*Report of the Maine Commission for the Feebleminded and the Survey by the National Committee for Mental Hygiene*, 1918, p. 53).

Consistent with the NCMH's expansionist, preventative, and extra-institutional emphases, the commission called for the "rapid expansion of the School," and the addition of housing units for both long—and short-term residents. Specifically, the state was urged to expand both the Maine School for Feeble-Minded and the Women's Reformatory "to twice or three times their present capacity" (p. 54) and operate the former as a dynamic "educational … rather than a custodial institution … [where] the primary function ... is to train the young and transformable of the high grade feebleminded from a mode of life leading to dependency into a mode of life leading to limited usefulness and moral rectitude" (*Report of the Maine Commission for the Feebleminded and the Survey by the National Committee for Mental Hygiene*, 1918, Bulletin 5, pp. 88–89). Since some "dependents" were considered curable, ideal residents were those whom the commission characterized as "in a formative period," of "somewhat higher grade of mentality" and capable of "parole to community life and a tentative assumption of self-determination" (*Report of the Maine Commission for the Feebleminded and the Survey by the National Committee for Mental Hygiene*, 1918, p. 26).

The commission saw younger, brighter residents who could be paroled as a way to expand the institution, meet its newly created mission of serving both short and long term residents, and curtail open-ended custodial expansion and its accompanying costs and professional devaluation. Facility officials would be granted expanded professional authority to identify and register targeted persons, remove children from their families, rehabilitate them within the institution, discharge them to their communities, and monitor them under psychiatric supervision. This would allow psychiatrists to greatly expand the numbers over whom they presided, increase their authority beyond the confines of the institution, reduce their custodial role, assume a more dynamic image, and serve a younger, higher functioning, and potentially more valued population.

Going beyond the state's well-established power to institutionalize certain groups, the commission promoted compulsory institutional commitment of all improperly supervised feebleminded, regardless of parental wishes. Relying largely on medical discourse to support their proposals, the commission argued for "quarantining carriers of the disease of feeblemindedness" (Carey, 2003, p. 419). Securing the power to remove children from their families against their parents' wishes, however, would prove controversial, to say the least, and require conjuring up more than medical rationales. Such a policy threatened to usurp the sacrosanct legal tradition of giving parents primary responsibility for raising their children, a tradition that the courts upheld except in cases where parents' incompetence or negligence could be proven (p. 419). Consequently, the commission set about the task of defining and discrediting families they termed "feebleminded" and "defective." At one point, the commission pointed out that "case studies here in Maine show plainly that one very large contributory factor to juvenile vice and dependency is the disorganization of the home. Child after child has been found to be dependent because of the failure of the parents to teach and control" (*Report of the Maine Commission for the Feebleminded and the Survey by the National Committee for Mental Hygiene*, 1918, Bulletin 5, p. 89). The commission went on to argue that some parents also posed grave danger to their children's safety, alleging that "feebleminded parents" were responsible for high childhood death rates. Although acknowledging that such statistics could also be attributed to poverty and poor medical care, the commission largely dismissed that possibility, asserting that in "feebleminded" households "accidents of fire and water and sickness which ordinary foresight and care would prevent, are unduly frequent. That defective mothers love their children no one should doubt; but that they know how to care for and rear their children, no one should believe" (*Report of the Maine Commission for the Feebleminded and the Survey by the National Committee for Mental Hygiene*, 1918, pp. 43-44).

Endorsing the case for strong marriage restrictions, the commission made some outlandish, even laughable, associations between mate selection and attributes such as intelligence, character, decision-making ability and productivity. Not surprisingly those considered feebleminded did not fare well:

> Decisions in the field of matrimony and family perpetuation, are … most vital and do form an important single index of adult intelligence and

> character.... Those who are whimsical and shiftless in their selection of a consort may be expected to be whimsical and shiftless in their occupational, religious and cultural decisions, and they are found to be poor farmers, and neglectful of religion, ethics and patriotism.... The point is that if these communities furnish poor consorts, parents and neighbors, they might be expected to furnish poor laborers, artisans, and producers generally. (*Report of the Maine Commission for the Feebleminded and the Survey of the National Committee for Mental Hygiene,* 1918, pp. 41–42)

One might wonder why the commission bothered to make such a dramatic case for marriage restriction laws when Maine had passed such legislation already, and even some of the staunchest eugenicists considered these laws impractical and ineffective. Perhaps the commission had a broader agenda in mind. By characterizing individuals and/or families as inherently incompetent, dependent, and/or deviant (criminal), the commission began using legal discourse (as well as continuing medical arguments) to deny full citizenship and its concomitant rights and protections to a widening array of people and recommend expanded social exclusion and/or control by a growing professional class (Carey, 2003, pp. 414–415). In addition, by promoting the idea of "feeblemindedness," as a blanket devaluation that spoke for itself, requiring minimal elaboration or assessment of individual or family skills, productivity, and/or criminal history (pp. 416–417), eugenicists could legalize compulsory institutionalization without parental permission, justify the expenditures for expanded segregation, and extend eugenic control to those outside the institution (p. 418).

The commission's paternalistic tone and social reforms reflected the best progressive ideals of the time, arguing that marriage restrictions were based on the best science of the day, that the proposed reforms were directed toward overall societal betterment, and matters such as marriage were best left to specialized professionals, namely psychiatrists, who should serve as the "final court of decision" for any appeals of marriage restrictions ((*Report of the Maine Commission for the Feebleminded and the Survey by the National Committee for Mental Hygiene*, 1918, p. 40.

Arguing that new power and wide-ranging discretion be granted to psychiatrists, the commission proposed that this group identify, treat, and dispose of all cases of feeblemindedness; and in addition hire, train, and supervise an emerging corps of social service professionals. This "small force" of field workers would include social workers, field investigators, probation officers and special teachers served as the mechanism for the commission's proposed community control of feeblemindedness (*Report of the Maine Commission for the Feebleminded and the Survey by the National Committee on Mental Hygiene,* 1918, pp. 38-40, 82). Field staff would conduct registrations of extra-institutional cases; process and transfer people between the community, institutions and/or schools; and monitor and control those on parole/probation, specifically concerning their work training or placement and their sexual activities (pp. 38–40). The commission also proposed that a state psychiatric board be the final judges on family and individual appeals of marriage restriction (p. 40).

Admitting "higher grade" residents for observation, but not prolonged retention, the institution could serve everyone in the state, rotating residents in and out as they would in a general hospital. Registration, expanded admissions of extra-institutional residents, and a liberal policy of parole was defended as fiscally responsible compared with the looming vision of an ever-expanding custodial plant. As the commission noted:

> Upon examination by the psychiatric staff, [residents] would be found to be sufficiently well equipped intellectually to keep industrially occupied or to have no character deviation which under supervision could not be corrected or tolerated. The reaching of this point will automatically put a stop to institutional extension. (p. 26)

Maine's survey represented and promoted an expanding eugenic agenda. Based on widening professional interests and authority to judge human potential, decide on societal membership, and assign suitable social roles, the commission confidently predicted short—term individual sacrifices for some and long-term societal gain for many. According to the report, "if the unfit be prevented from parenthood for a generation, and the rising generation be supervised and trained to limited usefulness, the diminution of dependency is accomplished" (*Report of the Maine Commission for the Feebleminded and the Survey by the National Committee for Mental Hygiene*, 1918, Bulletin 6, p. 93).

The commission also aspired to reach beyond the institution for an expanded array of clientele and authority. "Extra-institutional" individuals would not only be prohibited from marriage and parenthood, but rooted out of their "degenerate" communities where they tended to congregate, intermarry, and reproduce inferior offspring. Reporting on visits to three such communities, commissioners displayed genealogical graphs to illustrate how inter-generational degeneracy occurred within each location, scientifically verifying "the validity of the Mendelian Law"of genetic transmission (*Report of the Maine Commission for the Feebleminded and the Survey by the National Committee for Mental Hygiene*, 1918, Bulletin 6, pp. 40–41). Pointing to the Malaga Island settlers as examples of transmitted, inter-generational degeneracy, the commission praised the state for "ingeniously dispersing" the settlers in 1912 where "little hardship resulted" (*Report of the Maine Commission for the Feebleminded and the Survey by the National Committee for Mental Hygiene*, 1918, Bulletin 6, p. 42). Malaga Island had become the eugenicists' symbol for widespread "degenerate communities" in Maine," and a well recognized rallying cry for statewide alarm, more aggressive intervention, and widening government and professional control.

Commending the use of resident labor with the Maine School, the commission praised the retention of older, capable workers "in order to more economically care for the invalid and aged feebleminded … relieving communities, almshouses, and hospitals" (*Report of the Maine Commission for the Feebleminded and the Survey by the National Committee for Mental Hygiene*, 1918, Bulletin 6, p. 27). This apparently assured politicians and municipalities that facility officials would continue to accept troublesome referrals, minimize costs and pursue the elusive goal of institutional self-support.

One potential shortcoming of the commission's plan was that in proposing to discharge people considered ominous threats, it seemed to undermine its dire warnings about their danger to society. The commission recognized the seeming contradiction and addressed it explicitly:

> Those on probation would be under surveillance, and in failing or stopping work would be looked up and helped.... The greatest difficulty will be the training of the rising generation of defectives and deviates to habits of limited usefulness, and the prevention of their parenthood. Fortunately, however, the teaching and supervision required for training also tends to enable control of sexual propensity. (*Report of the Maine Commission for the Feebleminded and the Survey by the National Committee for Mental Hygiene*, 1918, Bulletin 3, p. 81)

In this regard, the commission appeared to pull back from the most alarmist rhetoric and punitive practices of its most conservative colleagues. Given the societal threat posed by Henry Goddard's "morons" and Guy Fernald's "defective delinquents," the commission's recommendations for community discharge and oversight seemed rather perfunctory. Could "a small force of field workers" satisfactorily monitor people's activities "in each city … and rural district and be in daily touch with the activities and manner of life of all found to be of limited responsibility because of mental defect or disease" (*Report of the Maine Commission for the Feebleminded and the Survey by the National Committee for Mental Hygiene*, 1918, Bulletin 3, p. 81 pp. 39–40)? Could potential "criminals, prostitutes, and degenerates" be safely discharged with minimal oversight, given their ascribed resourcefulness, social invisibility, sexual promiscuity and prolific birthrates?

Notably absent from the list of eugenic solutions offered by the commission was eugenic sterilization, a procedure that had been gaining some favor among state and institutional officials as a way to curtail procreation, ensure "safe" discharges, and reduce the escalating costs of large-scale segregation. Sterilization was never explicitly mentioned because of its unpopularity in Maine, the unsettled legal questions it posed and/or the state's growing Catholic population.

Although the NCMH never officially endorsed sterilization, it had many members who favored the approach. Some sterilization skeptics, like the influential Walter Fernald, did not think that the hereditary science behind the surgery was sufficiently complete or compelling to warrant widespread application (Grob, 1983, p. 173). Fernald had softened his early eugenic tone after his follow-up study revealed that most released residents led lawful, uneventful community lives. By 1918, he began distinguishing between "good and bad defectives' arguing that not all of them should be considered "criminalists and socialists and immoral and anti-social.... We have really slandered the feeble-minded" (as cited in Rafter, 1997, p. 190). Fernald also believed that sterilization removed whatever inhibitions existed for "illicit intercourse," such as pregnancy and having children, and that its aggressive application could produce a backlash against the institution by "right-thinking persons who are sympathetic to those who are "afflicted" (as cited in Largent, 2008, p. 89). Fernald began advocating for "progressive" mental hygiene practices such as selective discharges, state registration of those with mental deficiency, and family care vouchers, some of which were also included in Maine's survey report.

Another reason the NCMH may have been reluctant to publically endorse compulsory sterilization, was that one its most prominent benefactors, the highly prestigious Rockefeller Foundation, preferred to sidestep political and social controversy in favor of medical research and education and more benign public health information. Despite the fact that the foundation was headed by John D. Rockefeller Jr., who was an enthusiastic eugenicist, Foundation officials referred to eugenic sterilization legislation as "propaganda" (Dowbiggin, 1997, pp. 127–128). As the foundation began to change its funding priorities away from psychiatry and toward more laboratory research, it reduced its support of the NCMH, increasing the pressure on the Committee to conform (p. 129).

Eugenic sterilization would not be legalized in Maine for another six years, leaving Maine officials to negotiate between their own commitment to the "menace of feeble minds" and the NCMH's mental hygiene approach with its mixed message of menace and heightened segregation alongside expanded community discharge and supervision. Hedin conceded that not all of those identified as feebleminded could or should be incarcerated indefinitely if they could be controlled in the community by some state authority. He was, however, unable or unwilling to discharge many more residents, reiterating his menace message and arguing on economic, legal, and social grounds for a larger facility:

> Our inadequate accommodations for the great demand for admission of applicants and the overcrowded condition of the institution, have not enabled us to admit more than 38 per cent of the applicants … from October 1, 1916 to June 30, 1918…. From an economical point of view, however, there is no question in my mind that it would be a good investment for the State of Maine to erect this building, even under present war conditions. For as surely as the feeble-minded girl is allowed to be at large unprotected she will increase mental deficiency, immorality, crimes, and other social problems, for which the State must pay.
>
> In reference to the large number of uncared for feebleminded in the State, I cannot do better than to recommend for the State of Maine, in part, the admirable program for the care of the extra-institutional feeble-minded which Dr. Walter F. Fernald has already recommended to the state of Massachusetts, namely … that some State authority should have friendly guidance over all mental defectives in the state who are not cared for by their friends. Those who can lead wholesome, harmless lives in the community should be allowed to do so. (*The Ninth and Tenth Annual Reports of the Maine School for Feeble-Minded*, 1917-1918, p. 19)

During Hedin's last year as superintendent, the facility was ravaged by the influenza pandemic of 1918. Beginning at the Hill Farm in mid-October, 1918, and lasting for approximately 6 weeks, the disease was often accompanied by pneumonia, causing death and hardship. Operating with a staff depleted by war and unprepared for an emergency of this magnitude, officials were soon overwhelmed by a medical catastrophe, as Hedin admits:

> As soon as the disease was recognized, all cases were separated from the other patients, and every precaution was observed to prevent a spread, but as we have no hospital wards or proper facilities for isolation the disease spread rapidly to other parts of the institution…. The school was quarantined, the clothing and utensils used by the sick were kept apart and sterilized after use, and all known antiseptic precautions were observed. Vaccine was used, but the epidemic was at its peak before the vaccine could be obtained. (*Eleventh Annual Report of the Maine School for Feeble-Minded*, 1919, p. 5)

At the height of the epidemic, 166 people were being treated within the facility and those staff who were healthy enough were forced to work long hours, often in unfamiliar roles. The entire institution was quarantined and unable to function without outside assistance from nurses and doctors from the Bangor and Augusta State Hospitals, the Red Cross, and the city of Portland (*Eleventh Annual Report of the Maine School for Feeble-*

Minded, 1919, pp. 4–5). Before it ended, the disease infected a total of 238 residents and 25 staff, and caused the deaths of "one matron, one attendant, and seventeen inmates" (p. 4).

Before departing, Hedin complained about the institution's lack of "hospital wards or proper facilities for isolation" for preventing the disease's rapid spread *(Eleventh Annual Report of the Maine School for Feeble-Minded,* 1919, p. 4). The epidemic's toll and Hedin's complaints may have served as an early indication that the institution should be considered a self-contained community, requiring services comparable to that offered in a small town, including a fully functioning hospital. The hospital was eventually completed in 1931.

After serving for 6 years, Carl J. Hedin left the Maine School on July 8, 1919 to become superintendent of the Bangor State Hospital (Kleinberg, 1974, p. 34) At the time of his departure, the eleven year-old, Maine School had an enrollment of 275, a figure that was about to increase dramatically to about 370 with the completion of a new dormitory. With the new building came a new construction priority and an old rationale. The priority: another new building, this time for 140 girls and a separate unit for 70 "delinquent" women. The rationale: "Every uncared for feebleminded girl is potential, prolific breeder of dependent children" (*Annual Report of the Maine School for Feeble-Minded,* Report of the Superintendent, 1920). Although the NCMH commission had opened the door a crack toward a more community-based approach in Maine, it was accompanied by both the rhetoric of "menace" and the promise of institutional enlargement. Moreover, a rejuvenated campaign to legalize compulsory sterilization would soon return with the blessing of the Supreme Court, alleviating whatever legal reservations skeptics might have had. Apparently, the drive to eliminate human deficiency in Maine would not be satisfied until the condition was transformed into a cancer that required surgical exorcism.

CHAPTER 5

CONTINUING FEARS, LEGALIZED SURGERY, AND INSTITUTIONAL ACCELERATION

Just before the end of World War I, Stephen Vosburgh, a 38-year old Massachusetts-born physician became the third superintendent of the Maine School in 1919. Vosburgh quickly became a highly visible community presence, seeming to appear everywhere across Maine. An energetic public speaker, he addressed scores of civic and community groups, charitable organizations, father and son dinners, and state and regional conferences. Vosburgh was also elected president of the Cumberland County Medical Society and at one time, was rumored to be the Governor's choice for State Commissioner of Health and Welfare. He served for 18 years as superintendent, a time period exceeded by only one other official, and remained unsurpassed as an esteemed figure and influential force who tightly controlled the manner in which "mental sub-normality"—a term he preferred to feeblemindedness—was defined and applied. The media portrayed Vosbugh as a reluctant empire builder and true humanitarian who wished that "there was no need of [the school], and that soon Maine will be relieved of [it]" (Lord, 1930, p. A–1). According to the superintendent, he continued his mission of facility expansion only because "his daily mail

Voices of Pineland: Eugenics, Social Reform, and the Legacy of "Feeblemindedness" in Maine, pp. 103–124

brings ... pathetic letters from people who present cases for admittance, cases that desperately require such care as this state school gives" (p. A–1). His record as superintendent, however, shows far more enthusiasm than reticence for institutional expansion.

Like most of his medical colleagues, Vosburgh was a committed eugenicist, promoting wholesale segregation, marriage restrictions, institutional expansion, minimal parole, and ushering in Maine's sterilization era. Immediately after replacing Hedin, Vosburgh renewed the call for a larger institution despite a just-completed dormitory for 105 boys. Between 1919 and 1939, he built up the Maine School in every conceivable way. Institutional enrollments nearly quadrupled from 271 to 1,069; staff more than tripled from 40 to 125 and buildings increased from 12 to 56 ("Dr. N.S. Kupelian Brands Connelly's Charges " 1938, p. A1; *Superintendent's Annual Report of the Pownal State School*, 1939, p. 4).

Vosburgh called for facilities to house 140 women, double the number awaiting admission. At one point, he recommended constructing an entirely separate institution for women that would hold 1,200 individuals, hardly the work of a reluctant empire builder. Defending his idea, he argued that:

> It is a sad fact that the tendency of feebleminded females is to lead dissolute lives.... A feebleminded girl has not sense enough to protect herself. Usually of sunny disposition; ignorant of shame; sometimes physically attractive, they go on either to marry and bring forth in geometric proportion and with amazing regularity defectives to continue the strain, or to become irresponsible sources of debauchery and disease in their communities.... What Maine needs is accommodation for 1,200 of such feebleminded women in a central institution. ("Maine's Problems in Sub-Normals," n.d., in *Clippings Pownal State School, 1909–1946*,1989, p. 105)

Eventually Vosburgh dropped his campaign for a separate women's facility, but with new estimates showing that 23,000 people with feeblemindedness resided in Maine, he called for aggressive institutional expansion (Maine's Problems in Sub-Normals," n.d., in *Clippings Pownal State School, 1909–1946*,1989, p. 105). In 1926, Vosburgh proposed to increase enrollments at the Maine School from 670 to 1,200 persons (Vosburgh, 1926, p. 46), a call he repeated in 1932 when the facility had 780 residents (*Twenty Fourth Annual Report of the Pownal State School*, 1932, p. 8). By 1933 he had raised his enrollment goal 25% to 1,500 (p. 5).

In June 1925, Vosburgh began a vigorous campaign to thoroughly medicalize mental sub-normality, solidify it as the cause of incompetence, dependence and deviance, and promote its control by physicians. Addressing the Maine Medical Association in 1925, he presented a paper titled, "The Problem of the Sub-Normals in Maine" (later published in the *Maine*

Medical Journal, 1926). In the address, he used Goddard's classifications, describing "idiots" as "so deeply defective in mind from birth or early age that they are unable to guard themselves from physical danger"; "imbeciles" as capable of only guarding themselves but incapable of earning a living due to their mental defect; and "morons" as "capable of earning a living under favorable circumstances but incapable of competing on equal terms with their normal fellows, or of managing themselves and their affairs with ordinary prudence" (Vosburgh, 1926, p. 43). Going beyond their incompetence and dependency, Vosburgh pointed to their inherited criminality, terming them "defective delinquents" with "serious deviated, perverted character traits" that require the oversight of physicians "in locating and putting under control this type of case" (p. 44). He criticized "the well meaning but destructive actions of philanthropists, overzealous lawyers, and misguided researchers," whom he accused of undermining existing beliefs and the correct treatment of sub-normality in Maine (p. 49). According to the superintendent, the stakes were high, determining no less than the "mental capacity of the nation's entire citizenry" and requiring no less than total victory by medicine over other pretenders for professional legitimacy and authority:

> There is an amazing lack of correct information regarding the sub-normal.... There has been a tendency during recent years for psychologists to emphasize the sociological at a sacrifice to the medical.... The medical application goes much deeper and treats more particularly the fundamental heredity and physical factors entering into causes.... Few of the legal profession, with their exact stereotyped procedures, recognize the limitations and individualities of medical testimony, particularly expert testimony.... It is sincerely to be desired ... that judges seek special advisory medical council rather than have lawyers formulate the hypothetical question.... Occasionally, a well-disposed philanthropist may believe that certain sub-normals of pleasing appearance who seem not too dull should never be sent to an institution. In general, the higher types of feebleminded, such as the morons, are the most dangerous to the community and posterity. (pp. 43–44, 48–49)

Central to Vosburgh's control of mental sub-normality was the state institution, which he increasingly presented as a dynamic, professionalized medical center, reflecting cutting-edge science and expert diagnosis and treatment of the disease. Without the institution serving as the state's central source of problem definition and treatment, the superintendent would have to compete for legitimacy and authority with the courts, philanthropists, and psychologists. Growing a dynamic institution became a critical ingredient in the battle for professional supremacy.

In 1925, Vosburgh announced that the institution was being renamed the Pownal State School, a title he described as less offensive and retaining an optimistic, educational image. Lest anyone misinterpret the defined problem or its solution, Vosburgh clearly emphasized that regardless of what it was called, the facility was essentially a medical center treating a physical disease:

> This [name change] eliminates the undesirable term "feeble-minded" so objectionable to relatives and friends of our pupils. It also emphasizes the educational function. However, it should be understood that as mental deficiency is a result of faulty brain development, the entire problem is a medical one. Improvement by educational training is dependent on the physical health of the individual. (*Seventeenth and Eighteenth Annual Reports of the Pownal State School*, 1926, p. 1)

By 1932, the superintendent had added to his medical construction, indicating that:

> The disturbances of the secretions of the endocrine gland have been found to be responsible directly or indirectly in a large number of cases admitted and studied. Indicated treatment has been given and it is anticipated that a further study of glandular disturbances will be made. (*Twenty-Fourth Annual Report of the Pownal State School*, 1932, p. 14)

LEGALIZING STERILIZATION IN MAINE

Eugenic surgery remained controversial in Maine, as did the seemingly uncontrolled growth and escalating costs of the Pownal School. One editorial argued that if the current admission rates continued, "there will be nobody to deny [admission to] ... and once they are there, it is extremely difficult to secure their discharge," creating an "indefinite charge upon the State" ("Filling Up the State Hospitals," 1925, p. A8). Thus, at the same time that the eugenics movement was encountering more scientific skepticism and prominent medical superintendents in the mental hygiene movement were moving away from large-scale sterilization and advocating for heightened community parole, adjustment and adaptation, the surgery was acquiring a new life, identity and momentum as a fiscal instrument for regulating institutional enrollments and size.

In 1925, State Senator Alexander Spiers proposed a sterilization law, using both fiscal and alarmist rationales:

> There are now over 2,000 such persons in the State of Maine who cannot be accommodated in our institutions for lack of buildings.... Would [sterilization] not be more humane and do we not owe something to our

> citizens to whom this class is a constant menace and expense, caused by bringing into this world children who are feeble- minded and inflicted with inherited disease?
>
> Even with the splendid management which the State now has at Pownal, the cost of caring for the number of inmates ... is nearly one quarter of a million dollars per year.
>
> To segregate all the feeble-minded we now have in Maine would necessitate the erection of at least 15 buildings at a cost of $180,000 each or $2,7000,000 with an increased maintenance of $600,000 per year. ("Urges Sterilization Of The Feeble-Minded," 1925, p. A2)

Calling the surgery both "humane and economically wise," Spiers minimized its discomfort and effects, calling it "very slight," producing "no harmful results," and producing "no pain or discomforts," while maximizing its need for those he described as chronic failures, barely human:

> A visit to this institution would go far to convince one of the necessity of the State taking steps to check the ever-increasing number of unfortunates; considering the matter either from a humanitarian or economic standpoint, as many of these beings are of such low mentality that they can do little else but breathe in a normal way.
>
> They are controlled entirely by the lower passions causing them to be very much more prolific than the normal person, and every child born of such parents is certain to be feeble-minded. (p. A2)

Summing up his case, the senator called sterilization the "most humane way ... to prevent reproduction of all moral imbeciles; to permanently improve the human race, to enforce in a simple way sound, decent, and efficient human beings [in place of] unsound, indecent, inefficient and the depraved" (p. A2).

On July 11, 1925, Spiers' bill became law, and permitted "vasectomy and fallectomy in certain cases of mental disease and feeblemindedness in order to prevent reproduction of further deficiency, or to treat certain forms of mental disease" (Rep. No. 1925, p. 198).

Maine's law was one of those classified as "voluntary" in that consent was required, although it could be secured rather easily from the nearest relative or guardian in cases where an individual was declared to be intellectually incompetent and following the approval of a committee of three physicians from the Pownal State School. Legal scholars and historians consider the term "voluntary" a misnomer when applied to eugenic sterilization and a gross misrepresentation of the process experienced by designated "patients." Targeted people were often coerced to undergo the surgery for numerous and varied reasons and threatened with permanent incarceration by institutional, prison, and/or health officials (Gould, 1996, p. 366; Largent, 2008, p. 6; Scheerenberger 1983, p. 155).

Despite its legalization, sterilization was vigorously opposed by the Roman Catholic Church, opposition that resonated with increasing numbers of Mainers. One third of the state's population were now first or second generation Americans; about 12% were foreign-born, and another 22% had at least one foreign born parent. The largest percentage of these were Catholics, most from French-speaking Quebec (Condon, Eastman, & Allin, 1995, p. 512).

Religious affiliation was not the only source of concern about eugenic surgery. Even a staunch eugenicist like Superior Court Justice Lauren Sanborn, harbored reservations about the legality of the surgery. Calling "segregation and sterilization" the only viable remedies, Sanborn preferred the former as "the only practical solution," since the surgery was "too great an invasion of personal liberty" (as cited in "Kiwanians Elect Officers," n.d., in *Clippings Pownal State School, 1909–1946*, 1989, p. 51). Apparently, however, eugenic arguments, propelled by the linkage of biologically inferior immigrants and inherited sub-normality; by a continuing fear and antipathy toward rural "degenerate" clans such as those evicted from Malaga Island; and by a vigorous campaign by the state's medical community, were sufficiently persuasive for passage of Maine's sterilization law in 1925.

This was a rather tumultuous period in Maine. The state was marking 50 years of changing state demography and experiencing ethnic-religious tensions that often ran high (Condon, Eastman, & Allin, 1995, p. 512). Following the Civil War, the Ku Klux Klan established a foothold in the state and by 1924, claimed 50,000 members, openly operated "an impressive Portland headquarters," exerted considerable political influence in the legislature, and marched and burned crosses across the state, spreading virulent anti-Catholic sentiment (p. 512). The Klan's power waned as the state's population became more Catholic and by the early 1930s, the Klan's influence was described as "moribund" (p. 512). By then, however, the legislative damage had been done. In fact, the majority prejudice against Catholics, particularly French Canadians, during that period undoubtedly helped eugenic sterilization advocates legalize the surgery. New England states with high Catholic populations like Massachusetts and Rhode Island never passed sterilization laws.

Some Protestant denominations joined the Catholic Church in opposition, others supported legalizing sterilization. A Universalist minister from Portland argued that the best legislation a state can pass is "a code of law sterilizing stupidity and stabilizing high physical and mental quality" (as cited in "Portland Clergy Differ With Pope On Birth Control," 1931, p. A16). The Anglican Bishop argued that it was a moral obligation "to protect society from the very real menace of physical, mental, and moral degeneration" (p. A16).

Newspapers generally favored legalizing eugenic surgery and some worried that the new law was too timid and overburdened by permissions and safeguards. One editorial, for example, characterized sterilization as a vaccination and wondered why it should not be ordered routinely by a physician like other medical treatments, ("Our Imbeciles and Insane," n.d., in *Clippings Pownal State School, 1909-1946*, 1989, p. 96).

Superintendent Vosburgh lauded the newly passed law, citing the dangers of inheritability, the futility of marriage restrictions, and the increasing threat of "degenerate communities," the last which he referred to as "tribal aggregations and ... scattered hamlets throughout the State peopled by sub-normals in ancestral shacks ... the most notable of which is Malaga Island [along with Athens and China, Maine] ... lead[ing] to illegitimacy rates approaching 20%" (Vosburgh, 1926, pp. 44–45).

Two years after Maine legalized eugenic sterilization, the U.S. Supreme Court endorsed the practice as constitutional, removing the legal inhibitions and opening the door for previously reticent practitioners to perform the surgery. Although it is difficult to accurately report the total number of eugenic sterilizations performed in Maine, and specifically at Pownal, due to inconsistent and diffuse accounting methods, it is clear that few if any eugenic surgeries were performed in the state prior to the *Buck v. Bell* decision in 1927. Before the Supreme Court's ruling, Harry Laughlin at the Eugenics Record Office (ERO) in Cold Springs Harbor, New York, an organization that reportedly kept meticulous records, recorded no eugenic sterilizations in Maine until 1928 (Black, 2003, p. 122). Other sources indicate that a few surgeries were done in 1925 (see Largent, 2008, p. 79; Paul, 1965, p. 370). Vosburgh's successor, Dr. Nesib Kupelian, recorded 72 sterilizations performed at Pownal between 1927 and 1940 (Kupelian, 1939, p. B1). For the same period, the ERO recorded 190 eugenic sterilizations in Maine (Black, 2003, p. 122). The discrepancy may reflect operations performed in other locations and for reasons other than mental sub-normality. As Black has noted, eugenic sterilizations were justified for varied and amorphous reasons that included insanity, criminality, moral degeneracy, medical unacceptability, and "other" (p. 123).

In the early 1970s, Julius Paul, a New York State political science professor, compiled what appears to be the most comprehensive data on state sterilization figures and policies across the country. According to Paul (1965, pp. 367, 370), Maine sterilized 326 people between 1925 and 1963, of which 189 were recorded at Pownal/Pineland. The peak period for Maine's sterilization occurred during the years 1933–40, most of which occurred under Vosburgh's direction when 149 individuals were sterilized (p. 370).

Combining U.S. Census data for 1940, and comparing them across several New England states provides some context to Maine's sterilization record (U.S. Census Bureau, State and County Quickfacts (n.d.). New Hampshire, with a population in 1940 roughly 60% of Maine's, legalized sterilization from 1910 through 1959, sterilizing a total of 679 individuals (1 in every 785) (Largent, 2008, pp 78–79; Paul, 1965, p. 418). New Hampshire performed no eugenic sterilizations before 1921 and, like Maine, did few surgeries until *Buck v. Bell* in 1927 (Largent, 2008, pp. 78–79). The other northern New England state, Vermont, had a population in 1940 of 359,230, legalizing the operation from 1931 through 1957 and sterilizing 253 citizens (1 in every 1,493 people) (Largent, 2008, pp 78–79; Paul, 1965, p. 494). Before the eugenic surgeries ended in New England a total of 1,815 people were sterilized. To the Maine, New Hampshire and Vermont figures, Connecticut added 557 individuals. No sterilization laws were passed in either Massachusetts or Rhode Island and no recorded eugenic sterilizations were performed in either state (Largent, 2008, p. 72).

Across all of the northern New England states, the vast majority of these eugenically sterilized were women and individuals deemed to be "feebleminded." In Maine, 86% were women, while in New Hampshire and Vermont the percentages were 90% and 67% respectively (Kaelber, 2009). In Maine, 72% of those sterilized were considered "feebleminded," 6% were classified as insane, and 22% were not labeled as either. In New Hampshire, 56% were identified as "feebleminded," 37% as "insane," and 17% as "other" (p. 418). Of those sterilized in Vermont, 80% were labeled as "mentally deficient" (Kaelber, 2009)

While not all of Maine's eugenic surgeries were performed at Pownal, the institution served as the "custodian of all papers and records of eugneic sterilization performed under these [legislative] acts, and up to the present time there have been thirty-four operations" (*Twenty-Fourth Annual Report of the Pownal State School,* 1932, p. 13). Between 1927 and 1963, 58% of the state's eugenic surgeries were performed at Pownal (Paul, 1965, p. 370), some on residents who were transferred in from other state facilities such as the Hallowell State School (a woman's reformatory) and Bangor State Hospital (a psychiatric institution) (*Superintendent's Annual Report, Pownal State School,* 1940, p. 9; Superintendent's Logs, October, 9, 1930, p. 14).

In 1931, Maine amended its 1925 law by: (a) the increasing the power of state physicians to authorize the operation; (b) extending sterilization to any state institution, including reformatories, penal institutions, and so forth; and (c) enhancing the appeals process for individuals, relatives and guardians. A notable addition to the law was the explicit, mandatory linkage of sterilization and discharge. Any resident who institutional officials defined "as likely, if released without sterilization, to produce a child or children who by reason of inheritance would have a tendency to serious mental disease or mental deficiency" could now be sterilized (Rep. No. 1931, p. 308). This determination could be implemented after 50 days with approval of the board and two hospital superintendents. Individuals slated for the surgery had the right to appeal to the state superior court (Rep. No. 1931, p. 308).

While proponents of the bill reiterated their promise of preventing feeblemindedness throughout the state, they began to give equal weight to its fiscal benefits: "Sterilization would permit institutional authorities to release some of the high grade inmates" and make room for "many others who should be in our institutions" ("Smith is against prize fighting films … Dr Tyson opposes sterilization bill," Rep. No. 1931, p. A6). Once again, it is interesting to note how eugenic sterilization, initially proposed as a societal vaccine against the spread of inherited medical pathology, was gradually promoted as a means to control institutional size and combat escalating costs. This poignantly illustrates how the mechanisms of social control can be set in motion by one rationale that over time may recede in importance, but is merely replaced by another that serves to legitimate and perpetuate the desired control (Trent, 1994, p. 223).

Legislators likely anticipated that widening the law and increasing the number of sterilizations would heighten the number of attempted institutional escapes and elicit sympathy from the general public and even some law enforcement officers. Thus, in addition to passing a new sterilization bill, lawmakers also increased the penalties for aiding and abetting the escape or concealment of any inmate from any state institution. Such penalties were previously reserved only for those who assisted escaped criminals.

Vosburgh never wavered publically in his support for eugenic sterilization, arguing that the surgery would lead to more institutional releases, reduced numbers, and decreased costs. He recommended that sterilization be considered for every resident who was proposed for discharge. Coercively sterilizing even a small number of people should be considered a gross miscarriage of justice, and no superintendent in Pineland's history ordered more eugenic sterilizations than Vosburgh. Overall, however he discharged relatively few people and sterilized even fewer, revealing that he was more cautious than might be predicted either from his harsh rhetoric or from national trends that favored sterilization-for-discharge as the antidote for unending institutional growth.

On the question of resident discharge, Vosburgh's (1926) rhetoric far outstripped his actions. He recommended two types of "extra institutional care" (p. 48). One consisted of self-supporting colonies, maintained by the larger institution, located 20–50 miles away, and inhabited by "adult men in good physical condition." According to the superintendent, the colonies, while still affiliated with the larger institution, would allow for a "greatly increased number of cases at a minimum cost to the State." In addition, he proposed a policy of home care, or boarding out, that followed "successful institutional training and discipline." Placements would be followed-up and supervised by an expanded Community Services Department that had been started under Hedin. This department would also conduct "heredity and special investigations ... of cases and communities" (p. 48).

Despite these proposals, Vosburgh's "extra community placements," never materialized much beyond the on-grounds farms at Pownal although the Community Services Department expanded its activities under Vosburgh. It's duties were described as performing "examinations of inmates" of the boys' and girls' reformatories, the Skowhegan Reformatory, and "those committed to the Bureau of Social Welfare" (*Twenty-fourth Annual Report of the Pownal State School,* 1932, p. 16). In addition, the department conducted "investigations of home conditions," and provided "information and advice to relatives and friends and representatives of any charitable agency regarding the medical condition of any person, particularly in reference to prevention and treatment." The department also completed "hereditary charts which are made in every case" (pp. 15-16).

There is little subsequent mention of self-supporting colonies in his reports and, based on his own figures, home care or boarding-out placements were seldom used. Vosburgh was recording discharge rates (excluding transfers, escapes, etc.) that hovered around 3%, slightly less than his predecessor. The average number of official annual discharges between the mid-1920s and mid-1930s was about 18. Adding in those who were absent, escaped, and/or had gone on home visit, roughly doubled the total, which would still be relatively modest.

Vosburgh defended his expansionist vision of Pownal, arguing that eugenic sterilization was an impractical primary strategy for controlling feeblemindedness, but left unchecked, the problem would grow rapidly throughout Maine. Citing heightened incidence figures showing that 3% of the state's population—about 23,000 citizens—were mentally sub-normal, the superintendent claimed that the feebleminded were four times more prolific at producing children and should not be expected to migrate away from their current locations. He estimated "conservatively" that "131 children are born each year with feeble-minded parentage" (Vosburgh, 1926, p. 44), and asserted that since the "widespread application of these operations [sterilizations] cannot be expected," the solution called for the "permanent segregation ... for idiots, imbeciles, defective delinquents, and feeble-minded women of child-bearing age, excepting those who can be safely released after operative procedure" (p. 45). According to Vosburgh, "it is not to be believed that defectiveness can ever be entirely eliminated, care for large numbers will always be necessary" (*Seventeenth and Eighteenth Annual Reports of the Pownal State School*, 1925–26, p. 2).

Vosburgh was not the only eugenicist cautioning about large-scale sterilization and favoring expanded segregation. He joined a prominent list of icons of that period such as Maine natives, Walter Fernald and Henry Goddard, and Cold Springs Harbor Laboratory Director, Charles Davenport, all of whom had varied reasons for their reservations about sterilization, but were united in urging caution.

Following passage of Maine's sterilization law, Vosburgh carefully threaded his way between sterilization critics and advocates, arguing on one hand that the surgery would cut costs by "permitting the discharge of certain types of mental deficiency;" reduce proliferating, inherited forms of the disease by decreasing "the numbers of sub-normals born of

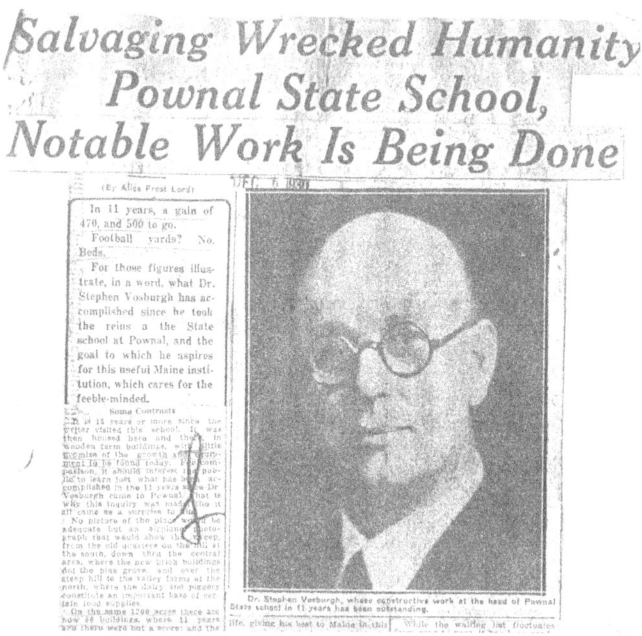

Salvaging Wrecked Humanity
Pownal State School,
Notable Work Is Being Done

(By Alice Frost Lord)

In 11 years, a gain of 470, and 500 to go.

Football yards? No. Beds.

For those figures illustrate, in a word, what Dr. Stephen Vosburgh has accomplished since he took the reins a the State school at Pownal, and the goal to which he aspires for this useful Maine institution, which cares for the feeble-minded.

Some Contrasts

Dr. Stephen Vosburgh, whose constructive work at the head of Pownal State school in 11 years has been outstanding.

Figure 5.1. Superintendent Stephen Vosbergh. From newspaper article circa 1930 contained in *Clippings Pownal State School, 1909–1946*. (1989). New Gloucester, ME: Pineland Center. Norma Higgins collection.

defective parents;" and, combining with "the many health activities and better understanding of prenatal and child care, eventually lessen the [total] number of defectives" (*Seventeenth and Eighteenth Annual Reports of Pownal State School*, 1926, p. 2). On the other hand, he warned that the surgery could not be considered a "cure-all," should be administered "selectively" with "the interests of the individual carefully protected" and given only to "certain higher types who have moral twists" (p. 2).

Vosburgh's use of the term "selective sterilization" was neither original nor accidental. This term was increasingly being used by professionals across the country to describe a policy of sterilization restraint. What it meant in actual practice, however, was unclear. For example, in 1930 Harvey Watkins, superintendent of the Polk (Pennsylvania) School and future president of the American Association on Mental Deficiency (AAMD), offered what seemed like a ringing endorsement of large-scale sterilization that he claimed benefitted all parties. Watkins contended that after 10,000 reported surgeries, it was clear that sterilization "saved thousands of taxpayer dollars," was a "blessing" to the community "freed from worries about future defectives," and but also benefitted "mental defectives, who could now be paroled, freed from the constraints of parenthood" (as cited in Trent, 1994, pp. 200–201). The title of Watkins's paper: "Selective Sterilization." A 1933 White House Conference on Child Heath and Protection also used the term, although it is difficult to discern what specific limitations were being proposed:

> There are at present no legal, surgical, or humanitarian obstacles to the extensive practice of selective sterilization of the adult feebleminded; these facts should be impressed upon the consciousness of every responsible citizen.... When adequately safeguarded, little individual or social danger attends sterilization ... and ... selective sterilization may be regarded as a highly desirable, although perhaps not indispensable, adjunct to any program of prevention. (as cited in Paul, 1965, p. 71)

According to Paul (1965, pp. 171–172), "selective sterilization" referred to targeting individuals identified by physicians as "clearly" having a hereditary form of mental deficiency, excluding those who would likely be incarcerated for life (and not require surgical "protection"), and parents afflicted by "secondary feeblemindedness" who had normal children (pp. 171–172). Whether or not attaching the qualifier, "selective," to sterilization was merely a professional strategy, justifying its continued use while tacitly acknowledging some obscure limits in response to scientific criticism, by the mid 1930s, Vosburgh added some new, powerful allies cautioning against widespread eugenic sterilizations and favoring expanded segregation.

In 1932, J. H. Landman published a widely respected and circulated book criticizing the overuse of sterilization. Two years later England's Committee on Sterilization challenged the evidence behind widespread sterilization, calling for "more science and less speculation, especially regarding compulsory surgeries (as cited in Paul, 1965, pp. 73–77).

Around the same time, even America's medical community began looking more seriously into the use and validity of widespread sterilization, leading the boards of both the *New England Journal of Medicine* and the *Journal of the American Medical Association* began to slowly retreat from their pro-sterilization views, particularly surgeries considered "mandatory" (Sofair & Kaldijian, 2000, pp. 316–317).

Perhaps the most influential study on sterilization was conducted by the American Neurological Association (ANA) which appointed a group titled the Committee for the Investigation of Sterilization. The organization selected a nationally known critic of the surgery, Tuft University Professor Abraham Myerson, to head the committee. Issued in 1935-36, the report was highly critical of eugenic sterilization practices, debunking claims that feeblemindedness or other forms of social deviancy were a proliferating and genetically-based social threat that required widespread involuntary surgery to wipe out. (Largent, 2008, p. 122; Paul, 1965, pp. 77–78; Sofair & Kaldijian, 2000, p. 316). The report was also instrumental in reducing the most egregious sterilization practices and beginning the gradual demise of the surgery across the country (Sofair & Kaldjiian, 2000, pp. 316–317).

Before chairing the ANA committee, Myerson came to Maine to address the state's Conference of Social Welfare. His presentation was covered extensively in local papers that announced his message with headlines such as "Feeble Mindedness Not a Great Threat To Society—Myerson" (1930, p. A1). While in Maine, Myerson offered a preview of the ANA report as he challenged the inheritability of mental functioning, argued that mental deficiency should not be linked either with higher birthrates or criminality; and indicated that feeblemindedness is not a great national threat and would never become one (p. A1). Although still largely opposed by Maine's medical and political establishment, Myerson was supported by one prominent state medical authority, Dr. Forest Tyson, Superintendent of the Augusta State Hospital. Tyson's dissent may seem surprising given his position, but he consistently opposed the surgery dating back to the original 1925 law. According to Tyson, "we do not know enough about heredity to take the step of sterilizing inmates of institutions (as cited in Dr Tyson Opposes Sterilization Bill," 1931, in *Clippings Pownal State School, 1909–1946*, 1989, p. 275).

Although Myerson's visit to Maine and the subsequent ANA report may have bolstered Vosburgh's policy of "selective" sterilization, he did not stop eugenicists in Maine from criticizing Vosburgh or calling for a more aggressive policy. In 1933, Leroy Folsom, legal counsel for the State Health and Welfare Department, excoriated Vosburgh's discharge record and claimed that the existing emphasis on segregation was expensive and inadequate. Folsom told a local Rotary group that the number of "grown, sub-normal people with less than a fourth grade mentality" was between 3,000-3,500, a figure he termed "amazing." He asserted that ridding the state "of the menace of sub-normal adults and children" by segregation alone was "nearly an impossibility" that would require "a second institution three times the size of the Augusta State Hospital" and cost 5 million dollars (as cited in "Says State Needs Second Institution for Feeble-Minded," n.d., in *Clippings Pownal State School, 1909–1946*, 1989, p. 441). Citing several cases he investigated in northern Maine, where one woman had 23 children, 7 of whom were confined to the state institution, Folsom reiterated the threat women posed to society, asserting that men are "undersexed," while "oversexed" females are the most dangerous, and accounted for "the exceptionally large families among sub-normal people." According to Folsom, sterilization was the solution, if only state officials would pursue it more aggressively using the existing statutes (p. 441).

Even before Folsom's public rebuke, Vosburgh acknowledged his low discharge rate, emphasizing in 1930 that discharges were "limited" to those who were discovered to be "normal," or "finished school and learned manual training or some occupational work," enabling them "to take positions in homes where they can be safeguarded" (Lord, 1930, p. A–1). In 1932, he assured state officials that "consideration for sterilization is given at the time of discharge of every case, and in general those who are fitted by training to be at least partially self-supporting are recommended for the operation" (*Twenty Fourth Annual Report of the Pownal State School*, 1932, p. 13). Following Folsom's criticism, Vosburgh continued to warn against accelerating discharges that resulted in "hurried decisions" placing people into "unfit surroundings" (*Twenty Fifth Annual Report of the Pownal State School*, 1933, p. 3). Defending his "selective" approach, Vosburgh emphasized his record of "safe" discharges:

> A continuous, consistent effort to return to the community some of the older, less hazardous cases has produced some results. A larger number of cases who were of advanced age or who have been protected by eugenic

> sterilization have been placed in families. (*Twenty Sixth Annual Report of the Pownal State School*, 1934, p. 3)

Vosburgh also had very practical reasons for not sterilizing and releasing large numbers of residents. For one thing, doing so meant losing the facility's most capable residents without whom he could not run his expanding, underfunded, and understaffed institution. Like his predecessors, Vosburgh touted resident labor as therapeutic and cost effective. In 1930, he claimed that each resident cost as little as $6.27 per week and that Pownal operated more efficiently than comparable institutions within the state. Attributing much of this success to the facility's farming operation, which provides "over half of all that is consumed on the place," representing a savings of $82,000, and added revenue of $86,000 per year, he cites the importance of keeping "the children employed," as both good facility management and rehabilitation: "Busy children give little trouble, is the slogan" (Lord, 1930, p. A–1).

The superintendent reported that residents were performing a wide variety of institutional jobs beyond farm work, like maintaining building supplies and furnishings; furniture making; tin ware manufacturing and repair; mattress rebuilding; and linen, underclothing, and frock cutting, sewing, and conditioning. He expressed "astonishment" at "what excellent quality of workmanship in carpentering, caning chairs, tin smithing, painting, and sewing is to be seen here- all the work of these feebleminded children under competent supervision" (Lord, 1930, p. A–1). By 1932, Vosburgh boasted that resident labor made Pownal nearly self sufficient, an exaggerated claim, but attesting to the importance of this work to Pownal's operation:

> Behind the administration is the unwritten law that there shall be no idleness.... The by-product of keeping all inmates busy is that the school is largely self-supporting. Over $100,000 of earning power was produced last year, $40,000 of which represented vegetables that made up one half of the food supply. ("Dr. Vosburgh Describes Work," n.d., in *Clippings Pownal State School, 1909–1946*, 1989, p. 392)

To avoid giving the impression that residents might function as effectively in society, Vosburgh argued that, while they may appear competent, they had multiple impairments beyond low intelligence that rendered them productive only within the institution and successful largely because of the facility's skilled and patient staff.

> Many of those cared for in institutions actually have superior intelligence, but are so lacking other qualities as to be unable to live normally. The Pownal

> institution, commonly termed a school for feeble-minded, is in reality a school for feeble personalities.
>
> A person whose character is sub-normal can, for instance, be of far greater damage to a community than a so called feeble-minded person whose character may be normal. (*Twenty Sixth Annual Report of the Pownal State School*, 1934, p. 392)
>
> Many of the children cannot be depended upon to carry on by their very own initiative, no matter how long in training. They work only under constant direction and repeated instruction. If they were not sub-normal they would not be here for exactly that patient and persistent guidance. (p. 392)

Resident workers were critical to the facility's operation, not only because they were productive and cheap, but also because they replaced the paid staff who Pownal could not attract and retain. This problem was not new, dating back decades and enduring throughout the Great Depression and beyond. Vosburgh attributed the ongoing problem to low salaries, the facility's isolated location, and the strenuous demands of resident care (*Twenty Fourth Annual Report of the Pownal State School*, 1932, p. 8).

In 1914, staff turnover was reportedly 205% (Lord, 1933, p. 2–A). Hiring rates and turnover improved greatly during the depression but still persisted, ebbing and flowing as work opportunities in other occupations fluctuated. As the depression deepened, employee turnover was *reduced* to 64.5%, and Vosburgh reported that "the general conditions of [statewide] unemployment give opportunity to engage individuals [staff] of a higher type, and at present the personnel of the School is highly satisfactory" (p. 8). In 1933, however, while reporting an improved rate of attrition to 34.6% (*Twenty Fifth Annual Report of the Pownal State School*, 1933, p. 7), he indicated that due to reduced salaries, the quality of staff and resident care had dropped, and previous gains in the nursing department had been lost. While reporting that reduced staff salaries were "better received than might be expected," the superintendent pointed to low pay as a primary and worsening problem. According to Vosburgh, facility salaries, were already "below financial returns in other kinds of work," and "there are indications of [staff] returning to other employment where remuneration is greater (p. 7). By 1934 the turnover rate had increased to over 40%, and the superintendent was not optimistic, relating that "with the increased opportunities for trained citizens in commercial work, and the continued salary deduction, it is evident that this turnover will further increase during the coming year.... Only by a return to the normal salary schedule will this situation be permanently corrected" (*Twenty Sixth Annual Report of the Pownal State School*, 1934, p. 7).

While the Great Depression undermined the arguments supporting the genetic superiority of the rich and successful, and weakened the case for large-scale sterilization and incarceration of the poor (Ludmerer, 1972, p. 127), it also increased the pressure from local municipalities and some families to provide institutional relief (Trent, 1994, p. 218).

Large state institutions served as prominent places of employment and the same fiscal pressures exerted on municipalities and families bolstered calls for more work, serving as another rationale for expanding state facilities. In a sinking economy, institutional construction and Pownal's expanding need for goods and services offered desperately needed employment. As the governor called for building "more institutions of its kind," officials and the press reverted to more alarmist rhetoric in making a case for a bigger facility ("Gardiner Deplores Crowded Conditions at Pownal School," n.d., in *Clippings Pownal State School, 1909–1946*, 1989, p. 176).

Despite the expanding institution, waiting lists and overcrowding continued and Vosburgh's need for resident labor remained. The surrounding economic picture, in fact, offered him an additional reason to retain valuable resident workers, claiming that it was more humane to keep them in productive institutional pursuits than releasing them to communities where officials, neighbors, and families did not want them:

> the reduced circumstances of families having sub-normal children needing care ... for which accommodations are lacking result in immeasurable distress. Likewise the same circumstances have prevented the discharge of many older boys and girls who under normal conditions could be partially self-supporting. Consistent efforts to arrange the discharge of many harmless, older cases have met opposition, though several have been discharged. A waiting list ... of 59 males and 165 females increases daily. (*Twenty Fifth Annual Report of the Pownal State School*, 1933, p. 3)

Through the economic depression, Pownal's enrollments nearly doubled. In 1930 there were 698 residents (*Twenty Third Annual Report of the Pownal State School*, 1931). Two years later, that total had reached 809 (*Twenty Fifth Annual Report of the Pownal State School*, 1933, p. 4). The same year, the superintendent recommended a facility for 1,500 (pp. 3–5). In 1935, the campaign to build and expand more state institutions accelerated further as the voters approved a $2,000,000 bond issue, out of which Pownal was allotted two 150-person dormitories, one for males, and one for females, as well as a laundry building and an addition to the nurses' quarters. This expansion eventually increased the capacity of the institution to 1,120 (Connor, 1937, p. A16). After the new dorms were finished, the waiting list of 406 was reduced to 106, but not eliminated (p. A16).

One particular construction project that brought Pownal multiple advantages was its on-campus medical hospital. Described as one of only a few "fully functioning hospitals located on the grounds of State institutions across the country" ("$210,000 Hospital Being Built For Feebleminded," 1931, p. A2), the hospital proved to be as important economically, politically, and professionally as it was medically. It offered local construction work and additional facility jobs and, following completion, served as additional dormitory for an overcrowded institution. Begun early in the depression, the hospital was constructed primarily with private funds from the estate of Ms. Kate Anthony, dedicated in 1931, and intended for residents described as "bed patients, the cripples, and the sick of the Pownal State School" (p. A2). Besieged by demands for admissions, institutional officials immediately filled it to its capacity of 110 "patients," but not because of any reported wave of new illnesses.

Beyond its physical, economic and political benefits, the new hospital also served important professional interests. Having a fully equipped, on-grounds hospital conferred on Pownal the identity and image of a typical, self-standing community, a metaphor not lost on state and institutional officials who declared at the hospital's opening that the institution had "all the needs of a town" ("$210,000 Hospital Being Built for Feebleminded," 1931, p. A2). Towns typically had departments for building, street and park maintenance, fire and police protection, and recreation and religious facilities, all of which were eventually provided at Pineland, overseen by a corps of professional administrators, and staffed by dozens of employees.

Having an on-grounds hospital also increased the medical legitimacy and professional prestige of the institution as a modern scientific facility. Portrayed in the media as a magnificent achievement, the new facility surrounded mental sub-normality and its care with a heightened medical aura, lifting Pownal's image from that of a bleak, custodial institution to a dynamic medical-research setting, staffed by highly trained and professional personnel who were conducting cutting-edge research that informed their treatment practices. Needless to say, the facility's heightened medical identity and activities brought glory and prestige to its director, staff, and state politicians. According to one newspaper account:

> The hospital building itself will be a work of splendid architecture and a credit to the State of Maine. It sets imposingly on the spacious campus overlooking a broad countryside. Because of the elevation of its site naturally the air is of the highest purity.... In addition to the airy wards for the inmates with their attached solariums, where patients may enjoy the benefits of the sunshine, will be private rooms for critically ill patients, suites of sick employees, x-ray, drug dispensary, and emergency rooms.
>
> Dr. Stephen Earle Vosburgh, head of the institution, will direct the activities at the hospital through assistants, [and] anticipates great work to be done towards the study and aid of those afflicted with feeblemindedness.... There will also be ... the best in medical men and hospitals, and the best ... in science.... Laboratories for research into every channel of feeblemindedness

> are at the disposal of scientists. ("$210,000 Hospital Being Built for Feebleminded," 1931, p. A2)

Revealing the numerous treatments that were routinely performed within Pownal's hospital, Vosburgh collectively listed treating bruises, doing dental work, and conducting varied types of surgery, including eugenic sterilizations ("Pownal School Improves Services for Weak-Minded," 1932, p. A6). Presenting sterilization on a list of routine treatments, Vosburgh normalized the operation, bestowing on it not only medical legitimacy, but typicality, portraying it as no different than treating injuries or removing tonsils. In this way, institutional officials transformed sterilization from a controversial, moral dilemma to an everyday medical procedure. As Trent (1994, p. 224) notes, frequently the most effective social controls are those considered "day to day care."

Medicalizing sterilization to enhance its legitimacy and reduce its controversy in Maine made perfect sense to Vosburgh, who, like most other physicians, seemed to earnestly believe that mental deficiency was an inheritable disease infecting human fitness and social order. But enthusiasm for human fitness now extended well beyond the medical profession. A remarkable editorial, attributed to the *Portland Evening News,* appeared during the last years of Vosburgh's superintendency, reminding us how deeply entrenched eugenic ideology had become, even to the point of praising some of Hitler's early efforts:

> The proposal of Oklahoma's state health director, Dr. G. N. Bilby ... probably will evoke cries of protest from sentimentalists and the "sob sister" element everywhere.... Yet it cannot be said that everything Hitler has done ... is completely wrong. His sterilization law, applying to society's misfits, is winning the applause of eugenicists, pathologists, and psychologists throughout the world. These scientists do not admire Hitler, necessarily, but they are in sympathy with any system which may attend to reduce the number of physical, mental, and moral degenerates.
>
> If the fear of emasculation at the hands of the law should not deter such criminals from further acts of violence, the penalty itself would at least prevent them from reproducing others of their kind in other generations
>
> Had some such system been in place thirty years ago, had the mentally unbalanced and the moral degenerates of the early nineteen hundreds been subject to such a "brutal" and "inhuman" law as Dr. Bilby and others are advocating, the world would been afflicted with fewer misfits of the John Dillinger and the Machine Gun Kelly type. ("To Stamp Out Crime," n.d., in *Clippings Pownal State School, 1909–1946*, 1989, p. 459)

Vosburgh never publically recanted his views on segregation or sterilization and while his actions seemed consistent with his professional beliefs, he was also able to bend and manipulate his policies and practices as he was influenced by and responded to numerous and powerful professional, fiscal, political, and/or economic forces. Vosburgh remained a popular and admired figure in Maine until his death in 1939 and was able to survive and prosper, expand his authority, and affirm his professional legitimacy in part because of his ability to successfully thread his way through the maze of competing interests and parties, convincing politicians, state officials, and the media of his moderation and judiciousness.

Vosburgh and other state officials did not appear quite so moderate and reasoned when their actions were described in rare media accounts. In one highly publicized case, Vosburgh and other state officials illustrated the extent to which they would go in defending the idea of inherited feeblemindedness, asserting their coveted legal and professional authority, and displaying their socioeconomic and gender biases and professional self-interests.

The case involved a young woman, Eleanor Chase Libby, who was a 23- year old woman accused of being mentally sub-normal, assigned to Pineland where she spent 3 years, and arrested with her husband and two other people in Portland following her escape. According to the newspaper account, "the most unusual feature of the case was" that her husband is indicted on a charge of "harboring and concealing" his own wife ("Two Men and Two Women are Held" 1937, p. A1). This charge against the Libbys could only have been made because Mrs. Libby was identified as feebleminded, an escaped Pownal resident, and prohibited by Maine law from marrying. State officials voided her out-of-state marriage, which opened up her husband to criminal charges (p. 1A).

Heralding the beginning of the trial, large headlines on page one of the *Portland Evening Express* read: "Court Battle Over Bride Begins" (1937, p. A1). Called "one of the strangest cases ever tried here," the newspapers portrayed the state in the persons of Superintendent Vosburgh and the state attorney as standing between a poor, uneducated woman, and a normal life with her husband and relatives (pp. A1–A2). Supporting her continued incarceration, Vosburgh declared that Mrs. Libby is feebleminded, as indicated by tests showing she had "the mentality of an eleven year old child" (p. A2).

> "I am not feeble-minded," Mrs Libby declared. "Have you a wedding ring?" Sullivan (her lawyer) inquired. "Yes," she answered, "but Mrs. Vosburgh took it from my finger last night." She said, "I wasn't married." Replying to additional questions, Mrs. Libby said she was able to read and write, and

> had passed through the eighth grade at the State School in Pownal, and had never been kept back in a class. (p. A1)

Mrs. Libby explained that she escaped from Pownal, because, "I knew that I would never get out of there" (p. A2).

In attempts to demonstrate her cognitive impairment, the prosecutor for the State asked her geography questions that might be asked as general information items on standardized IQ tests. "Where is India? Where is England?" Failing to respond correctly, she replied that she did not remember, and that she had been out of school a long time ago. In explaining that she was placed at Hallowell [reformatory] for school truancy and staying away from home, she acknowledged that her previous actions "were not right" and promised to "make good if given the chance" ("Court Battle Over Bride Begins," 1937, p. A2).

Several days later, an agreement was announced whereby Mrs. Libby was released from Pownal, "free to enjoy her liberty" ("Mrs. Libby Released After Compromise,"1937, p. A1). Those who assisted in her escape and/or concealment were not so fortunate, having been prosecuted and sentenced to short jail terms under the 1931 law prohibiting aid and abetment of Pownal fugitives (p. A1).

Mrs. Libby subsequently filed charges against the institution and sued Vosburgh for civil damages. She reported that as a resident she was forced to have her head shaved several times, and that following her escape she had been placed in a strait jacket that was only removed prior to her court appearances. She also charged that she had been unconstitutionally denied due process when she was transferred to Pownal without a hearing and kept there after age 21, which was a violation of state statutes ("Pownal State School Head Sued For $25,000,"1937, pp. A1–A2).

Libby and her family come across as neither passive, menacing nor incompetent, but as active and assertive agents on their behalf who were treated unfairly. Contrasting sharply with the image of feeblemindedness and immorality painted by Vosburgh and the state's lawyers, Mrs. Libby appeared quite ordinary, not very different from an average citizen with whom many people might easily identify. Eventually Mrs. Libby dropped her lawsuit against Vosburgh, and the incident caused no immediate, discernible changes in state policy, law, or practice, despite revealing the legal and political vulnerabilities of targeted individuals. In the process, however, the public heard a voice of "feeblemindedness" that was far different than the official version they had been served. In addition, the "problem" here was recast, perhaps for the first time, as a legal/civil rights issue as much as a medical question. And Mrs Libby was cast more as a victim than a threat. While such discourses and perspectives would remain dormant for decades, they would reemerge as compelling rationales for broader social change and eventually for Pineland's demise.

CHAPTER 6

RECEDING EUGENIC INFLUENCE

Persisting Policies

In August, 1937, Stephen Vosburgh became seriously ill with what doctors termed a coronary occlusion. He took a medical leave, but never recovered, passing away on Christmas Eve ("Dr. S. E. Vosburgh, Supt. Of Pownal Dies at 2:46 A.M.," 1937, pp. A1–A2). Due to his long tenure, high energy, forceful personality, and community visibility, Vosburgh was one of the most influential superintendents and a powerful force in shaping and applying eugenic policies toward people considered mentally sub-normal through the 1920s and 30s. Eulogizing the superintendent on December 28, 1937, the *Portland Evening Express* described Vosburgh as a public servant "whose place [the State] may never be able to quite fully replace (p. A4)." The article also emphasized his administrative skills, pointing out that "Dr. Vosburgh ... has saved the State money in many different ways outside of his routine duties," and under his direction the institution was "not an increased expense but an economy" ("Dr S. E. Vosburgh, Supt. Of Pownal Dies at 2:46 AM," 1937, p. A4).

Whether or not Vosburgh saved the state money, certainly he was a skilled and intrepid advocate for the institution, expanding it in every direction.

Voices of Pineland: Eugenics, Social Reform, and the Legacy of "Feeblemindedness" in Maine, pp. 125–141

Envisioning Pownal as a highly professionalized medical, research, and treatment center, replete with a fully functioning hospital, Vosburgh was able to firmly establish mental sub-normality as the treatment domain of physicians and transform Pownal's image from custodial to medical. As the eugenic movement receded following World War II, Vosburgh's medicalized institution, with its social and economic benefits and its continuing image as a viable clinical setting would endure.

Succeeding Vosburgh was the school's assistant superintendent, Dr. Nesib S. Kupelian, who had been a physician at the facility for 12 years and served as acting superintendent during Vosburgh's illness. As the last avowed eugenicist, Kupelian served from 1938–53, a transition period in Pineland's history when community discharge became inevitable and the accumulated abuses of previous decades were dramatically revealed, but largely ignored.

Before the beginning of World War II, Pownal was overcrowded and underfunded, but following the outbreak of war, was decimated by fiscal cutbacks and staff departures. During this period, institutional officials continued to indict people as societal menaces, sterilize a receding number of Pownal residents, support the expansion of the surgery to those living in the community, warehouse people in unprecedented numbers, and propose expanding the institution by almost 800% to 9,000 ("Need Accommodations for Mentally Defective," 1940, p. A14).

Almost immediately after his appointment, Kupelian faced allegations of institutional abuse, enduring blaring headlines in the *Portland Press Herald* such as, "Charges Of Neglect At Pownal State School To Be Filed," (1938, p. A1). The accusations were made by a Portland attorney and former State Superior Court judge named Joseph Connolly and led to a state investigation that eventually exonerated the state. The press vigorously defended Kupelian, although the incident raised some serious questions about conditions within the facility that lingered and reemerged later in the superintendent's tenure.

Superintendent Kupelian continued to perform a few eugenic sterilizations in the early 1940s, although by 1939, he was disappointed that marriage restrictions were apparently ineffective in reducing illegitimacy and that sterilization laws were being inadequately applied:

> The marriage of feeble-minded in the State ... is prohibited ... but the element of illegitimacy greatly overshadows such control. An act was also passed in 1925 relating to the sterilization in certain cases for the prevention of the production of feeble-mindedness... Since then there is the record of 72 eugenic sterilizations in Maine. Considering the fact that the sterilization law in Maine has been in effect for thirteen years, this comparatively small

> number of cases is disappointing, and apparently a widespread application of these procedures cannot be expected. (Kupelian, 1939, pp. B1, B15)

By 1940, Kupelian claimed that Pownal's "quarters are cramped [but] ... overcrowding does not exist," although he was confronting a waiting list of 300 of "the most urgent cases" and sounding increasingly desperate ("Need Accommodations for Mentally Defective," 1940, p. A14; *Superintendent's Annual Report of the Pownal State School*, 1940, p. 3). Addressing a local Kiwanis group, Kupelian turned up the eugenic rhetoric in an effort to stem Pownal's escalating enrollments, declaring that: "One of the greatest causes of it [mental deficiency] is heredity, and the only instrument to combat this cause is the authority to sterilize, granted in Maine in 1925. At Pownal, 65 to 70% of the inmates have abnormal heredity" ("Need Accommodations for Mentally Defective," 1940, p. A14).

In the absence of massive sterilizations, and faced with a long waiting list, an overcrowded facility, and likely demands for new referrals due to the continuing depression and increasing possibility of war, Kupelian called for a whopping increase in facility size, from 1,100 to 9,000 residents—big enough to incarcerate between 50–60% of the state's "mentally defective persons" ("Need Accommodations for Mentally Defective," 1940, p. A14). This was far in excess of the waiting list, surpassed the most grandiose expansion proposals of his predecessors, and considered fiscally unacceptable to state lawmakers, even legislators wishing to promote employment opportunities in a depressed economy. The impracticality of sterilization and ever-larger institutions was turning other states to alternative solutions such as foster care. Kupelian, however, dismissed this option as too expensive and time consuming, pointing out the difficulties of investigating and securing a sufficient number of satisfactory homes, providing more clothing, and offering community medical care (*Superintendent's Annual Report of the Pownal State School,* 1940, pp. 3–4). Rather, he pointed out the need for more family and community visits and more intensive, institution-based instruction:

> It is difficult for children who have had a relatively long period of institutional care to adjust themselves properly to community life. We are endeavoring to overcome this by bringing as many children as possible into contact with everyday family and community life. In addition to these contacts, we have planned for the girls a class in cooking. In the elementary grades a course in everyday shopping for boys and girls has been added. (p. 3)

It seems unlikely that Kupelian was unrealistic or naive enough to believe that his proposal to expand the facility to 9,000 would be approved by hard-pressed legislators. More likely, he was attempting to dramatize the overcrowded conditions and admissions pressures that he was facing in a attempt to persuade state politicians of his desperate need for assistance.

A response came in January, 1941, when State Senator Neil Bishop of Bowdoinham announced that he would sponsor a bill to establish a state eugenics board comprised of the directors of the state's largest institutions who would be empowered to sterilize Maine citizens who are not residents of its state institutions but considered by municipal officials to be "defective" and "a menace to society" (as quoted in, "Sen. Bishop Proposes Sterilization of the 'Defectives At Large,"1941, p. A1). According to Bishop, "There already is a law ... causing sterilization to be made of defective persons when or if they are released from our state institutions, but my measure would seek to take care of that individuals [*sic*] at large in our communities" (p. A1). As with the 1925 and 1931 laws, Bishop' legislation was described as "voluntary" but contained no additional safeguards. Seeking to blunt growing opposition, Bishop insisted that "the bill does not make sterilization compulsory, but only by consent either from the person himself, or his parent or guardian" (p. A1).

Kupelian, along with Bangor State Hospital superintendent and the former head of Pownal, Carl Hedin, enthusiastically supported Bishop's bill, citing some well-worn, discredited eugenic alarms, such as "there are 50 percent more births in the families of mental defectives than in normally healthy families," and assuring legislators that "sterilization is more humane than locking them up" ("Sterilization of Maine Defectives Is Advocated ," 1941, p. A1). The superintendents were joined by a Colby College professor of biology, who underscored the central issue underlying Bishop's bill—the continuing and escalating cost of incarcerations—an issue dramatically illustrated by Kupelian's oversized request for a facility of 9,000. The Colby professor stated simply that: "I am rather unwilling ... to continue to pay more taxes for the upkeep of this population" (p. A1). For his part, Bishop elected to emphasize the hereditary theories and ring the eugenic alarms that he hoped would still resonate with his constituents colleagues. According to one newspaper account:

> Bishop said he recently had accompanied members of a legislative committee on an inspection tour of state hospitals and institutions. "Every person should see what I saw," he said. "If they could, they would feel differently on this touchy subject of eugenics."
>
> He asked his colleagues "to put out the fire of feeble-mindedness before civilization is lost."
>
> "We have spent millions on the improvement of animal breeding, but we have done nothing for the human race-we have let people marry without

> any thought to what kinds of children they would produce." (Sterilization of Maine By Maine Senate 28 To 4," 1941, p. A11)

As reflected in Bishop's comments, eugenic sterilization remained controversial and opposition to his bill was stiff. A leading opponent again was Augusta superintendent, Forrest Tyson, who rejected the inheritability myth, offered a contrasting view of mental functioning based on human difference rather than medical pathology, and proposed an alternative perspective on community assistance that was emerging but still ahead of its time:

> Instead of sterilizing the feeble-minded, society should help the poor and unfortunates to establish themselves in the community. The feeble-minded is the most substantial group in the world.... They do your housework and dig your ditches. All but a fifth of the children of feeble-minded parents have been found to have a higher intelligence than their parents. In contrast, children of brilliant parents often do not reach the same mental plane. ("Dr. Tyson Opposed To Sterilization," 1941, in *Clippings Pownal State School, 1909–1946*, 1989, p. 756)

Legislative opposition to Bishop's bill was led by Senator Francis Sullivan of Cape Elizabeth who indicated that the bill was opposed on religious grounds by 200,000 Catholics in the state who would not subscribe to a law which would allow the state to touch a person's body except for punishment for a crime. Sullivan warned that, if enacted, the law too easily could lead to mistakes in judgment ("Sterilization Bill is Aired," n.d., in *Clippings Pownal State School, 1909–1946*, 1989, p. 746).

Terming the proposal a "viscous and unchristian bill," Catholic clergy urged parishioners to flood their legislators with protests and according to the *Lewiston Daily Sun*, extra clerks had to be added at Western Union offices to handle the extraordinary traffic ("Bishop McCarthy Urges Parishioners To Protest," 1941, p. A1). In an interesting reversal from previous decades, the protestors characterized the bill, rather than its targeted victims, as the "threatening evil . . . the moral evil . . . to be protected from" (p. A1). Scorning selective breeding and the application of animal husbandry to human beings, opponents pointed out that most people with mental deficiency were already residing in the community without threatening the existing social order or prolifically reproducing themselves ("Sterilization Bill Rejected by Maine Senate 28 to 4," 1941, pp. A11).

The proposed legislation passed the Senate Judiciary Committee but was roundly defeated in both of Maine's legislative chambers ("House Agrees to Rule Out Sterilization," 1941, p. A1). Accounts of the debate regarding this bill indicate that while some support persisted for the inheritability of social pathology and eugenic-era solutions, this was the last legislative proposal to expand eugenic sterilization, demonstrating that the real power of the eugenics movement to move social policy in Maine was diminished. The movement's effects remained, however, as the state's marriage restrictions, eugenic sterilizations and large scale segregation at Pownal continued for decades.

WORLD WAR II: MASSIVE OVERCROWDING, STAFF REDUCTIONS, AND ADMISSIONS PRESSURES

The nation's entry into World War II in December of 1941 changed all employment patterns, economic priorities, and social policies and dashed whatever hopes Kupelian had for significant fiscal assistance. Writing in June of 1942, the superintendent related how the war decimated his staff:

> Since the beginning of the war we have lost many of our employees. Some have been inducted into the Army, and others have secured employment at the shipyards and other defense work with considerably more pay.... We have had considerable employee turnover, and it is expected that this situation will grow very serious as the war continues. If we are to run the institution efficiently, it is imperative our employees should receive more in wages. (*Superintendent's Annual Report of the Pownal State School,* 1942, p.10)

Kupelian also claimed that the onset of the war greatly increased family referrals to Pownal and expanded an already long waiting list. He argued that the national need for industrial help required all family members to work, leaving "no one to care for the defective member" (*Superintendent's Annual Report for the Pownal State School,* 1945, p. 33). In 1944, Kupelian cited a waiting list of 434, rising to 464 the following year (p. 35), and expanding in 1946 to 513 (*Superintendent's Annual Report for the Pownal State School,* 1946, p. 3).

More than the waiting list was expanding, however, as an already overcrowded institution became a scandalous human warehouse. Connor (1944) reported that residents' slept in Pownal's dormitories "with their beds placed so close together that it is necessary to walk sideways to pass between them; there can be no successful argument that the institution is not overcrowded" (p. A1). By the end of the war, enrollments reached 1,120, a level even Kupelian now described as "crowded to its capacity" (*Superintendent's Annual Report of the Pownal State School,* 1946, p. 3).

Adding to the superintendent's personnel shortages and bulging enrollments was the loss of "working" residents to carry out essential institutional tasks. At one point, the superintendent related that, "during the war years we have discharged quite a few patients who have made sufficient progress to take their places in the community" (*Superintendent's Annual Report of the Pownal State School*, 1946, p. 3). Some residents left Pownal and joined the armed forces where they reportedly performed admirably, attesting to both their capabilities and the injustice of their incarceration. In what must be considered a most ironic revelation, Kupelian noted:

> It is gratifying to note that as far as could be ascertained about 25 of our discharged boys served in the United States Armed Forces during World War II. Of these, 20 were in the Army, 3 in the Navy, 2 in the Marines. The ranks ascertained were as follows: 3 Privates, 1 Technical Sergeant, 2 Sergeants, 1 Corporal, and 1 Seaman Second Class. The boy attaining the rank of Technical Sergeant ... was one of the Paratroopers landing behind enemy lines on D-Day. (*Superintendent's Annual Report of the Pownal State School*, 1945, p. 40)

One resident who served during World War II was Richard Turcotte who was admitted to Pineland after being orphaned at age 3 when his mother died (Philbrick, 2001). Placed with a neighborhood family in Lewiston, Turcotte was sent to Pineland when that family could no longer care for him. He remained institutionalized for 25 years, serving honorably in the Aircraft Warning Service before finally leaving Pineland in 1950. During his time at Pineland, he compiled a 23 page album of "meticulously cared for and well labeled photographs" of his time there. Turcotte lived and worked in Lewiston following his discharge and died in 2001, leaving no family. His remarkable photos have been preserved as part of the Richard Turcotte Collection at the Maine Historical Society.

Some of those who might otherwise have been sent to Pownal during the war found community jobs. Like his predecessors, Kupelian (1939) complained that this left the institution's applicant pool with a greater proportion of lower functioning individuals who required more care and were less productive:

> It has been our policy to admit all levels of mental deficiency in proper proportion. This has been impossible during the war as the morons were employed in various defense work; and ... admissions of low grades have been out of proportion to the admission of middle and upper groups of defectives. [Unless remedied] the Institution ... will be an infirmary for the care of low grade mental defectives. (p. 33)

The superintendent was also upset with the Juvenile Defective Deficiency Act, legislation passed in July, 1941 requiring that juvenile delinquents with the measured intelligence of a 12-year old or less be admitted to Pownal. While facilitating the admissions of more intellectually capable residents, the law also opened the doors to residents who required more staff and supervision, were not considered dependable institutional workers, and created publicity nightmares for the institution with their frequent escapes and acting-out behaviors. Reacting to the escape and multiple barn burnings of "a defective delinquent and a pyromaniac" whom reformatory officials sent to Pownal, Kupelian repeated many of Vosburgh's complaints about having to admit too many people he considered too troublesome:

> The presence of defective delinquents in this institution is not conducive to the proper care and training of defective children. Contrary to the general belief, the definitely defective child is not a criminal child. Delinquency increases in proportion to the higher degree of intelligence. It would be an ideal arrangement if the defective delinquents could be cared for in a separate institution. (*Superintendent's Annual Report of the Pownal State School*, 1945, p. 35)

By 1943, the Pownal farm became a central focus of the institution as a way to demonstrate support for the war effort, save the state money on food supplies, and serve as a needed training ground for area farm workers. According to the superintendent, residents who demonstrated farm work proficiency were placed on community farms, where "they are making excellent adjustments" ("Educating Boys in Farm Work," 1943, p. A11). He explained that some residents were hired as farm hands or granted extended placements, but only if their "services, behavior and conduct warrant, and after careful investigation of the home conditions ... and trial visits" (p. A11). Kupelian related that under the state's farm-placement program an individual might secure final release from the institution if "at the end of one or two or three years, they are able to earn their own living and adjust themselves to community life" (p. A11).

Kupelian's efforts to find farm placements had every reason to succeed. For years, residents had been engaging in farm, manual, and maintenance work at Pownal and were likely attractive employees for area farmers in need of farm help. Kupelian's idea was far from new, since 30 years earlier in upstate New York, Charles Bernstein had proved the worth of many institutional residents as workers on farms and in domestic settings.

Despite the favorable job market for farm hands and other workers, the evident success of residents in community and military occupations, and Pownal's overcrowded state and escalating waiting list, there was no apparent large-scale effort to discharge residents to community employment. Based on the superintendent's annual reports for the decade of 1940–50, the facility's enrollments continued to rise—from 1,106 at the beginning of the period to around 1,290 at the end, an increase of about

14%. Official discharges averaged about 13 per year for the years 1940–47, ranging from 3 in 1945 to 20 in 1943, spiking to 25 in 1950 (see Table 6.1). The waiting list for that period ranged from 317 to 520, so even doubling the number of "discharges" by including those who had died or were transferred, still leaves a relatively small number compared with those awaiting admission.

These totals, however, reveal only the surface of the real discharge story. Embedded within Kupelian's annual reports were larger numbers of ongoing releases that were termed "home trial visits" (see Table 6.1). Such visits had been a long-standing but modestly recorded classification, initially included as early as 1919 as one of several types of "dismissals," along with deaths, escapes and miscellaneous discharges (*Eleventh Annual Report of the Pownal State School*, 1919, p. 1). Later the visit/trial visit category was dropped as a separate category and included under the term "absent" from Pownal. It is not entirely clear how the term "visit" translated into actual time away from Pownal. Were those on visit eventually discharged? Were individuals "on visit" counted as part of the official institutional census? As shown in Table 6.1, in 1940, 13 residents were officially discharged, but 141 children were allowed to go on home visits (*Superintendent's Annual Report of the Pownal State School*, 1940, p. 8). The following year the number of visits increased to 172. Figures were not available for the next three years, but in years 1945-47, home visits totaled 164, 171, 169 respectively. (*Superintendent's Annual Report of the Pownal State School*, 1945, p. 34; *Superintendent's Annual Report of the Pownal State School*, 1946, p. 5; *Superintendent's Annual Report of the Pownal State School*, 1947, p. 8).

Apparently, Pownal officials, in their desperate efforts to manage an overcrowded facility, reverted to a release policy that permitted many more resident discharges than Pownal administrators cared to publicize overtly. This process alleviated some of the overcrowding, reduced costs, and obscured Pownal's actual enrollments. Likely most of those discharged were younger residents, allowing the superintendent to retain as many mature and capable resident workers as possible to run the crowded institution, especially as paid employees and some of the best resident workers left for war.

The idea of paroling residents on visit/trial visit and retaining them on the rolls had been discussed at Pownal as early as 1913 and carried out "selectively" since the late 1930s. Kupelian was accelerating the practice, however, to a point that was clearly at odds with his alarmist public pronouncements. Like his immediate predecessors, Kupelian, the last overtly eugenic superintendent, had no problem contradicting himself and ignoring his own warnings about the "societal menace," as he assured any

Table 6.1. Institutional Enrollments, Discharges, and Home Visits: 1940–50

Year	*# in instit. (+ absent)*	*Total Enrllmts*	*Wait List*	*Visits/ Home/Vsts*	*Official Dischrg**
1939–40	1,086 +20	1,106	317	141	13
1940–41	1,077 +30	1,107	349	172	10
1941–42	1,065 +45	1,110	unavail	35	11
1942–43	1,075 +35	1,110	unavail	unavail	20
1943–44	1,072 +41	1,113	434	unavail	3
1944–45	1,079 +38	1,117	464	28 (164)#	13
1945–46	1,080 +40	1,120	513	33 (171)#	19
1946–47	1,059 +48	1,117	520	39 (169)#	10
1947–48	1,058 +48	1,114	unavail	unavail	unavail
1950–	1,240 +48	1,290	unavail	unavail	25

* includes only figures listed under "discharge" category which may not always be calculated consistently between years.

figure in parenthesis not included with this category in annual report but in a separate section of the report.

skeptics of the nearly flawless selection and monitoring process that Pownal staff conducted around such visits:

> As there has been an increase in the Home Trial Visit Group Program it has become necessary to make special investigations as to the advisability of certain patients going home. Attempt also is being made to place certain improved patients for outside employment. It is gratifying to state that there has been practically no failure in this group. The community services supervisor visits at stated intervals all home wage children and records in a special book the result of her investigations. The patients in the care of relatives receive a modified social supervision. (*Superintendent's Annual Report of the Pownal State School*, 1940, p. 15)

Despite heightened home visits, Kupelian reiterated the need for a greatly expanded institution due largely to heightened admission demand. Clearly, the waiting list was growing during the war years, going from 349 in 1941 to 525 in 1947 (*Superintendent's Annual Report of the Pownal State School*, 1941, p. 7; *Superintendent's Annual Report of the Pownal State School*, 1947, p. 4). Kupeliam attributed the burgeoning lists to the growing economic burdens imposed on families. Many of these admissions, however, were initiated by municipal and court sources following the 1941 "defective delinquent" law. Certainly some families requested admission for their son or daughter due to war and financial hardship, perhaps termporarily. Most did not, however, and, likely many families requested discharges for a member to help at home. Kupelian acknowledged that some individuals avoided incarceration at Pownal by finding employment in the accelerated wartime economy, a situation that economically benefitted families in need of additional income to replace a departed, disabled, or deceased member. In their efforts to defend the overcrowding and bolster the case for enlargement, Pownal officials appear to have exaggerated the extent to which families were demanding institutionalization. Pownal's records indicate that families were actually requesting more discharges than admissions and that Pownal administrators were granting less than half of these requests. In 1940, families and friends made 329 requests for resident visits/trial visits but only 164 were approved (*Superintendent's Annual Report of the Pownal State School*, 1940, pp. 13–14). The following year requests totaled 372 of which Pownal granted 172 (*Superintendent's Annual Report of the Pownal State School*, 1941, p. 7). As reflected in Table 6.1, between 1945–47, over 500 residents were released under the visits/trial visits rubric, although officials stopped reporting the total number of requests for such visits (*Superintendent's Annual Report of the Pownal State School*, 1945, p. 33; *Superintendent's Annual Report of the Pownal State School*, 1946, p. 8; *Superintendents Annual Report of the Pownal State School*, 1947, p. 8).

During the war years, the superintendent was operating a grossly overcrowded and understaffed institution with people who were considered more difficult to manage. Kupelian complained bitterly about the type of residents he was admitting and he lobbied incessantly for a large increase in space, money, and staff to accommodate this trend. In the face of such fiscal shortages, however, everyone was looking for places to send people they considered troublesome. Portland municipal authorities, for example, complained they had "missed the boat" in 1941 when they failed to lobby hard enough for a bond issue that would expand Pownal enough to take more of the city's "mental and old age cases" ("Mental and Old Age Cases Confront City With Problem," 1943, A11).

At the request of Governor Sumner Sewall, the commissioner of the Department of Institutional Services, Harrison Greenleaf, called for expanding all of the state's 13 institutions, particularly Pownal and the two psychiatric facilities at Augusta and Bangor ("Greenleaf Sees Expansion," 1941, p. A1). Greenleaf termed facility expansion "as imperative if Maine is to meet the demands for institutional care and relieve local communities and family groups of serious problems ... [and] accommodate the anticipated post-war increase in patients (p. A1)."

Added to the humanitarian rationales, and embedded within the commissioner's proposals for expanded segregation, were economic arguments that had never been so explicitly used to help justify institutional expansion. According to Greenleaf:

> The 13 Maine institutions ... care for some 5,000 inmates and patients, and in normal times afford employment for 1,200 persons.... Beyond the fact that such projects will provide useful employment to many returning veterans and men discharged from lucrative defense industry employment ... there exists now a real need for enlargement of certain state institutions. (Greenleaf Sees Expansion, 1941, p. 1A)

In September 1944, Governor Sumner Sewall requested legislative authorization to build two large (200 person) resident dormitories in order "to expand the over-crowded Pownal State School" (Connors, 1944, p. A1), "relieve human suffering in the family burdened with defective children" ("Pownal School, Fish Station Work Urged, 1944, p. A1) and "practically clean up the waiting list (Connor, 1944, p. A1). As in 1941, state officials added that an expanding institution supported the returning troops and defense workers by offering good construction jobs and stable institutional employment. According to the governor: "this will be the year that the greatest number of our veterans will be returning ... [and] the year therefore when it will be tremendously important to have abundant business and employment opportunities for our veterans" (p. A8). Institutional expansion had not only become patriotic but a growth industry and good for the state's economy.

As understaffing and overcrowding reached unprecedented levels at all state institutions, scandal erupted and with it, the first major public expose'. Following the death of a man discharged from the Augusta State Hospital with multiple fractures of his ribs, Maine's Attorney General, Frank Cowan investigated and found instances of residents being punched, beaten, kicked in the face and stomach, choked, tied up by the wrists and ankles, bound to objects and bed rails, and so forth ("Cowan Charges Abuse at State Insane Hospital," 1944, p. A1, A5). He concluded that a clear and extensive pattern of physical and verbal abuse existed within the institution, dating back years before the onset of the war (p. A1). Although Cowan's report was vigorously challenged, its findings were sufficiently disturbing to warrant investigation of other state institutions, including Pownal.

At the request of the governor, the Maine Federation of Woman's Clubs investigated Pownal in 1946–47. Ironically, this was the same group of social reformers who 40 years earlier had been so instrumental in establishing the Maine School in order to improve the circumstances of persons considered feebleminded. The women's report excoriated the institution's leadership and staff, characterizing employees as resistant to the women's inquiry, the facility as a place where "physical neglect and abuse [were] nearly commonplace" (Hood, 1968, p. 22)." and the superintendent as clueless, or "not ... aware of some of the conditions described" (p. 23).

Kupelian blamed residents and the state legislature for Pownal's disgraceful condition, complaining in 1946 that "new admissions ... have been mostly low grades who will always require custodial care. If this ratio of admissions continues, the time will arrive when dismissals will be few. It is therefore recommended that new admissions be equalized" (*Superintendent's Annual Report of the Pownal State School*, 1946, p. 3). The following year, Kupelian, the same superintendent who a few years before had proposed enlarging the institution to 9,000, argued that "the original purpose of the School, which is not to be an infirmary for the physically and mentally helpless and a convenient dumping ground for the troublesome but an institution for training the mentally handicapped to return to community life (*Superintendent's Annual Report of the Pownal State School*, 1947, pp. 5–6).

The Federation women were outraged when officials excused the conditions as merely reflecting the nature of custodial care. In a stinging rebuke to Kupelian and other state authorities, they pointed out that "merely custodial care-however clean and sanitary-is not too great an advance from the old Bedlam and for any who think that statement extreme I recommend their spending some time in Yarmouth Hall at Pownal" (Hood, 1968, p. 23).

Pownal officials argued that without increased capacity, staff, appropriations, and more capable residents, conditions would not improve (*Superintendent's Annual Report of the Pownal State School*, 1947, p. 5). They heralded Pownal's new dormitories as the solution for overcrowding, improved living conditions, and decreased waiting periods. Apparently, the only thing that changed regarding the facility's living conditions was that they had become even worse. Moreover, the solutions now being proposed were identical to those that were offered, and failed, in the past. The prospects for improving Pownal through expansion and more selective admissions seemed dim. Moreover, as Pownal officials persisted in expanding the facility and admitting more people, they worsened their staffing shortages resulting in the continued retention of unpaid resident workers, many of whom the most feasible for immediate release.

One possible option for Pownal officials was to perform more eugenic sterilizations, although the surgery continued to be publically and scientifically controversial and its proposed application to noninstitutional populations had been defeated in the legislature only a few years before. Nevertheless, sterilization was still legal in the state, remained generally supported by Maine's medical community and Pineland officials, and would continue to be performed legally through 1963.

The advent of war, a lack of physicians, and the 1942 *Skinner v. Oklahoma* Supreme Court decision (a case in which sterilization was determined to involve a basic human right and Oklahoma's compulsory sterilization law of all habitual criminals was found to violate the constitutional right to equal protection (Elkins & Anderson, 1992, p. 19; Nourse, 2008, pp. 15), operated to depress the number of eugenic sterilizations performed nationally during World War II (Paul, 1965, pp. 86–87). Although it is often claimed that after Nazi atrocities were exposed to worldwide view during, and immediately after World War II, there ensued a quick end to the eugenics movement and its practices. In fact, despite Deutsch's (1949) research that discredited the inheritability myth by concluding that 89% of children with intellectual disabilities were born to parents with normal intelligence, the number of eugenic surgeries actually increased during the decades after World War II. According to Largent (2008), "from the end of the war through the 1960s" (p. 117) there was little popular recognition of a link between the American eugenics movement and the Holocaust, and that revelations about the Nazi genocide during and following the war did not lead to immediate cessation of the harshest eugenic practices in the United States. Beginning in the mid-1960s, and continuing through the 1980s, sterilization laws were under widespread attack, yet until the early 1980s, sixteen states still had sterilization laws for persons with intellectual disabilities that were based on the same eugenic assumptions that fostered *Buck v. Bell* (Elkins & Anderson, 1992, p. 20).

Eugenic surgeries in Maine peaked between 1933 and 1940 when an average of about 21 individuals per year were sterilized (Paul, 1965, p. 369). During the war years, 1941–1945, the surgeries declined to a total of 14, or about 3 individuals per year (Paul, 1965, p. 370). From 1946 until 1963 (the year the last eugenic sterilization was recorded in Maine) sterilizations rose again as 106 people underwent the eugenic surgery, an average of almost 6 per year. Although these figures never reached their prewar levels, the post war numbers indicate that nearly one third of all the persons sterilized in Maine were operated on after 1946.

Despite the enormous distractions of war, it is difficult to defend the post World War II era with its ongoing sterilizations and incarcerations in the face of discredited rationales and deplorable institutional conditions. Even though Pownal officials accelerated resident discharges and embarked on the first serious parole effort in its history, their activities were largely covert and they soon reverted to their expansionist policies, justifying them as responding to the demands of Maine families, the requirements of the postwar economy, the employment needs of returning veterans. It was clear by this time that individuals who continued to be targeted for institutionalization posed no threat to society, showed themselves to be capable community workers and soldiers, and were referred by their families in far fewer numbers than was reported.

While the women's federation expose of 1947 was the most serious scandal to ever hit Pownal, revealing terrible conditions and abusive treatment, it apparently had no discernible effects on the way the institution was administered, perhaps due to the absence of the lurid visual images that would accompany later scandals. Kupelian survived the Federation's investigation and stinging rebuke and continued as superintendent into the post-war era. In early 1953, however, four residents set fire to the dairy barn, devastating the institution's dairy operations and leading to Kupelian's resignation on May 1, 1953 (Hood, 1968, p. 24).

The barn burning incident, although treated in the press as a predictable act of lawlessness by a group widely considered to be socially deviant, could also be interpreted as a dramatic sign of protest from within the facility by some of those subjected to the unbearable conditions reveled by the women's federation. Conceivably, embittered and disempowered residents acted out in their own behalf, using whatever means available to rebel in numerous ways such as setting fires, derailing trains, and/or escaping. Early institutional records and newspaper stories record such incidents, although first hand accounts and descriptions are nearly non-existent. One exception are the interviews conducted with Mr. Charles (Charlie) Wyman, a Pownal resident in the 1930s during the tenures of Vosburgh and Kupelian, who shared his experiences as a resident and escapee. Admitted to the facility at age 7, Wyman spent 11 years at Pineland, escaping three times and returned twice by people seeking the $25 reward, which he noted, "in those days was a lot of money" (Williams, 2000, A11; Wyman, personal communication, August 21, 1999). Describing how and why he was sent to Pineland, Mr Wyman recalled:

> My father and mother lived in Troy (Maine) and he had a small farm and he owned it. He sold vegetables ... up in Pittsfield and he did some work around and with what he could pick up, we got by all right.... And one day when our mother took us to school, someone came in and put the place [home] on fire.... The place was burnt flat.... When we got burnt out, we lost a lot of things and it made things difficult.... And then they [town officials] came out and got us and took us to the town farm in Troy. And then they come out and got me and put me in a foster home in Sidney and they got to strappin me and I didn't know what to do. My mother never did that, so I ran away. They picked me up and took me back to Augusta and the state woman put

> me into Pineland. She said, "I'll put him where he'll have to stay," and they locked me up. (Wyman, personal communication, August 21, 1999)

Speaking with a reporter, Wyman related that he learned from records years afterwards that he was classified as a "moron" but that he and others he knew "were not mentally retarded," just "poor or orphans" (Williams, 200, p. A11). As an "inmate," he was physically abused "whipped with a two inch leather belt after first being soaked in bathtubs of ice in order to hide the bruises" (p. A 11). For 10 years, he reported being taunted and bullied, forced to work in the fields before he was 13, and threatened if "he didn't keep his mouth shut" (p. A11)." According to Wyman, "Those attendants were big and rugged and they could get away with it" (p. A11). When the school's trustees came to the campus, Wyman was warned, to say nothing about what he saw or experienced or else "'we'll just tell them you're retarded. Then after they leave, we'll beat you to death' " (p. A11).

Escaping twice, Wyman was returned the second time, by the Pownal scoutmaster who received his reward money and left Charlie to face angry employees:

> So that night, they [Pownal staff] said, "When you get out it'll be in a pine box." I said, "No, I'm not gonna go in no pine box. I'm gonna go on my feet and legs." They said, "Well, you can't do it. There's bars on the windows and they lock your coat up in the hall at bedtime. You have to go in your night clothes." I said, "That's ok I got a plan." [But] someone told [on me] and they cut my hair right off ... because they said if you run away ... they'll know you run away from school. They said, "Are you going to run away?" I didn't say nothin.
>
> We was under surveillance all the time, just like prisoners. And this old fella come back and locked the door. He was trying to get his key in and when he did that, I went right on through. I stayed at the end of the line. I planned that, you see.... I didn't realize they'd seen me but there was a lot of bushes right there ... and he said, "Oh, a fellow's run away." And the other two attendants they was lookin all around and while they was lookin' I was laying there. And while I was laying there I said, "Oh Lord, don't let 'em find me." I wasn't a born again Christian then but I believed ... there was a God up above somewhere. And they almost stepped on me but they didn't. And they said, "Well we got to get these kids going or they'll be more of 'em running away. We''ll blow the whistle" [escape alarm].
>
> Well, I was about two miles from school and I had been running awfully since the time I had gotten away from school. And I walked along the river . . . and I saw a set of buildings, and I said, "I don't know who lives here but I got to get in." So I opened the door ... and I got up in the hay. So I thought to myself, "Before he comes out to do his chores I'll wake up and get of here" 'cause they posted it [the escape] all around. They'll give 'em $25.... They posted all the farms around.... Now I woke up kinda late and I could

> hear him out there milkin' his cows. I planned when he went out to dump his can of milk, I'd go. My timing was off. He was on his last cow. When he dumped that pail of milk , he came [back] and saw me coming down the ladder. He said, "Well, we have a transient." I said, "Yes ... I was huntin' with a group and got separated." He said, "Well, I'm goin' in to have breakfast. Why don't you come along?" I said no because if I took off my hat, he'd see my head shaved. He had hired help who could've held me until he called the school and had 'em come and get me. So I got up there probably about 100 yards and when I got to the road, I ran like a deer because I figured he might change his mind and come after me.
>
> In no time at all [I] came into Danver Junction.... So I see this man walkin' along and it was daylight. I said, "Excuse me, could you tell me where Route 1 is?"... So he says, "Well, where are you going?" I says, "I want to go to Bangor." He said ... "I'll introduce you to my wife, and get you some breakfast and you can ride through with me to Bangor."
>
> So they never got me. They had four posses after me but they never got me. I could run like a deer through the woods. Now you know God was with me because you run through the woods at night you could fall with no light or nothin'. God I believe led the whole thing. He didn't want me there no more (Wyman, personal communication, August 21, 1999).

Large-scale segregation at Pineland would continue to expand until 1958. Even when enrollments began declining in the late 1950s, deplorable living conditions would be documented for decades. Residents like Mr. Wyman remained incarcerated, not only because they were needed to run the facility efficiently and cheaply, but also because their presence prevented the facility from being identified as a strictly custodial institution for only "the most chronic cases." The 1950s in Maine could be called the beginning of the end of eugenic practices, but the end was not yet assured.

CHAPTER 7

INSTITUTIONAL EXODUS AND EXPOSÉ

PETER BOWMAN AND EMERGING INSTITUTIONAL REFORM

Hood (1968, p. 24) describes Pownal as "sinking to a new low" under Kupelian's tenure, marking the end of a 45-year tradition of custodial care and the beginning of a more humanitarian, rehabilitative emphasis. Certainly the period of the 1940s and early 1950s was a disgraceful chapter in the institution's history, illustrating how the continuing indictment of a targeted group could be conducted for newly invented reasons and proceed in spite of discredited scientific rationales, institutional scandal, and viable and proven alternatives.

In 1953, Dr. Peter W. Bowman took over as superintendent. A 33-year old psychiatrist who emigrated to the United States in 1949 from Germany and settled in Massachusetts, Bowman was a forceful and intimidating individual. According to those who knew him, he was respected more than liked and feared more than anything. Some employees described him as the most controversial, visionary, and autocratic superintendent they had ever worked for. A long-time employee and former social worker remarked that:

Voices of Pineland: Eugenics, Social Reform, and the Legacy of "Feeblemindedness" in Maine, pp. 143–178

> I admired him but was afraid of him. He was a dictator.... Once he reprimanded [my husband] for not properly caring for me during my pregnancy. He [Bowman] was always right and not someone to argue with.... He used to tour the grounds at all hours of the day and night and scare people who were working and catching people sleeping on the job. (Rogers, personal communication, September 24, 1998)

Some considered him the primary reason for Pownal's turnaround from a place of custody to one of rehabilitation, a lightning rod for change, and a maligned figure who was never given sufficient credit for his pioneering work. Another veteran employee who later became acting superintendent, described Bowman as "very controversial ... but the initial force behind those dramatic institutional changes.... I have great respect for that man who I think was a real catalyst for change early on" (Kohler, personal communication, August, 19, 1998).

Bowman was the first Pownal superintendent since Bliss with no history of involvement in any of Maine's institutions and he apparently felt little obligation to defend previous practices. He commanded media attention and used the advantage well, surpassing even past masters like Bliss and Vosburgh in delivering carefully crafted accounts of the facility and its needs; projecting desirable images of himself and his plans; boldly criticizing existing conditions; and campaigning aggressively for public and legislative support. Bowman also pursued direct public access by developing the institution's first brochure, beginning the facility's in-house newsletter, the *Pineland Observer,* and instituting a Department of Public Education.

Terming his first year as "the most trying of 47 years in the history of Pownal State School," he reported an ongoing outbreak of infectious hepatitis, inadequate prevention and treatment of tuberculosis, a hurricane that caused a power outage and paralyzed food and water supplies and laundry services, and the indictment of the institution's director of education and scout leader for sexually abusing young male residents (*Annual Report of the Superintendent of the Pownal State School*, 1955, p. 4; Hood, 1968, p. 29). Announcing a full-fledged investigation that uncovered an even broader pattern of sexual and physical abuse within the facility, Bowman reported firing all those responsible, but warned legislators that future scandals would occur unless they increased Pownal's funding, facilities, and staff. According to the superintendent, 155 new staff were required immediately to substantially reduce the excessive use of solitary confinement and restraints and markedly improve patient cleanliness, poorly prepared meals, unsanitary conditions, inferior medical and psychiatric services, and inadequate recreational and educational facilities (Hood, 1968, p. 29). Bowman's actions impressed local politicians, and the newly formed Pownal Parents and Friends

Association. The latter would grow to be an influential group, consisting largely of parents of Pineland residents who actively promoted the institution, often volunteering time and money, lobbying for legislative support, and resisting any efforts to reduce its prominence, funding or size.

The legislature granted Bowman a robust funding increase the following year (Hood, 1968, p. 29) and that was only the beginning. During his tenure, the superintendent expanded and upgraded the institution's physical facilities through new construction and renovations. He built a new school, hospital wing, employee apartment units, a girl's dormitory, a resident cottage, a treatment and speech clinic, a 130-bed infirmary, a 70-person children's psychiatric hospital, and a vocational rehabilitation workshop (pp 32–53).

In 1956, Bowman took full advantage of a well-publicized visit by Governor Edmund Muskie by preparing an 18 page document in which he proposed to expand the institution to 2,500 by 1970, but warning that growth beyond that figure "under present conditions would create grave administrative problems which make it doubtful ... [to] plan on a larger institution" (Bowman, 1956, p. 1). Unlike his predecessors, Bowman was willing to sharply and publically criticize the facility, initially describing Pownals's living conditions as deplorable:

> In fact there is not single chair in any dormitory, neither a table nor a single locker for patients within the Institution. In other words, our patients have to put their dresses, shirts, trousers, stockings, etc, under their beds on the floor.... I sincerely believe that the present condition is not in accordance with customary provisions for hospital patients in the Country. There are no curtains in either dormitories or day rooms. Both dormitories and day rooms are either overheated or too cool.... Consequently, our patients are constantly suffering from colds.... We must give serious and immediate consideration to expansion to relieve the present overcrowding. (pp. 13–14)

Giving varied accounts of the institution's enrollment, Bowman (1956) reported an enrollment of 1,622 versus a capacity for 1,500 residents (p. 1). In the same document, he indicated that Pownal had certified dormitory space for 913 residents but was housing 1,486 (p. 14). The latter figures seem most accurate, as the larger totals appear to include discharged and/or paroled residents who were living elsewhere but were still officially counted as facility residents.

Early on, Bowman proposed discharging residents, starting with those he considered the most severely disabled—individuals whom he neither believed were productive within the institution nor consistent with his vision of a more dynamic, cost-effective institution. Exactly where these individuals would go remained unclear:

> Since we have several hundred patients whose severe mental limitations excludes them from participation in academic and vocational class work, in physical education, and in many cases even in occupational and recreational activities, one should think of relocating these patients elsewhere in existing adequate buildings, presently and presumably permanently vacant—<u>if available</u> [Bowman's emphasis] in order to create space at Pownal State School for those who can benefit from the existing facilities and services in terms of treatment, education, and training. This would delay the need for costly new construction. (p. 1)

The superintendent also urged discharging residents "who can function adequately and gainfully in community life" (Bowman, 1956, p. 2), and expanding the institution's authority and control into the community in order that released residents "receive constant and proper supervision, for they do not command the judgment necessary to manage their own financial affairs, or raise a family" (p. 2). He went on to propose that carefully monitored placements could be implemented in lieu of eugenic sterilizations, the latter still legal as an institutional option. According to Bowman:

> Sheltered workshop conditions on farms and similar employment situations under supervision is probably the best and most economical answer and will appeal to all those who have mental reservations regarding eugenic sterilization or who reject such a procedure as a matter of principle or of religion. Such a placement program would again relieve the School, and would be economical as the supervised patient would maintain himself. (p. 2)

Legalized sterilizations continued in Maine through 1963, although it appears that the last operation performed at Pineland was in 1960 (Kaelber, 2009; Paul, 1965, p. 369). Bowman's record on sterilization is decidedly mixed. From 1953, the year he began at Pownal, through 1960, he approved sterilizations for 64 people, 45 women and 19 men (Paul, 1965, p. 369). In addition, to the evident gender imbalance, these surgeries were done well after their scientific legitimacy was widely discredited. Moreover, while Maine may have had a record of "moderation" in conducting eugenic sterilizations, Bowman approved a relatively high number of the surgeries in a relatively brief period. The number of individuals sterilized on Bowman's watch equaled almost 20% of the total number of individuals sterilized in Maine since the surgery was legalized in 1925 (p. 369). There was also an alarming surge in eugenic sterilizations during the middle years of the 1950s when in just 2 years, 1954–55, 15 and 26 people were sterilized respectively, exceeding the total of all those sterilized at Pineland for the remaining 8 years of the 1950s (p. 369). It remains unclear why so many operations were performed in this short period since there is no mention of the sudden increases in the superintendent's annual reports. Releases from Pownal did not accelerate until 1958, so it is unlikely that Bowman conducted a campaign of "sterilization for discharge" at that time. That eugenics practices such as sterilization continued, even accelerated, in Maine during this period, is a disturbing, but far from isolated, trend. A similar surge occurred in New Hampshire in the early 1950s when 79 people were sterilized from 1950–53 (p. 418), although no such increases occurred in Vermont where only two people were sterilized after 1950. New Hampshire ended its eugenic surgeries in 1959, while the last documented sterilization occurred in Vermont in 1957 (pp. 418, 494).

Bowman continued to approve sterilizations for several years after both New Hampshire and Vermont ended the practice, although his policies were described by Paul (1965, p. 367) as judicious—low in number, very selective, and carefully monitored. Commenting on his eugenic surgeries, Bowman (Bowman, personal communication, October, 14, 1960, as cited in Paul, 1965, p. 367) said:

> I am not at all concerned with legal provisions, external and internal provisions, but rather with scientific, sound, professional standards to indicate when eugenic sterilization should be performed and when not. Neither the American Medical Association nor the American Psychiatric Association has set up such standards, and having traveled throughout the Country, I am horrified about the approach either because it is promiscuous [sic] or influenced by religious concepts neither of which, in my opinion, is a scientific approach.

Bowman's claims of strictly adhering to a "scientific approach" seems dubious given the amount of scientific evidence that had now accumulated to justify halting the practice completely. The superintendent, however, was not the only professional who was slow to reverse course. Although the prolonged and active opposition of the Catholic Church likely muted the number of surgeries performed in Maine relative to other states, the advocacy of the state's medical community, along with the support of Maine's legal, and political community, helped to perpetuate the surgeries until the early 1960s. In Maine and elsewhere, institutional officials presented the surgery as ordinary, routine, medical care, obscuring and largely removing it from public scrutiny.

In his 1956 report to Governor Muskie, Bowman also called for expanding Maine's special education efforts, reflecting the growth of these programs following World War II. Specifically, Bowman (1956) recommended increasing "special education classes at the community level for mildly and moderately retarded children as part of the local school system [to] spare many children the limitations of institutional life, and again relieve the Pownal State School and the State Government Budget" (p. 1).

Since the superintendent was proposing to discharge residents with the most serious disabilities and those who could function successfully with community supervision, one might ask why he would need a facility as large as 2,500 people. Apparently the answer lay in his short-term desire to reduce overcrowding by increasing capacity and his long-term vision of creating a cutting-edge, medical-teaching hospital.

Bowman was proposing a revitalized institution along the lines envisioned by Stephen Vosburgh 20 years before, but on a grander scale. A reconceptualized medical-research facility would subsume the institution's small on-grounds hospital and contrast sharply with the static, custodial image of the surrounding Pownal State School. Gone would be residents with severe and chronic impairments, replaced by short-term in-patients and expanded outreach services to the 25,000–27,000 people suspected of being mentally deficient across Maine (Hoffman, 1982, p. 3; Hood, 1968, p. 31).

From the beginning of his tenure, Bowman worked hard to more thoroughly medicalize and professionalize the facility's staff, emphasizing therapeutic credentials, developing health-related departments, and providing scientific research. Modeled on the medical teaching hospital and the progressive ideal of cutting-edge science informing social policy and clinical practice, the facility would treat mental deficiency as a non communicable disease as opposed to the eugenic perspective of genetically transmitted social pathology. According to Bowman, residents should be considered patients and receive professionally delivered treatments aimed at "ameliorating, improving, even curing," and then discharging them to re-enter society (Hoffman, 1969a, p. viii). Medical professionals would run the organization and the name of the facility would be changed to reflect its new identity. In 1957, the institution was renamed the Pineland Hospital and Training Center.

Unlike Kupelian who expanded parole and discharge as a temporary step to remedy a burgeoning waiting list and alleviate staff and funding shortages, Bowman viewed institutional discharges as integral to Pineland's new medical/training image, role and function. Aligning mental deficiency as closely as possible with biomedical pathology, Bowman would recast discharge as integral to typical hospital treatment, followed up by an expanded corps of community placement and supervisory professionals. In actual practice, however, discharges would occur at unprecedented levels but community supervision, services, and supports would not.

Bolstering his in-house resources more than his community-based capacity, Bowman hired Pineland's first full time dentist, pathologist, public education director, and volunteer services director. He established departments of psychiatric social work, clinical psychology, laboratory services, and physical, occupational, and recreational therapies and argued that these professionals would eventually save money. According to Bowman, more physical therapists would allow "40 crippled children who would only get worse to successfully walk;" more social workers would enable "cured" patients to be discharged; and "three to four good psychologists could prevent mental retardation, and mentally disabled children from ever having to go to an institution" ("Bowman takes over," 1953, p. 1A). According to the superintendent, true institutional reform could only occur with more professionals and funding to hire more medical and health-related professional staff.

Also integral to Bowman's vision of a rejuvenated institution was an infusion of medical and scientific research to uncover the causes of mental deficiency, prevent "such human disaster in the future," and avoid the expensive custodial care they required (Bowman, 1956, p. 3). Bowman appointed Dr. John Hoffman, a sociologist, as Pineland's Director of Research, to conduct in-house studies. He also encouraged corporations to conduct medical research using residents as subjects in return for institutional donations. Two studies that were mentioned in the superintendent's 1957 annual report involved drug testing, where Pineland residents were used as uninformed, involuntary subjects. Including institutionalized persons as research subjects was common practice throughout the country, although the egregious human abuses discovered as part of research at facilities like the Jewish Chronic Disease Hospital, Tuskegee Institute and the Willowbrook State School led to the beginning of federal human-subjects regulation in the mid-1960s. In one of the Pineland studies, the state and a major pharmacology company collaborated to test experimental antibiotics on victims of dysentery who served in both the treatment and the "no treatment" control groups:

> One greatly disrupting feature was a widespread epidemic of Bacillary Dysentery of the Shigella type ... accounting for about 400 clinical cases. The State Laboratory and the District Health Officer were at all times ready to co-operate. Smith, Kline and French Laboratories provided hundreds of bottles of their Sulspansion to compare with other medications for many of our cases, both as prophylactic and treatment measures. (*Annual Report of the Superintendent*, 1957, p. 1)

In another study on the effects of Thorazine, a powerful tranquilizer, the same company donated some furniture to Pineland in exchange for access to residents who were

> drawn from all-female dormitories and some ... transferred to other buildings to concentrate the research project in one building.... [I]t involved a great

> deal of work, many transfers, and much time.... [T]he newly furnished day room at the generosity of Smith, Kline, and French has been a source of pleasure and pride to personnel and patient. (p. 2)

In 1957, Pineland's Medical Department reported on the expanded and effective use of drug therapy, ignoring the irony of the alleged "improvement" and underscoring the widespread appeal of the approach and its potential for abuse.

> Tranquilizers of various types were used more freely this year and although destruction of property and assaultiveness [*sic*] have continued in some cases, many other cases have shown marked improvement. One patient camisoled for years now sits quietly and without restraint but interestingly enough in a position as though still restrained. (*Annual Report of the Superintendent*, 1957, pp. 1–2)

Throughout this period, Bowman was garnering medical accolades. In 1956, the American Psychiatric Association awarded Pownal one of its three national awards for "outstanding improvement in patient care and treatment" (Hood, 1968, p. 33). The crowning achievement, however, occurred in 1963, when, as Bowman proclaimed, the institution, "in its 56th year of existence and after ten and one-half years of sustained efforts," was granted full accreditation by the Joint Commission on Accreditation of Hospitals (*Annual Report for the Pineland Hospital and Training Center*, 1964, p. 2).

Around the time he changed the name of the institution, Bowman published what may have been Pineland's first official brochure promoting the institution's new role, emphasis, and activities. Sharply contrasting with typical promotions of this kind, the document expressed the superintendent's ongoing frustration with the state's fiscal stinginess and likely did not endear him to the state's politicians. Promoting his accomplishments and criticizing the facility's custodial character of the past and its current state of disrepair, Bowman described "completely outmoded, inadequate overcrowded and unsafe conditions," adding that "every effort is being made to replace and bring up to acceptable standards this type of facility" (*Pineland Hospital and Training Center*, n.d., p. 4). Although Bowman's enrollment figures and various resident statuses (e.g. trial visits, temporary employment, etc.) were somewhat confusing, tending to obfuscate rather than clarify enrollment figures, he claimed in his brochure that all buildings except Sidwell Hall were operating over capacity and that Pineland was over-enrolled by 361 residents (p. 5).

In addition to pressuring state lawmakers for more money, Bowman was waging a public relations campaign, presenting facility residents as largely harmless and pitiable versus menacing. He appealed for acceptance and sympathy (despite his disclaimer) rather than fear and detention, referring to residents as "patients" whom he characterized as victims of medical misfortune "who did not ask to be born," and who "don't want your sympathy—they want your understanding. And they NEED *(brochure's emphasis)* your help" (pp. 2–3). As with any medical hospital, the major goal was not permanent custody, but treatment followed by discharge, with the latter described as Pineland's high, but still uncertain, priority. On the brochure's first page was proclaimed: "The Mentally Retarded and the Mentally Ill Can Return—Somehow—Somewhere—" (p. 1). A later section emphasized that "the main objective" of Pineland had changed, focusing now on "the **eventual return** *(brochure's emphasis)* of as many patients as possible to their families and their communities" (p. 3). The last page reemphasized the changed mission and criticized the past with the slogan: "Training and Integration NOT *(brochure's emphasis)* Segregation and Detention" (p. 8).

Bowman acknowledged that there would always be some people for whom there was no feasible treatment and who would remain institutionalized for life. In the pamphlet he assured the public that staff would continue to offer the understanding required "to make at least a partially hopeful life for the patients," either within the institution for those who "will never return to society" and for those who may return to "their own homes, or placed in boarding or nursing homes, or with relatives" (*Pineland Hospital and Training Center,* n.d., p. 3).

At the same time Pineland officials were emphasizing a new community vision and discharge policy, they were admitting an entirely new population of residents: children identified as emotionally disturbed. This was a population whom officials previously rejected for their facility, insisting they required a separate, specialized mental health facility. Thus, as Bowman began promoting the discharge of some residents, he was expanding admissions for others who would offer him access to a new disability population that was more closely aligned with the expanding medical specialty of child psychiatry and consisting of a group not yet identified with custodialism.

Bowman also criticized the "excessive use of resident labor" ("Bowman Takes Over,"1953, p. 1A), which he attributed to unusually high staff shortages and attrition. He contended that a lack of ward attendants caused residents to work "15 hours per day to care for those who can't care for themselves" (p. 1A). Defending some unpaid, resident labor by arguing that the "job has to be done" and "they [residents] are willing and eager to help," Bowman also implied that they were being exploited since "they should be out, and could be out" if there were social service workers to assure their care and civilian employees to replace them (p. 1A). Sixteen years later, Bowman would escalate his rhetoric, referring to unpaid resident labor as "indentured servitude" (Hoffman, 1969a, p. vii).

Criticizing the use of unpaid resident labor was a bold move. The practice had become a well-entrenched policy that state and institutional officials had long considered an integral, desirable element of facility operations. Unfortunately, Bowman failed to heed his own criticism, continuing to rely on unpaid resident labor throughout his tenure, presumably because the state would not increase staff funding and the facility was heavily dependent on resident workers.

ORGANIZED PARENTAL ACTIVISM AND INFLUENCE

When Bowman began as superintendent, the Maine chapter of NARC—the Maine Association of Retarded Children (MARC)—was the state's only organized parent group for children with intellectual disabilities and consisted mostly of parents who did not send their children to Pownal. Soon after Bowman began, parents of Pownal residents, "aroused at reports of economy-caused evils" at the institution, took the first steps to form a state-wide parents' association in order to "blast the legislature" and support more adequate funding for Pineland and other state institutions ("First Steps Taken to Form Parents Club," 1953, p. A1). The smaller group eventually broke away from MARC, naming itself Pownal Parents and Friends (PP&F) and continued for decades as the institution's most visible and vocal supporter during its most turbulent years. According to Hood (1968) in April, 1954, only 6 months after it began, PP&F consisted of 85 members and elected its first president, Edward Berman, a Portland attorney (p. 28). By June, the group had added over 300 people from the Lewiston-Auburn area alone (Hood, 1968, p. 28), quickly becoming a political force to be reckoned with for the next 40 years.

The formation of an institutional advocacy movement by parent groups was not unique to Maine. Similar chapters formed across the country as the move away from institutionalization developed salience among parents. As in other states, the PP&F became a highly focused organization and Pineland's most ardent defender, even as the institution was bombarded with public revelations of abuse and neglect. PP&F parents often described themselves as young and naive when they had to make what they characterized as the most difficult decision of their lives. Frequently urged to institutionalize their child by their family doctors, community professionals, even family and friends, they recalled feeling alone, having few community resources or other service options available to them. Most often parents, especially mothers, also talked about experiencing the pressure of being the primary care givers and family decision makers for their children, feeling overwhelmed and unprepared for their role, expressing fears about disrupting other family members, and wanting to offer their children the therapy and educational services that they were told only the institution could provide. One mother described feeling alone, under pressure, and without any alternatives:

> When [son] was about 3½ we had an evaluation.... [T]he doctor there said that yes, he thought that the child did have some brain damage and he recommended perhaps that he would need to be in an institution. See, in those times, there was nothing in the community for people with problems like that, absolutely nothing.... At the time Pineland had a very good speech program and school. They offered a lot in the way of education and training, and he was educable at that time.
>
> My husband was away, and I just took the recommendation of [the doctor]. I felt that I really didn't have a choice at the time, because [son] was very, very active and, it was beginning to affect [our other children] in that they were quite stressed from his hyperactivity.... He had terrible seizures. Almost every time I would have to call a policeman who would take him to the hospital ... and very often he would be there overnight.... [My husband] did not want me to [admit him to Pineland] at all. I mean if I had said no, I don't know what life would have been like. (Dube, personal communication, April 23, 1999)

One couple referred to the cycles of fear and hope they experienced and shared with other parents in similar circumstances. They also described what they considered their inadequacies and eventually their deep disappointment at having to admit their son to Pownal:

> We belonged [to PP&F] for years ... [and] knew how hard it was to raise a son or daughter and have to fight for everything.... No one was trained to be a parent. For several years we were thinking about getting [son] out into the community.... We were filled with a great new hope that a focus on [son's] strong points rather than his deficiencies could lead to a more fulfilling life, but also fearful of how he could handle the new freedom, and what he might encounter in a normal community.... I believe that all parents felt these two urges—the fears and the hopes-in continual and severe tension, and both fueled strong emotions.... That was one of the parents' biggest fears. I think that parents who had the greatest objections to putting people in the community were those who had children with the severest problems. They just felt very protective.
>
> One time it took [husband] and his brother to control [son].... When [he] was 20, he had a terrible tantrum and [husband] had to wrestle him and I didn't think I could handle him. We had to call the police to help us.

> That's when we had to turn to Pineland. Never will I ever forget the day we committed him. (Biddle, personal communication, November 9, 1998)

One couple wept as they recounted the increasing difficulties they experienced caring for their child, heeding the recommendations of professionals, and recalling the emotional pain on the day the father took him to Pineland:

> After [child] was born, we knew something was wrong, but we didn't know what. But caring for her became very difficult. [Mother] would sometimes have get up at night and hold him because he was trembling so bad. We had another child, so it was a big problem. We ... consulted a doctor ... [and] after the exam, ... told us to put him in an institution and forget about him. We had no intention of forgetting, but we did decide to put him there.
>
> It was terrible thing to have to do. He was about 7 and I dropped him off when I was coming down for some work. We stopped at a restaurant, and when we got up to leave I forgot my hat, and when we got to the car [child] reminded me about my hat. He remembered my hat. When we got there, I brought [child] in and they accepted him. When I left, I heard him crying at the top of his lungs. I just felt terrible. Later that day during work meetings I broke down crying, and I told them (co-workers) why, and they were sympathetic. (Murray, personal communication, September 10, 1998)

Family members bitterly resented being characterized as neglectful parents or accused of abandoning their child because they placed him/her at Pineland. While acknowledging that there were parents who "dumped their kids at Pineland," one father pointed to "many loving parents who have stayed involved and should not be lumped with them" (Moore, personal communication, August, 19, 1998). Parents pointed out how actively involved they remained with their children under difficult circumstances. One parent considered her responsibilities and her relationship with her daughter as similar to that of any parent:

> One of the great myths of parenthood [is] people say you're different. No, I'm not. You know you are insulted everyday ... and the ones with the best intentions are the worst. I heard people say, "Oh, don't worry, ... there are lots of other people who will love [your child] and take care of her as if she was their own." Somebody else will love your child if you don't want to ma'am? Even though I put [daughter] in Pineland, I did not put her up there to just to get her up there. I visited. I brought her home. Our home was Pineland. On weekends [we stayed] in the old motel. It was pretty run down ... but they made it into units and [daughter] could spend the night with us [and] we

> could be a family there.... I just didn't put her there and forget about her. (Choate, personal communication, April 16, 1999)

Joining PP&F, parents reported feeling supported in a world where they often felt isolated, misunderstood, judged, and criticized from all sides. As one parent said, PP&F served as an important social network comprised of people who shared common experiences:

> I wasn't alone, and there were people I could talk to and they knew what I was saying, could hear and understand. Meant I didn't have to keep my guard up. I was told from them that once you have one of these children, its like you go into a different world. You can talk with people [who have typical children] but you're never really one of them again. I hate to say it but it's true. (Choate, personal communication, April 16, 1999)

For years, both MARC and PP&F supported a strong and viable institution. As time went on, however, PP&F continued to focus on expanded funding for Pineland while MARC, like other NARC chapters across the country, became increasingly disillusioned that an expanding and expensive state institution was operating at the expense of more desirable home-based and community options. Although continuing to fight for higher standards of institutional care, NARC called for more home-like residences, increased community programs, and a reduction in institutional construction (Lakin & Brunicks, 1985b, pp. 6–7). Presenting a united parental front for years, MARC became increasingly critical of Pineland by the late 1960s and the differences between MARC and PP&F grew more contentious.

Although Bowman enjoyed the support of Maine's parent associations through much of his tenure, gradually his relationship with both groups soured. MARC desired a less centralized, less institutional mental retardation system and grew increasingly impatient with conditions in and outside of Pineland. PP&F was also upset with the facility's deteriorating physical plant but was equally upset with Bowman's increasingly aggressive discharge practices that they believed would place their children at risk and eventually lead to the facility's closing. Pineland officials reacted to the changing, more activist, role of families with mixed emotions. On the one hand, parent groups wielded considerable power, eliciting legislative and media attention, and serving as indispensable allies in securing more funding. On the other, they could be sharp and visible critics, gaining widespread public attention and intruding on institutional authorities accustomed to operating independently and obscurely. Active parental involvement also signaled the beginning of the end of the "strong superintendent" who could dominate the media as the statewide expert, develop unchallenged treatment policies and practices, and rule the institution as his personal fiefdom.

THE 1960s: FROM PROMISE TO PURGATORY

While growing tensions persisted between parent groups and state officials, the decade of the 1960s began with great accomplishment, recognition and promise for Pineland. Hood (1968) described the prospects of this period:

> Despite the personnel problems due to low wages and difficult working conditions, Pineland was seeing some of its best days in the early 1960s. Dr Bowman ... had achieved an international reputation. The number of employees had nearly doubled since 1953, while the patient population reversed its upward trend and began to decrease in numbers.
>
> Many new buildings were constructed, and many new services started. The legislature and governors did provide money, however grudgingly, and Pineland had finally achieved accreditation.... Several visitors from Nebraska, California, and Australia had praised Pineland's facilities and treatment programs. (p. 46)

As reflected in Table 7.1, between 1953 and 1971, enrollments within Pineland underwent a dramatic reversal as the census dropped from 1,368 to 753, a decrease of 45%. This reduction would have been even more remarkable if institutional authorities had not initiated a new, 70-person children's psychiatric hospital in 1961 which offset some of the declining numbers. The decrease was surprisingly sudden and implemented under a superintendent who once called for nearly doubling Pownal's enrollment to 2,500. Clearly, something had changed. One long time employee credits Bowman for Pineland's dramatic turnaround:

> I had tremendous admiration for Dr. Bowman. Maine owes him a tremendous debt.... He believed people belonged in the community before it was popular.... Bowman's position was that you had to get people out into the community or the community will never accept them if they never see them. When Dr. Bowman left, enrollment was down to 800. Later superintendents took great credit for this lowered number, but it was Dr. Bowman who really did it. (Rogers, personal communication, September, 24, 1998).

In 1961 the census at Pineland was 1,400 with an additional 250 people in community living. Bowman, unabashedly, took credit for Pineland's reforms, declaring in 1969 what he proudly hoped would be his legacy:

Table 7.1. Pineland Enrollments for Years 1953–71

Year	*MR Pop*	*Children's Psychiatric*	*Totalt (1)+(2)*	*Other (Absent)*	*Total Enrollmnts*
(1)	*(2)*	*(3)*	*(4)*	*(5)*	*(6)*
1953	1,368	N/A	1,368	110	1,478
1955	1,445	N/A	1,445	121	1,548
1957	1,403	N/A	1,403	232	1,635
1960	1,316	N/A	1,316	268	1,584
1961	1,241	Not listed	1,241	252	1,493
1962	1,167	Not listed	1,167	293	1,460
1963	1,100	39	1,139	282	1,421
1965	1,100	51	1,119	369	1,465*
1967	900	50	950	471	1,421
1968	832	56	888	524	1,412
1970	737	57	794	660	1,454
1971	698	55	753	686	1,439

Enrollment figures did not always agree between or within annual reports. The above figures are taken from the superintendent's summary, and medical records sections. When sources disagreed by more than ten, the mean was calculated, indicated by (*).

When I was appointed superintendent of Pineland Hospital and Training Center, I was rudely introduced to an institution that was in many ways a typical exhibition case of the worst practices prevailing in the days of the older philosophies of custodial "care" for the "feeble-minded."

Patients were forced to work up to 16 hours per day, 7 days per week, without any form of remuneration. They in fact, occupied places of responsibility as assistant attendants, washmen, food service workers, cleaning women. Their employment was one of involuntary servitude in fact. They drank unpasteurized milk.... Raw sewage of the institution ran down hill in an open ditch. One unlicensed physician attempted to take care of 1,450 patients.... Inmates voiced their conviction that there was no way out of this place except in a pine box.

The institution was sexually segregated in every conceivable activity from attending school to social dances, and the patients were treated in an atmosphere that one would expect to find in a poorly run correctional institution.

In general, Pineland Hospital and Training Center in the mid 1950s underwent a complete change of direction by assembling a diversity of highly skilled and specialized professions and disciplines, all with definite relevance to the amelioration, cure, or improvement of a variety of problems presented by people with retardation syndromes.... Hundreds of patients who previously had been condemned without real reason to a lifetime of custodial

> confinement and deprivation here, based on work training experience, were discharged to useful and rewarding lives of self-support and various degrees of independence.
>
> The combined programs have resulted in a decrease of population at this hospital by some 48% over the past 15 years. (as cited in Hoffman, 1969a, pp. vii-viii)

Bowman indeed inherited an overcrowded, understaffed, and underfunded institution when he became superintendent in 1953 and he complained frequently and vocally throughout his tenure to state lawmakers and administrators about a lack of adequate support and resources. It was not until the deplorable conditions within Pineland were starkly revealed through dramatic newspaper photographs that ordinary citizens saw vividly what conditions were really like inside. To his credit, the superintendent also began large-scale discharges before most other institutional directors across the country. Pineland's enrollments peaked in 1958, nine years before institutional enrollments across the country.

Bowman's laudable actions stemmed neither from a consistently progressive philosophy, nor from the thoroughly innovative practices that he and his staff claimed. Although Bowman improved Pineland in numerous ways, he was inconsistent and selective with an eye toward enhancing his professional authority, image and circumstances. Discharging large numbers before it was popular, Bowman paid little attention to where people were placed following their release. Criticizing the use of resident labor as "indentured servitude," he continued the practice, retaining many of the best workers whom he needed to perform many tasks, some of which were Pineland's most unpleasant jobs. Characterizing the increasing numbers of residents with more severe impairments as largely helpless and hopeless, Bowman did little to improve their living conditions despite having in-house evidence that much could be accomplished with this group. Like many other superintendents, he worried that their growing numbers gave Pineland a custodial image and emphasis, which was a professionally unappealing prospect, inconsistent with a medical-research focus, and unlikely to reflect well on him or attract additional funding.

DRAMATIC PUBLIC EXPOSÉ OF CONDITIONS WITHIN PINELAND

The living conditions within Pineland were publically revealed in 1969 when *Maine Times* reporter, Hannah Kamber wrote a series of damaging articles, accompanied by explicit photographs, in which she described some units in the strongest terms, such as "snake pit" (Kamber, 1969a,

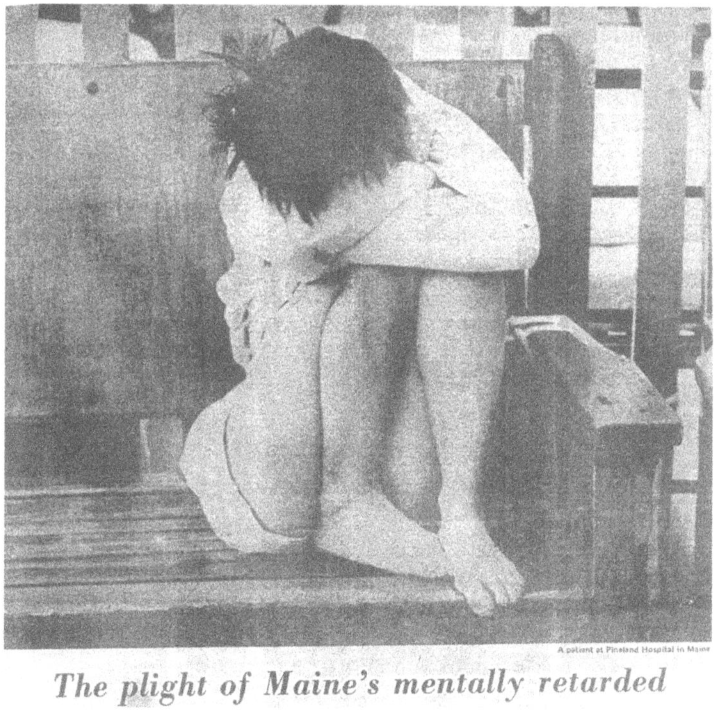

Figure 7.1. Kamber, H. (1969a, January 31). Inside Maine's snakepit. *Maine Times, 2.* Hannah Kamber, photographer.

p. 2) and "the land of the living dead" (Kamber, 1969b, p. 8). After visiting Kupellian Hall, Kamber referred to it as a place that could "shatter the nerves and wrench the stomach" and where "profoundly retarded children and adults are being kept alive under conditions that make the term " 'custodial care' a euphemism" (1969a, p. 2). Describing the overall scene, Kamber wrote:

> Anyone in doubt of the "snake pit" definition should tour Kupelian Hall. Yet anyone so inclined should also be prepared for pools of urine in the day halls and bathrooms, walls and ceilings stained by feces, and at least an occasional pile on the bathroom floor, for the odor of this human excrement mixed with that of the disinfectants, sprays, used to fight the filth and some further pollution hard to isolate.
>
> One should be prepared for the moaning, wailing, howling, bellowing roaring of the anguished; for the sight of children sick with flu, tied to their

> beds with rags both day and night; for the old women tied to their potty chairs.
>
> One must be prepared for the sores, the scabs where untied patients have brutalized themselves by constant head banging; for the scars, the tapes, the lesions where patients have torn, dug or bitten chunks of their own flesh, or have attacked each other.
>
> One must come prepared for the day hall, absolutely barren- except for the wooden benches and chairs which line the walls, here up to 60 patients spend all their days, sitting, sprawled or tied (sometimes hand and foot), with nothing to do, to feel, to see, to hear except each other, a TV which they ignore and on a really good day as many as four psychiatric aides.
>
> One must be prepared for the heaps of soiled clothing; for the nudity; for the sight of the drugged or withdrawn hunched on the floor; for the hands of the curious; for the gestures of the aggressive; for a spectrum of human misery that finally defied words. (p. 2)

A former secretary in the superintendent's office reported being shocked and angered when she saw photos of the conditions that existed so close to her office:

> I saw those pictures and I couldn't believe that in this day and age, two and a half miles from where I live and a heartbeat from where I work, that kind stuff was going on.... People were just not going to tolerate that stuff. (Holden, personal communication, October 23, 1997)

Employees who worked on the units verified Kamber's descriptions. One Pineland staff member described the nudity, overcrowding and human abuse he observed:

> A lot people in the '60s were not even clothed. You could walk into Yarmouth Hall which was for middle aged women and half the women wouldn't have any clothes so it was really kind of barbaric in that sense.... See when I first came, ... there were 2,000 residents here.... The beds were just stacked barracks style, people all slept in the same room; had open bathrooms and showers; it was pretty crude.... Residents would go out into these fenced areas and sit all day long and rock; it was like a playground in a school except these were adults.
>
> At Pineland you were essentially warehoused.... In some wards people were tied into camisoles and they would sit there and rock all day long; ... sometimes with no clothes on (Herbert, personal communication, April 23, 1999).

A former social worker and PP&F member recalled "horrible overcrowding" and "miserable conditions," describing Bliss and Kupelian [dorms] as "the worst" where staff-client ratios were 28–1 [and] they had tile floors with a drain in the middle and they would hose down residents when they soiled themselves" (Rogers, personal communication, September 24, 1998).

Working on a federal grant, Kevin Baack visited Pineland in 1968 and later became director of the Bureau of Mental Retardation. Recalling his first impressions of Pineland, Baack suggested that it was worse than other institutions he had known:

> I had been involved with [other] institutions, and in many ways Pineland was like that, but in some ways it was very different. I recall the use of pig wire and chicken wire that was used extensively as fencing-within the institution like an outdoor day room. Partially clothed people wandering around inside with some supervision but not much. They would wander around outside and then be herded back in. Now this wasn't in all the buildings, but enough to make an indelible impression on my memory 30 years later. (Baack, personal communications, September 5, 1997)

Ron Welch held several positions in the state's mental health and retardation system, eventually serving as acting commissioner. He related his impressions and experiences after he joined Pineland as a student intern in 1968:

> my first day on the job I could barely breathe because of the stench on the ward. The room was divided in half with chicken wire, on one side was 20-30 cots crammed together, with vinyl mattress and some ... blankets.... The forward part of the day hall was where people virtually lived their lives. Feces were smeared on the walls. It blew me away it was such an assault on the senses. We all had the same reaction: how could people live here? .... Many of the residents were naked. Some wore these stiff, brittle, and hot nylon clothing-same color. Very cold in the winter. We tried on the clothes, and saw how unbearable they were.
>
> People ate pureed food from a big bucket that was wheeled into the ward. People just reached into the bucket with their hands and ate what they could grab. Some got food and others didn't. Pureed food was used because a lot of people were missing their teeth. Dental problems were solved by pulling teeth without any anesthesia. (Welch, personal communication, August 31, 1998)

Parents who visited Pineland during Bowman's tenure were nearly unanimous in declaring the facility overcrowded, although as one PP&F member observed, "most "parents were terrified because it had taken them so long to get their children into Pineland and it [admission] had been so difficult. They also thought the community was not ready for their kids and they would be abused out there" (Rogers, personal communication, September 24, 1998).

Most parents believed that the staff was caring but harried, although several observed blatant abuse, some directed toward their own children. One mother recognized early that Pineland's overcrowding and understaffing led to abuse and neglect, and while praising most staff as excellent, she remained involved and vigilant:

> Let's face it, over the years the ... place [Pineland] went down hill.... [I]t was neglected.... Back then they called it custodial care.... [Daughter] was the type of child that needed 24 hour care. It is very hard for a parent to accept, when your daughter gets hurt, and the evidence is there. And supposedly she is being taken care of by staff people, ... and no one can explain how she got hurt.... I know she has some scars. There were suspicions; there was room for improvement up there.... Overall they had some super people that worked there.... There were several buildings on the grounds ... which I didn't like. Some ... staff had a lot of residents to get to, and ... I think that was why I became so involved, because you know how they say, that if the parent doesn't come around they must be satisfied.... I think what I saw was the morale was worn down. (Saylor, personal communication, April 12, 1999)

Another parent recalled the noise and overcrowding she observed:

> When we took [son] to Pineland, ... in the early 1960s it was very full with around 1,600 people of all ages. He was taken to the hospital building and [then] moved into Cumberland Hall which was full of larger, older, and rougher clients. The noise in that building was deafening. Being in a ward with so many others must have been bewildering. The aides were kind to him, I am sure, but they had a lot of care-taking to do for so many. Television watching was at that time the main activity, along with being out of doors in a large caged area. (Rusch, personal communication, December 12, 1999)

One woman described several incidents that deeply upset her and her husband, making them question the decision to admit their son:

> When [son] went to Pineland in [mid 1960s], they took me to show me where he was going to be ... and I was devastated.... It was one huge room partitioned off with chicken wire between the day room and the bed ward. When I looked back I don't know how I did leave him there in those conditions ... I mean, it was clean and most of the people were nice, but they had some people that were, maybe a little abusive. We had some incidents where we actually witnessed that, and I mean, I'm not sure what was going on when we weren't there.
>
> My husband and I were leaving one day and we heard ... [child] cry out and so my husband went to investigate and [attendant] was trying to change his clothes or something and [son] had finger marks on his face from where

he was hit.... He was only at that point in time about 5 or 6 years old. Another one of the residents could not have done that, and he was in the building with just the attendants. So we reported it ... and it was investigated, but you know how that goes.

In [early 1970s], I got a letter, not a phone call, a letter saying [son] had a rather severe seizure and that he was in [hospital].... So I went up and found [him] to be totally out of touch, lying in a bed, not even able to make eye contact or focus and I was just horrified.... Well, it was like the old [son] was gone and here we have this child who is very brain damaged and not able to do anything. He couldn't sit up, couldn't walk; couldn't do anything. He used to run, ride a bike.... So that was very devastating to us, so I tried to get information from people in the buildings and little by little I learned that what they surmised happened was that [he] had a severe seizure during the night, and apparently nobody had done the bed checks as they are supposed to do every hour, or whatever it was at that time. [Son] apparently fell out of bed ... and when they found him in the morning, about 5 o'clock he was under the bed and he was still convulsing, had a temperature of 107.... So, Looking back, we never made a big to do about it, and I regret in a way that I didn't. I don't know. The way he was at that point, and I guess we just kind of put all our energy into [moving on]. It was very, very difficult. (Dube, personal communication, April 23, 1999)

Several parents observed conditions that caused them to reverse their decision to admit their child. When deciding whether to admit her son, one parent described how observing a young child's neglect formed a lasting, negative image of Pineland:

In 1970, he was around 5, and I went to Pineland and it was disheartening. I walked into this big room where I expected to find a lot of children playing, but found a small child tied to a radiator, sleeping. When a nurse came by, I asked what was wrong, and she said that he was hyperactive. That was the dismal picture of Pineland I always carried. So it was always something lurking in the background as something to avoid. (Biddle, personal communication, November 9, 1998)

Another parent brought her son to Pineland because she thought he would receive special therapies that only Pineland could offer. After observing how the facility operated, however, she became disillusioned and brought him home when she discovered that the promised therapy would not be immediately available:

You know it finally dawned on me after awhile that the reason they had you stop at the office first [when visiting] was that they put the others on alert until they got things straightened out down there [in the dormitory]. So this one time I went right through and ... I walked in on `em that day [and] they were giving him pills. And that got the old dander right up.... And I said,

> "What's that for? Oh, just to keep him quiet." And I says, "He don't need any of them." "Well he flaps his hands." "So, he flaps his hands, he has to get rid of energy some where. He don't need drugs for that...." And I told them, "If I catch you doing that again I'm going to haul you into court."
>
> The aid said to me "How long you gonna be leaving him here, anyway?" I said, well he's only here for speech therapy and physical therapy. She says, "Yeah, well nothing's gonna happen for three months. The teachers are on strike." I told them, "Oh, okay, then put his clothes all back in the suitcase. I didn't have him down there for board and room. I can give him that at home..... " I didn't really like him being there, and.... I couldn't have him in an environment where there was no advantage.... I gave it my best shot. I don't think he improved a bit. He was glad to get home. (Cone, personal communication, June 21, 2000)

Not all parents spoke so negatively about Pineland's conditions and practices. A father acknowledged the overcrowding, noting that "they had around 1,700 people there, and the word warehousing was used to describe it, but ... that was limited to certain buildings" and that, otherwise, Pineland was an "excellent" facility (Moore, personal communication, August 19, 1998).

Having seen worse conditions elsewhere, one mother was impressed with some of Pineland's features and was especially pleased with its staff:

> It was clearly not utopia ... [but] Pineland wasn't as bad as it appeared to be. Better than most states.... Pineland looked like all the other institutions I visited ... [but] you got inside and the people were so different. In [another state] people weren't really making eye contact. They were calling them by diagnosis: "You don't bother with that one-hydrocephalic. This one over here's microcephalic.".... People [at Pineland] would scooch down to eye level for [daughter] and the first thing I noticed going back to visit her after lunch, her head ... was up in the air. She was very proud. And people were calling, "Hi," and she would smile in every direction.
>
> Inside it was certainly not nice and beautiful to look at, but the thing that really impressed me was that there was a play area in the front with a TV and some toys ... and the bathrooms were accessible.... And there was specialization.... You've got to realize I'd been hardened to the back dorms [in other facilities] where no parent knew what went on, where kids were naked and dripping water. (Choate, personal communication, April 16, 1999)

Bowman explained that the negligent conditions in Kupelian Hall were due to "the lack of funds to hire and keep qualified staff ... [and] to pay competitive salaries" (Kamber, 1969b, p. 3). Officials also pointed to the increasing numbers of residents with severe impairments as particularly problematic. Bowman described this group as human and medical failures, arguing that working with such residents demoralized staff, contributed to high employee attrition, and created the overcrowding and under-staffing that caused the deplorable conditions:

> In many buildings attendants have to handle soiling patients who are incontinent as to urine and feces. They have to handle soiled clothing, soiled linen, etc. They have to stand the smell associated with human excrement for the length of a working day. Many attendants have to handle children and adults with no power of mind. Many of these patients have to be fed. All have to be bathed constantly, and many are badly crippled and need to be carried around. In other sections, attendants have to deal with disturbed children and adults of higher intelligence. Their behavior might be erratic, unpredictable, sometimes threatening, and occasionally assaultive. These patients were brought here because their own parents, relatives, and social agencies were unable to handle them. (Bowman, 1956, p. 8)

Following the *Maine Times* articles, Bowman again emphasized "the growing numbers of the totally dependent retarded [who] lack any animal instincts for survival ... [and] in an earlier time many of [whom] would have died for lack of medical knowledge and treatment. According to Bowman, "they would starve to death in a grocery store" (Kamber, 1969b, p. 3)

The superintendent was not alone in blaming some residents for the surrounding conditions. His views were echoed, even trumped, by his superiors within the state. Responding to the media, Dr. William Schumacher, Director of Maine's Bureau of Mental Health explained that the state's priorities were not intended to be evenly distributed and that Pineland officials rightfully assessed human worth based on measured intelligence and apportioned the state's resources accordingly:

> Would you, be willing to double your taxes to clean this up? .... You expend Expend your maximum effort where the payoff is greatest. You can take care of the best first, then the middle group, then, if you have time or money or energy left you take care of the rest because the results are the poorest here in view of the expenditure of time and effort.... [Is it] worthwhile to teach someone to say five words when that same amount of effort could have raised the vocabulary of someone with a higher IQ from 500 to several thousand words? And what about the back wards of the other state hospitals? People in these wards ... being mentally ill rather than retarded, are potential wage earning, tax paying citizens, a better financial investment. (Kamber, 1969a, p. 8)

Although decades beyond social Darwinism and eugenic alarms, state officials' remarks sound eerily reminiscent. By asking if meaningful reforms were possible or desirable for certain residents and if there would be any tangible returns on improving their treatment, state authorities concluded there were virtually none. Changing the argument from one of moral culpability and social responsibility to that of economic pragmatism, officials constructed and promoted certain residents as impaired beyond hope. What seemed to be a moment of heightened public consciousness and social reform was muted by the state's characterization of some residents as so physically and cognitively helpless that they shared culpability for their own squalid circumstances. This argument would continue in numerous forms for decades. As public disenchantment with the institution grew and the facility was improved and grew smaller as more seriously impaired residents were discharged to community placements, officials continued to insist that there would always be people too impaired to live anywhere else.

As she reported on the conditions within Pineland, Kamber (1969b) discovered that not everyone within the facility considered residents with severe and profound impairments so hopeless. She (1969b, p. 8) pointed to the "one decent ward" for persons with multiple disabilities within a larger dormitory that was otherwise a "virtual pigpen." Kamber described the unit as having "immaculate bedrooms and beautifully equipped classrooms where "patients are cared for as human beings, ... a difference that "cannot be explained only in terms of higher or lower patient IQ, or by bricks and mortar renovation, or even by total funds and skill invested" (p. 8). The program she referred to was directed by Albert (Andy) Anderson, a psychologist, who, perhaps before anyone else in Maine, envisioned a world without Pineland.

THE EMERGENCE AND SIGNIFICANCE OF ALBERT ANDERSON

On the surface, Anderson's federally funded project focused on teaching self-care skills, such as dressing, eating, and toilet use to individuals with severe and multiple impairments. But as Kamber (1969b, pp. 2–3) described it, the project also signaled important changes to come:

> Prior to his {Anderson's] experimental project, conditions in [the project ward] were the same as they are today in the other three. Ninety percent of the 26 girls ages 8-22 were not toilet trained.... Sixty percent could not feed themselves. Up to twelve had to be tied ... to prevent them from harming themselves or others. They indulged in all types of psychiatric aggression .

> ... head-banging, biting, digging and hitting; and many would not touch a toy if it were placed in front of them.
>
> Yet Anderson, working with ... $17,000, ... ten college students, and three psychiatric aides, ... set out to prove that the untrainable could not only be trained in a group situation, but when given the opportunity to gain a measure of self-sufficiency, and could be made far, far happier.
>
> The summer staff left in September but there has been little regression to the state described above.... Soils and wets are under 10 a day; 30 percent of the non-feeders were taught to feed themselves in the first week alone; all can engage in strenuous recreation.... Some can play, even without supervision; three have begun to talk even without speech therapy; and the wailing is gone-just the sound of music in the background on the day I visited.
>
> And the current aides ... bought and decorated the Christmas tree ... with their own money, and painted the Christmas pictures on the walls. There was a Christmas party in the ward this year.... Perhaps more remarkable was the fact that 15 parents showed up for the party, about ten of whom had not seen their children in years. They came, they explained, because Anderson had written them a personal invitation, something that had never happened before.

In fact, nowhere was the conflict over change both within and outside of Pineland more dramatically illustrated than around the figure of Albert Anderson. As reflected in Kamber's article and in the reports of several staff members, Anderson's program stood in stark contrast to the medical- custodial approach that prevailed on Pineland's backwards where the line between treatment and abuse could be become blurred. After he began working at Pineland, Welch noticed that:

> Some [residents] got a reputation for acting out. They were put in straight jackets so often and for so long that their hands had atrophied away. Then when you checked their records to find out why they were restrained you couldn't even find a reason why they were restrained in the first place. (Welch, personal communication, August 31, 1998)

Welch, who served as an aid on Anderson's project, described Anderson's program as reflecting a new and controversial treatment philosophy imported from Scandinavia called "The Principle of Normalization" (Nirje, 1969; Wolfensber, 1972) in which the goal was to provide services that approximated, as closely as possible, the conditions, activities, and opportunities available to people in everyday society:

> [Anderson] gave staff a new way to think and act.... We started toilet training and rewarding [residents] with marshmallows. At the end of the summer, the training started to show some success. So we ... went on to the ADL [activities of daily living] skills" We also did some other

> humanizing things like getting them new clothes; we put together an outdoor place with a roof and.... People, for all practical purposes, never left the ward. We arranged for van trips to local recreational areas.... It didn't take long to know the nuances of their [residents'] personalities that came through and you began to understand what people were like and what they were saying and why they were doing what they were doing.... Andy's reforms laid the groundwork for the reforms that followed. (Welch, personal communication, August 31, 1998)

Margaret Bruns, Pineland's director of nursing in-service training and later superintendent, admitted that prior to Anderson's arrival at Pineland, "it never occurred to me that you can do anything with the severely and profoundly retarded" (Langley, 1973, p. 3).

Bruns was not alone. Anderson's unit, if only in its intent to actively engage a group of residents largely written off, illustrated that those considered severely and profoundly impaired could be defined very differently, more positively and optimistically, than was reflected in the existing medical/custodial approach that dominated Pineland's back wards. Contradicting Bowman's claims, Kamber (1969b, p. 3) concluded that the distinctions she observed between Anderson's unit and others had little or nothing to do with the attributes of the residents or the amount of funding involved, but with staff attitudes and treatment of those in their care. In contrast to the rest of Pineland, Anderson apparently experienced little trouble in finding and retaining eager and motivated staff or in securing the participation of families in back ward unit events.

Anderson was receiving very positive publicity about his program, but it was at the expense of many long time employees who intensely disliked him. Some staff considered him unorthodox and disloyal, resented his younger aids whom they considered troublemakers, and dismissed his program as a failure. Against the volatile and divisive backdrop of the 1960s with civil rights battles and Vietnam War protests often pitting younger activists with older authorities, long-time Pineland employees saw Anderson and his staff as unconventional and arrogant:

> Maybe the stupidest thing Bowman did was to hire Andy Anderson ... [who] came in here right after getting his degree with all these new ideas. He was what people referred to as a "rat psychologist." He got a grant to teach the profoundly retarded residents in Kupelian Hall to toilet themselves. This was referred to as the "marshmallow project" because every time someone used the toilet properly they were given a marshmallow. The project was a failure. Anyone who knew anything about mental retardation would know it would fail. I worked over there at the time and the grant was never continued, and people who worked there knew it failed. Then Andy went to Pownal Hall

> and completely renovated the building into a large more home-like group home. And he hired his own people to work on it. He was going to have a better staff-client ratio than the rest of Pineland. The project was also a staff training project. He hired a lot of hippies, is all I can call them. They were seen as undisciplined in comparison with the rest of the staff. They dressed informally and made other staff uncomfortable, and they were jealous of what they could get away with. I'm sure Dr. Bowman did not approve of what he saw. (Rogers, personal communication, September, 24, 1998)

Ron Welch also recalled the sharp distinctions between Anderson's and Bowman's styles and the conflicts that ensued:

> One small example was the end of the dress code. Under Bowman all the women staff wore white dresses, and the men wore white shirts, bow ties and black pants. Andy changed all that, and made the dress of the staff more like the residents, so that broke down one barrier, and that was coupled with a lot of training that started to make a difference. "Active treatment" was the name of the game ... not just warehousing people.
>
> During this time the administration was not supportive and even tried to hinder our efforts. We were told for example that we asked for the van too much.... We were seen as idealists, and I guess we were. (Welch, personal communication, August 31, 1998)

Bowmen's defenders pointed out accurately that conditions within Pineland differed little from those at other facilities across the country and that he did all he could to bring the facility's conditions and need for additional funding to the attention of state officials and lawmakers. Despite the reality that the terrible conditions within Pineland were replicated within most of this nation's state institutions, it is difficult to ignore Bowman's unwillingness or inability to acknowledge what Anderson was doing and to understand what *Maine Times* reporter, Hannah Kamber, apparently recognized in a few visits.

As time went on, Bowman's accelerated discharge policy began to adversely affect some of Pineland's operations that relied heavily on resident labor. One former social worker remarked that although many of the farm's workers should never have been placed at Pineland, eventually the superintendent began discharging them in such numbers that the on-campus farm had to be closed:

> At that time there were a lot of higher functioning people here; educable people who were put here because they had no family. There was no orphanage in Maine so people were dumped here; adolescents in trouble too—delinquents. There were a lot of people who got there because they got in trouble in the community, had little supervision, little family help, and had no training or help available to them. We had a lovely farm. Many

> of these people worked at the dairy farm that provided all the milk for the institution.... There was this theory that using residents in this way was slave labor, and if they could do this work so well, they should be out doing it on their own jobs. And that was Bowman's thinking.... As the smarter men were placed out, the dairy farm had to be done away with, and so was the other farm. (Rogers, personal communication, September 24 , 1998)

Clearly, Bowman was committed to increasing resident discharges through the 1950s and 60s, enabling many individuals to return to their families and communities and became valued workers and citizens. Unfortunately, others fared no better in the community than in the institution. Kevin Baack, former chief of the Bureau of Mental Retardation, describes some of the problems with the institution's discharge practices of that period:

> Bowman started an outpatient program. About 1,200 were in residence [at Pineland] and 600 were placed out in proprietary boarding homes run by a handful of operators who saw it as a business to make money on. Some were run by former chicken farmers [with] 60–70 people-just like a mini institution.
>
> When social security laws changed ... it was all federal money paid through the Department of Health, Education and Welfare to the state [to discharge residents]. Three employees, social workers, were responsible to oversee 600 people placed out, and it was an impossible task.... The boarding homes were ... not intended to replace the institution at all. They were intended to be annexes to the institution.... This farmer said to me: "Keeping boarders is like raising chickens. The more you have, the more money you make." That's a direct quote. (Baack, personal communications, September, 5, 1997)

Likewise, a long-time employee and later acting superintendent, pointed out that too many residents were discharged to continuing poverty, servitude, and sub-standard settings:

> Trial visits were for working boys/girls. The boys worked on dairy or poultry farms; the girls worked in private homes as housekeepers or mothers helpers or in nursing homes as kitchen help, or aides. Some people were placed in local resorts. Everyone received the same wage: $15 per week, and room and board.
>
> Prolonged visits [were for] people were deemed not capable of work and were placed in nursing or boarding homes where they received pretty infrequent follow up. Some of these places were fine, and people were treated well, but some were simply awful, the working and living situations were definitely sub-standard. All that changed after the lawsuit and the consent decree which also covered community placement conditions because, technically, people, though living and working in the community,

> were still [officially considered] institutional residents. (Kohler, personal communication, August 19, 1998)

A graphic account of one situation was provided by Sandra Ellis, who in 1965 discovered a former Pineland resident, Vincent Clukey, abandoned and nearly starving in the root cellar of her newly purchased farm house in the town of Monmouth. Ms. Ellis nursed him back to health and, despite having to care for her own young children, allowed Mr. Clukey to remain with the family until 1990 when he became ill, passing away in 1991 ("Vincent Clukey" 1991, p. A8).

Mr Clukey was paroled from Pineland in the mid-1950s to a farm with two other former residents, all of whom lived and worker there until the farm was sold. Mr. Clukey then began working for the farmer's relative who soon went bankrupt and abandoned both the farm and Mr. Clukey. Sandy Ellis bought the abandoned farm and described what followed:

> I know he [Vincent Clukey] was left there when we bought the farm from bankruptcy court in '65. I found him down in the boiler room eating jars of canned stuff evidently he'd taken out of the cellar.... He was filthy, filthy, filthy. I mean his toenails were actually grown in, curved around into the top part of his feet.... Well, he looked like an animal. He was very afraid of my husband at that time ... but between my two kids and I, we convinced him to get in the tub. He was terrified of the tub. I don't know why.... I scrubbed him and scrubbed him. That's when I saw his feet and they were so disgusting. So I had to take him to a podiatrist, cause I wasn't about to tackle that. After I got him cleaned in the tub, we took all his things to the laundry mat. It was disgusting. We threw out the bedding. And I finally got him to a doctor. I tried to call the state and they said they didn't have anything to do with it, that it was my problem as far as looking out for him.... I took him over to CMMC [Central Maine Medical Center] to see about his hearing and they said he was totally deaf.... And he was also blind in his right eye which the doctor said was due to heavy scar tissue from an old injury that had happened to him.
>
> I tried to find his family, cause I found his birth certificate. And I was told by a [court appointed] lawyer ... they [family] didn't want anything to do with him. It was so sad when that woman from California called me to say that the family had looked for him for years. (Ellis, personal communication, April 22, 1999)

Part of Bowman's discharge campaign occurred within the broader context of dramatic national changes in the treatment of institutionalized persons stemming from the heightened use of tranquilizing medications. and later, changes in federal policy toward individuals with mental retardation under Presidents Kennedy and Johnson. As part of the federal reforms under the Johnson administration in the mid-1960s, was a change in Social Security regulations that permitted states across the country to declare institutional residents "totally and permanently disabled," and discharge them "into suitable and more or less sheltered community situations" (Hoffman, 1982, p. 4). Reclassifying Pineland residents in this way would increase discharges, free up space within the institution, and transfer much of the cost of care from the state to the federal government. Unfortunately, what federal officials conceived of as social reform in practice contributed to what a former Pineland superintendent described as callous treatment of vulnerable people:

> The first wave of people who left the institution in the early '60s were those who could work and be put out on trial visit. Then came the people who qualified as PTD [permanently and totally disabled] and could be placed in boarding and nursing homes.
>
> Prior to the early '60s, there was no funding to receive care outside the institution. The first funding to offer this was what was called Aid to the Disabled-the first program offered through Social Security. To receive this you had to be determined to be permanently and totally disabled. We did some very cruel things to people in those days in order to prove that they were PTD and eligible for this assistance. Once they qualified, we could discharge them for prolonged visit. But in order to substantiate their eligibility, we would place them out and they would fail and have to return to Pineland. Then we would place them out again, knowing full well that they would fail again, and they would. Then we could verify that they were PTD. (Kohler, personal communication, August 19, 1998)

The effects of the federal legislation were quite dramatic. Between 1953 and 1965 Pineland's census went from 1,368 to 1,119 a decline of 249 people, or 18.2%. Following passage of the legislation in 1965 until 1971, the census decline was about 366 residents, or 32.7%. Although some of these releases undoubtedly were duplications that inflated the number of releases, clearly facility enrollments were diminishing rapidly.

Releasing institutional residents into the community was certainly not a novel idea. As early as 1913, institutional officials such as Charles Bernstein in upstate New York demonstrated the efficacy of such releases. Fifty years later, anthropologist Robert Edgerton conducted larger follow-up studies in the 1960s of discharged residents, many of whom did well with and without support. In 1969, John Hoffman, Pineland's Director of Research, received a federal grant to study the community adjustment of discharged Pineland residents. Meticulously, Hoffman traced 560 former Pineland residents released between 1952 and 1961 and concluded that following discharge they assumed "useful and rewarding lives of self support and various degrees of independence" (Hoffman, 1969a, p. vii). According to the study's conclusions, 57.2% of the men and 40%

of the women, or an average percentage of nearly 48.6% were found to be either fully self-supporting or the main or equal source of family support (Hoffman, 1969b, p. 68). Hoffman reported no evidence of people living in the impoverished private settings, boarding facilities, work situations, and/or nursing homes described by Baack, Kohler, and Ellis, and reported little evidence for the kind of community support recommended by Edgerton.

The dearth of community services and support offered to discharged Pineland residents continued to plague Maine officials long after Bowman's tenure. In the 1980s, they were accused of "dumping" individuals into communities with minimal support or resources. As late as 2009, the State remained under legal oversight from Pineland's consent decree (finally released in March, 2010), due in part to its inadequate community programs (Sundram, 2000, pp. 99-115).

While Bowman discharged many more residents than his predecessors, he also retained many competent workers as unpaid resident laborers. This was a practice that he publically condemned, as unjustly relegating capable "working boys and girls" to "indentured servitude" when they could be "achieving rewarding community lives of self-support" (Hoffman, 1969a, p. vii). Defending his actions, he argued that he received inadequate funding and experienced great difficulty in finding and retaining enough paid attendants to allow for more resident discharges. Given the changing enrollment and personnel picture at Pineland, however, this explanation does not seem entirely satisfactory. As reflected in Table 7.1, the numbers of people recorded as living at Pineland between 1960 and 1970 declined by almost 40%, a period that also saw its staff size nearly double (Hood, 1968, p. 46). The annual reports for this period showed that the numbers of residents and staff were inversely related from the middle of the decade into the early 1970s. In 1966 there were 550 employees, and 1,031 residents (*Annual Report of the Superintendent, Pownal State School*, 1966). In 1969, 577 staff and 837 residents were counted (*Annual Report of the Superintendent, Pownal State School*, 1969, Statement of Facts), and by 1970 and 1971, the personnel-resident figures had reached 602/737 and 620/699 respectively (*Annual Report of the Superintendent, Pownal State School*, 1971, Statement of Facts).

As more residents were discharged, the reduction in resident enrollments and subsequent staff increases should have allowed officials to replace all resident workers with paid staff, or at least pay residents the prevailing rate for their work. The latter seems even more desirable in light of the attendant staff retention problems that historically existed at Pineland. Apparently, Pineland officials, despite their rhetoric of reform, were unable or unwilling to recognize residents as qualified employees, capable of being paid equally to perform essential and often difficult work. In fact, based on their experience alone, residents could be considered as qualified as anyone to perform many of the institution's jobs.

In 1972 a federal class action suit, *Jorthberg v. U.S. Department of Labor and Augusta State Hospital*, was filed seeking an end to unpaid labor or subminimum wages for institutional residents. The *Jorthberg* decision in favor of the plaintifs barred states from paying institutional residents less than minimum wage for their work. Unfortunately, Pineland officials responded to the ruling by terminating most residents from jobs they had been performing for years. One of those laid off was a young man named Marti Wuori, whose name would soon become integrally linked with a class action lawsuit against Pineland that would change the treatment of persons with intellectual disabilities forever and eventually culminate in the institution's demise.

With media reports suggesting that Pineland's living conditions, low salaries, high staff attrition, and inadequate funding were creating a crisis that may result in its loss of accreditation (Kamber, 1969c, p. 8), Bowman warned that such a loss would lead to a withdrawal of federal funding and the further erosion of staff and services (p. 8). He lashed out at state authorities and politicians in his annual report, revealing the palpable tension and looming legal threat that now surrounded Pineland's operations.

> After conscientious, serious, and sometimes exhausting attempts to bring up the standards of medical care and treatment and general care at Pineland Hospital and Training Center, I have come to the inescapable conclusion that the present system of funding and administrating of the professional and non professional funding does interfere ... with the dispensing of specific treatments and general care, and that this system ... must be re-examined by those in authority for the purpose of making it the servant of the patients rather than their anonymous master.
>
> In other words, irrespective of consequences to patient care and treatment, a law was written that prohibits general [personnel hiring] adjustments if and when needed in order to provide the treatment that our patients are in need of.
>
> At the same time the body who represents those making statutes of the State of Maine deny the person who by statute is the responsible <u>authority</u> to assert, accept, and make this responsibility meaningful.
>
> Whether or not there is a constitutional conflict that perhaps should be presented to a high court is not as important as the fact that patients have been in fact deprived of prescribed therapy and the type of care that is considered essential. (*Annual Report, Pineland Hospital and Training Center*, 1970, Introduction)

Bowman's frustration was rising as fast as his power was waning in the face of increasing competition to control the mental retardation system. In this regard, perhaps the least heralded but most significant event of

1969 was the creation of the state Bureau of Mental Retardation (BMR). A pitifully underfunded department, BMR was conceived by the legislature as a division of the Maine Department of Mental Health and Corrections, was designed to oversee Pineland, and was intended to provide a wider array of services to families and individuals beyond the institution (Kerry, 1972, p. 4). Initially, the new bureau posed no threat to Bowman's authority and power. It's staff was skeletal, consisting of three people who included Albert Anderson as director, Kevin Baack as his assistant and an office secretary. Although it was a rather anemic entity, it represented an important milestone and a symbol of change to come. For one thing, BMR's existence signified the beginning of the end of Pineland as the hub around which all the state's mental retardation services revolved. One former administrator recalls the bureaus's long term impact and how much it reflected the views of its first director:

> The real change in philosophy probably began in the early 70s when BMR was created by state statue and Al Anderson became bureau chief. Anderson had a much more current philosophy than everybody else. He was a follower of Wolf Wolfensberger and other advocates of normalization and deinstitutionalization. Andy was a man before his time. He believed that anyone with MR [mental retardation] could learn and grow.... At worst, an institution was for only a very for a few. Actually, he thought that probably an institution should not be needed for anyone. (Kohler, personal communication, August 19, 1998)

The newly created BMR also illustrated the political arrival of the parent advocacy group, the Maine Association for Retarded Children (MARC) as a powerful political force that according to its executive director, Donald Allison, had become "the primary spokesman for the retarded" (as quoted in Kerry, 1972, p. 4). Most MARC members were caring for their sons and daughters at home and receiving little or no state assistance, following their graduation from special education programs. Unlike PP&F parents, most MARC parents viewed Pineland as a largely unacceptable choice and protested the lack of state financial support for family assistance and community programs that forcing them to consider institutionalizing their children at Pineland or develop their own community programs. According to Allison:

> We have denied the retarded people in Maine the right to be just like us.... The only difference between the retarded individuals and the rest of us is that they need some specialized help to enable them to accomplish their goals. They can do the same things we do; they do things more slowly but

with the same degree of efficiency and often times more effectively. (Kerry, 1972, p. 4)

For MARC, the newly established BMR symbolized their successful campaign to develop an umbrella state organization that would serve as an ally from which to launch both institutional reforms and program alternatives. Allison described MARC's expectation for the new state agency:

> The major purpose of MARC is to improve the welfare of the mentally retarded wherever they may be-at home, in schools, or institutions. Although our views basically coincide with those of the Bureau of Mental Retardation, we ... just do not have the funds or necessary capital to initiate the necessary programs. Someone has to do it. We have been trying to get the State and other organizations to do it.
>
> It has been estimated that 85% of the mentally retarded can function effectively in the community. They can hold jobs, raise families, and pay taxes-be an asset to the community-not a liability.... The thrust of the programs for the mentally retarded is trying to "normalize" each individual within the community and to enhance his full potential as a person.
>
> It's a matter of rights. The mentally retarded are people; they have rights. Their rights are being denied them. (Kerry, 1972, p. 4)

As reflected in Allison's comments, an emerging disability rights movement was transforming disability from a medical impairment to a civil rights issue. Reform was being discussed in terms of legal action rather than voluntary improvements, as class action lawsuits were being drawn up across the country on behalf of institutional residents.

With Anderson's appointment as head of BMR, Bowman's days as superintendent were numbered. Disengaging a well-entrenched official who was appointed virtually for life and determined to retain his authority, however, would not be easy. In contrast to the fledgling bureau and its novice director, Bowman wielded considerable power. As the head of what still comprised the bulk of Maine's mental retardation system, he directed an operation that included 630 employees, a $5.5 million budget, 13 buildings, and 1,400 acres. Baack indicated that Bowman had made a career of running Pineland, and could use the institution's dominance to resist change and erosion of its authority:

> The numbers on waiting list at the time were in the three digits—well over 100. If you had a child or adult you want institutionalized, you take that person to Pineland and have them evaluated and then decide whether they should [be admitted].... That decision [was] done exclusively at Pineland ... without the involvement of any other community organization.... [A]ll the information was at Pineland and they [Pineland administrators] didn't

> want to release that information. They didn't want to tell anyone about demand.... They didn't want to ... change, or ... tell [family] physicians that there might be another way to do this. You really can't fault the physicians. They don't specialize in MR and were told by people they thought were experts that this [institutionalization] was best. (Baack, personal communication, September 5, 1997)

Although controversial and leaving a mixed legacy, Bowman remained popular with a large number of Pineland employees and their powerful unions who welcomed his efforts to increase funding and retain/increase staff. Bowman was also supported by some key PP&F members who saw him as a much better option than Anderson. In fact, after state officials announced that Bowman would not be reappointed, the officers of PP&F made the remarkable offer to purchase and run Pineland as a private entity rather than turn it over to Anderson's BMR. To PP&F members, Anderson was an unremitting ideologue, who had overseen Pineland's physical decline and caused the resident exodus they so ardently opposed.

Despite their critics, Anderson and his superior, Commissioner William Kearns, were persuaded by MARC and the growing threat of litigation to assert BMR's authority. Bowman had to go. Baack defended the decision as the only way to stem growing criticism of Bowman's community placements, obtain the compliance of Pineland staff, and refocus the mental retardation system:

> Three employees ... to oversee 600 people placed out ... could not be done. We held the administration of the institution accountable for that. And that was one of the reasons that the law got changed. We got the Governor and a friendly legislator to sponsor the change, [and] ... make the superintendent more responsive to the Department of Mental Health & Corrections.
>
> Once he was out, supporters of Bowman knew that it was over and they became much more amenable to playing ball so to speak. And there were other people working there that [*sic*] wanted to see some change and this allowed them to have their voices heard better. And so that [Bowman's termination] was the event that turned things in a different direction. (Baack, personal communication, September 5, 1997)

In July of 1971, Bowman's career abruptly ended when Commissioner Kearns announced that the superintendent would not be reappointed due to reforms within the civil service system ("Outspoken Pineland Super Out Of A Job," 1971, p. A1). Some former employees saw the situation differently:

> Bowman was not too popular with some people around the state.... Parents were very upset with him too.... Bowman was a great one for going to the newspapers to get what he wanted from the legislature.... Bowman did not

> get along with his commissioners because of the way he went around them.... Bowman was finally pushed out, because one of the parents he annoyed was Catherine Carswell from Portland who was also an influential legislator. And the legislature was fed up with Bowman's demands. (Rogers, personal communication, September 24, 1998)

Never again would a physician serve as Pineland's superintendent, nor would any superintendent enjoy the power, autonomy, and longevity of Bowman and his four predecessors. Marked by remarkable stability and continuity, the institution was led by just five superintendents—all physicians—in its first 63 years of existence. This was half as many as held that position during the decade of the 1970s alone, attesting to the tumultuous changes and diminished superintendent authority that would ensue. With Bowman's ouster, the state conferred on an outside entity—the newly created Bureau of Mental Retardation—the power to direct Pineland's day-to-day operations. Although initially weak and ineffectual, BMR dramatically illustrated that Pineland had lost control of itself and its future.

CHAPTER 8

FROM MEDICAL TO LEGAL

Class Action, Consent Decrees, and Controversy

Following Bowman's dismissal, Pineland became an "ideological battlefield" (Hoffman, 1982, p. 5), characterized by some as evil and others as essential. One office secretary and a third generation member to work at Pineland, likens the internal conflict to a "civil war, with brother against brother and daughter against mother," and staff divided between those who believed that "Bowman should have stayed forever" and others who wanted change and "wondered why they didn't get rid of him years earlier. So you could feel the tension" (Holden, personal communication, October, 23, 1997).

Predictably, as Baack reported, the atmosphere in Maine grew as tumultuous as it was elsewhere:

> This was a real time of change, not only in Maine, but throughout the country in terms of institutions.... It was a really exciting time, but for the people going through it, it was terrifying.... Physicians were saying: "Put them in institutions" and other people saying, "No".... You had people pulling and pushing, and it was hard to describe. It was chaotic.... You had concerned parents and the unions trying to protect their interests. Also ... boarding

Voices of Pineland: Eugenics, Social Reform, and the Legacy of "Feeblemindedness" in Maine, pp. 179–212

> home operators who were making a lot of money who didn't want change either. (Baack, personal communication, September 5, 1997)

With the establishment of BMR, the state had a centralized entity for obtaining funding and controlling mental retardation services. Given Bowman's dismissal, heightened staff and parent discontent, and continuing media scrutiny, BMR was under pressure to show tangible results at Pineland. The bureau, however, was working in uncharted territory:

> We said that we were going to reduce the size of Pineland; ... how much reduction was unclear. That became clear when the consent decree came in, but at the time we didn't have a clue as to how much money the legislature was going to fork over. We were working off vision here. We were [also] going to upgrade community services. The only people who would go to Pineland would be those who really needed to, and we left the definition of "really needed to" deliberately vague, because we saw that as changing over time, and ... [eventually] zero people would meet that definition. Twenty-five years ago there were no alternatives [to] Pineland. (Baack, personal communication, September 5, 1997)

Switching from an institutional to a community focus proved to be a formidable task due not only to a scarcity of community agencies to serve people with intellectual disabilities, but also to the fear and uncertainty that accompanied such change. As he began to centralize control and de-emphasize Pineland as the sole provider of state mental retardation services, Albert Anderson came under withering criticism from PP&F, unions, and politicians. "Normalization" became an epithet, dismissed by unions as a guise for massive institutional downsizing and staff layoffs, and excoriated by parents as an excuse to discharge more residents, neglect Pineland's physical plant, and turn the facility into a chaotic and permissive place where residents learned to swear, have sex, practice poor hygiene, and misbehave.

Anderson's views were considered radical, his communication style was reportedly blunt, and his new ideas frightened and angered many Pineland supporters. Marcel Morin, a past president of PP&F was quoted as saying that "[Pineland staff] let residents] do their own thing," meaning in his son's case, "not taking baths, not cutting his nails, not brushing his teeth." According to Morin, "permissiveness is the worst thing ever done at Pineland, and it's all Al Anderson's doing" (Langley, 1973, p. 2). Even his admirers acknowledged that Anderson could be loose-lipped. Ron Welch related that Anderson's candor was his undoing as he unnecessarily antagonized politicians, parents, employees, and union officials by making statements like: "People do not need to be here. We should bulldoze Pineland" (Welch, personal communication, August 31, 1998).

Walter Hichens, a state senator from Kittery, took up PP&F's cause, making a series of accusations against BMR, and calling for Anderson's immediate resignation. He proposed legislation that would restrict BMR's activities by placing Pineland under the authority of a board of trustees consisting of mostly parents and by prohibiting further discharges without parental approval.

Among Hichens's most highly publicized charges was that BMR was undertaking a massive evacuation of Pineland and that Anderson's policy of normalization was promoting sexual promiscuity throughout the institution (Austin, 1972, A24; Brunnelle, 1972, p. A20):

> Segregated housing was discontinued and the young men and young women housed in the same buildings.... The patients were not only allowed sexual freedom but encouraged to exercise such freedom.... When they [residents] disappeared into the wooded areas together, state employees were warned not to question their activities nor time of return.... Parents became aware that their daughters were having sexual relations, were being given the pill, and as recently as two months ago, one patient was sent to New York for an abortion at the taxpayers' expense. (Austin, 1972, p. A24)

To students of history, the idea of the sexually charged, "feebleminded" menace was a familiar refrain, easily conjured up, along with accompanying eugenic fears. Under the new banner of institutional "permissiveness," it served to justify continuing segregation. Ironically, it was now state officials arguing against punitive social separation and sexual quarantine and defending themselves against charges of moral permissiveness that they had directed at others for decades. Reporter Brunnelle (1972) related that:

> Hichens ... would like to see Pineland make a special effort to prevent sexual activity of any kind at the Center. How? "They used to get after them and punish them," he says. "Oh, I don't mean real harsh punishment, but enough to discourage them.... " [A]nother legislator offered a prompt, sure

reply when asked what could be done about the mentally retarded youth who has suddenly developed an awareness of sex: "I'd lock him up." (p. 20A)

A SECOND EXPOSÉ OF PINELAND

Pressure on BMR intensified as a second media exposé revealed ongoing abuse and neglect within the facility and reported staff and union disputes that portrayed Pineland as riddled with internal dissension and low morale. In the spring of 1972, a Catholic weekly publication, *Church World,* published a series of articles that replicated the findings of the 1969 *Maine Times* investigation. Describing conditions in a building termed the "infirmary," *Church World* reporter John Kerry (1972) wrote:

> One's first impression of the infirmary is one of cold, dehumanizing sterility.... The floors, walls, and furniture in the foyer are highly buffed, brightly colored and friendly in introduction, but the door of the human cage will not even be closed before one realizes that one has entered a concrete pen.
>
> Unit I contains approximately 36 patients, most of whom are tied with rags to bare, wooden chairs or wheelchairs.... Others, tied to walls and make-shift restrainers, sit or lie in solitude on the bare, concrete floors and writhe uncontrollably-sometimes in their own feces or urine, and sometimes in their food. While still others sit in abject silence staring blankly into space or crouched in a fetal position with heads and hands hidden in a bundle of arms and legs.
>
> Filtering through the stench of excreta, one can hear the seemingly inhuman cries and wailing of certain patients. Shivering solitary laughter from some; whimpering heart-rendering crying from others. Every so often one hears someone calling, "mama, mama." (p. 2)

In the *Church World* article, Dr Saul Niedorf, Director of Psychiatry, and Richard Bogh, Director of Social Services, confirmed that terrible conditions continued to exist within Pineland, blaming the situation on staff, "who are mostly dedicated and conscientious, but oftentimes institutionalized themselves;" and on a lack of resources "promised by the legislature (which they have refused) to secure qualified staff and offer adequate care" (Kerry, 1972, p. 11). Nierdorf concluded by declaring that, "I'm a physician and I believe in the medical model ... I think we should be indicted for malpractice. I will welcome the day when someone sues us for the type of care and treatment our patients are getting here" (p. 11).

Parents, staff, and union representatives expressed outrage at such remarks, countering that Niedorf and other state officials, including Anderson, created an atmosphere of "general confusion and lack of

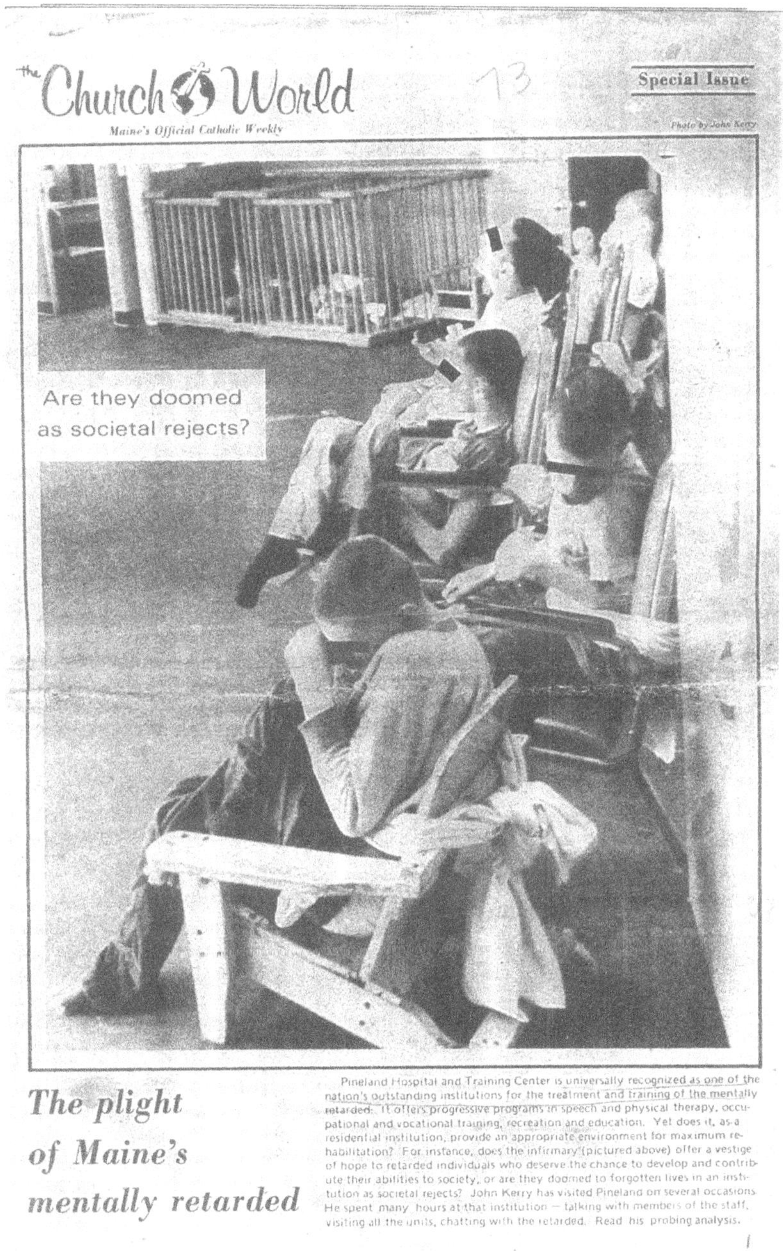

the Church World

Maine's Official Catholic Weekly

Special Issue

Photo by John Kerry

Are they doomed as societal rejects?

The plight of Maine's mentally retarded

Pineland Hospital and Training Center is universally recognized as one of the nation's outstanding institutions for the treatment and training of the mentally retarded. It offers progressive programs in speech and physical therapy, occupational and vocational training, recreation and education. Yet does it, as a residential institution, provide an appropriate environment for maximum rehabilitation? For instance, does the infirmary (pictured above) offer a vestige of hope to retarded individuals who deserve the chance to develop and contribute their abilities to society, or are they doomed to forgotten lives in an institution as societal rejects? John Kerry has visited Pineland on several occasions. He spent many hours at that institution — talking with members of the staff, visiting all the units, chatting with the retarded. Read his probing analysis.

Figure 8.1. Kerry, J. (1972). The plight of Maine's mentally retarded. *The Church World*, Special Issue. Portland, ME: Roman Catholic Diocese of Maine. John Kerry photographer.

communication" resulting in low staff morale and inconsistent treatment of residents (Langley, 1972, p. 28). PP&F and other institutional proponents characterized the news accounts and the new bureau philosophy as clear signs that the state was allowing Pineland to deteriorate as part of a long-range plan to shut it down (Gallant, 1981, pp. 10–11). Anderson's prospects of closing Pineland, or moving even faintly in that direction, were remote. Even *Church World* reporter Kerry believed that Pineland's most serious flaw was not its existence, but its failure to properly function. He pointed out that conditions at Pineland had noticeably improved since 1969 and that the major obstacle to further progress was more state funding. While calling for expanded community services and residences, Kerry saw a continuing need for "a single residential center [that] would provide a highly specialized program of treatment for retarded individuals with multiple or extraordinary disabilities" (Kerry, 1972, p. 16).

For his part, Anderson may have talked about bulldozing Pineland, but his actions reflected a different, more politically expedient direction. In 1971, acting on local pressures and federal funding incentives, BMR opted to build several, small, regional institutions, apparently to eventually replace the larger facility. Thus, at the same time BMR officials were laboring to reduce Pineland's size and influence and develop a series of competing local agencies, they were supporting the construction of new smaller versions of the large institution around the state. Baack explained the inconsistency:

> Part of the diversion was to get folks to look at alternatives to Pineland. One was the 80 bed pediatric unit, that was on the drawing boards—the Levinson Center-which we limited to 40 beds. And the other was a facility up in the County that would serve the educational and vocational needs of people up there. They deflected people away from Pineland. (Baack, personal communication, September 5, 1997)

Paul Tabor, long time employee at DMR-now part of Maine's Department of Health and Human Services—recalled that the Elizabeth Levinson Center in Bangor was approved by the legislature in 1969, at the same time BMR was created. The idea was to begin with 80 people, who would range from 2-year-olds to adults, and potentially expand facility enrollments to 300, "becoming a northern counterpart to Pineland." According to Tabor, Anderson modified the plan to admit only children and limit enrollments to "no more than could be intensively served by the staffing and funding available." Tabor described the original emphases at Levinson as "respite and short-term evaluation and program development, "with maximum admissions set at 36." He noted further that the numbers of residents "may have been briefly higher due to respites," and that "many children ended up staying longer than expected" (Tabor, personal communication, December 21, 2002).

Although it was surprising that Anderson would propose constructing new, mini-versions of Pineland, the bureau was doing what had become common across the country—build more modern, smaller institutions. In the 1960s, the number of public institutions for people with intellectual disabilities nearly doubled from 108 to 190, while their average size dropped from 1,500 residents in 1960 to 1,000 in 1970 (Ingalls, 1978, p. 426). Thus, in spite of its escalating costs, evidence of its harmful human effects, and increasing pressures from the largest parent groups for community alternatives, institutionalization continued as a well—entrenched practice. It enjoyed ongoing federal support and funding, provided jobs and business for local economies, and received vigorous political support from some parent groups and unions.

Following Bowman's termination, there were several interim appointments before BMR officials hired Dr. Conrad Wurtz as Pineland's new superintendent in the fall of 1973. Wurtz was educated as a school psychologist, had been the director of Iowa's Bureau of Mental Retardation Services, and was the first non physician to serve as Pineland's permanent superintendent. To say that Wurtz inherited a difficult situation would be a gross understatement. Not only was he faced with implementing BMR's unpopular, untested ideas and policies in the face of vocal opposition, but he also had to rely on many skeptical, angry and fearful institutional staff to carry out the new plans. One long-time employee described the anxiety and confusion she witnessed following Wurtz's arrival:

> When Wurtz came he changed a lot of things, and it seemed that people were on edge. People just didn't know what was going to happen.... People couldn't settle down. They knew they had things to do but they couldn't decide what they were. At that time they were saying that ... chronic people shouldn't be just housed, but they did that for years, and, you know, when you herd them all in one area you know where they are ... I mean they fed them and kept them clean but there wasn't much training going on.... A lot of people felt that those people were not trainable .... A lot of people were wondering how ... are we going to take care of them? Are we going to keep our jobs?
>
> Can we do what they expect ... and if we can't, are they going to replace us with people who can? (Holden, personal communication, October 23, 1997)

Wurtz's arrival did not pacify PP& F members who were now calling BMR a "tangled dictatorship" but were not sure "whether the dictator is the superintendent or Albert Anderson, or possibly Anderson's immediate supervisor" (Langley, 1973, p. 2).

Living conditions within the facility seemed little improved, staff morale plummeted, parents were fearful of more discharges or even facility closure, and the threat of litigation loomed larger each month. In April 1975, newly elected Governor James Longley replaced Commissioner Kearns with Jack Rosser as head of the Department of Mental Health and Corrections. Three weeks after his appointment Rosser attempted to dispel any rumors about Pineland closing, declaring: "To my knowledge there has never been any plan to close down Pineland" (Thompson, 1975, p. A1). In response to parental concerns, however, Rosser, "flatly refused to declare a moratorium on community discharges" (p. A1), further fueling parental suspicions.

That same year, Albert Anderson became the first major casualty of the de-institutional/reform era. His replacement was assistant, Kevin Baack, who explained Anderson's departure:

> Changes occurred due to politics. Anderson made a lot of enemies especially with the parents of Pineland. He wanted to get rid of the institution, and this went against the interests of the employees, and the parents, who had been led to believe that the only place to get services for their children was at the institution. Many Pineland employees lived in the Lewiston area, more even than in Portland. [Governor] Jim Longley was an insurance man who lived his whole life in Lewiston, had many business friends there, some of whom had children at Pineland. And these people told Longley that this guy Anderson was a loose cannon who was disrupting my family life, and on and on. So Anderson saw the writing on the wall. (Baack, personal communication, September 5, 1997).

Despite his continued state employment, Anderson would no longer be directly involved in determining Pineland's fate. Before and during his brief tenure as BMR director, however, he was a major catalyst in changing Pineland's role within the state's mental retardation system and developing broader possibilities for people once considered capable of only life-long incarceration. Although Anderson did not stop efforts to reinvent Pineland in varied forms, he voiced unpopular, controversial, often incomprehensible, ideas before they became well understood or accepted. Albert Anderson died at 54 in the summer of 1989 before he could witness Pineland's closing,

WUORI V. BRUNS

On July 3, 1975, Neville Woodruff, director of the Legal Services Corporation in Portland, formally changed the argument about Pineland and its residents from a medical—clinical matter to a civil rights case. That day Woodruff filed a class action lawsuit in U.S. District Court in Portland, Maine on behalf of current and previous Pineland residents, some of whom were living in the institution, and others who had been released as outpatients (Levine, 1986, p. 279). The plaintiffs were described as individuals seeking to lead normal lives through the provision of safe, healthful care, education, and training. The suit charged Pineland with offering its occupants only "acute boredom, physical deterioration, social regression, psychological debilitation, severe depression and low morale" (*Wuori v. Bruns*, 1975, p. 1), and argued that despite efforts to change, the institution continued to violate residents' constitutional rights to due process, freedom from cruel and unusual punishment, treatment, and freedom from harm at the hands of the state. According to Levine (1986):

> [Woodruff] concluded that the level of care fell far below any conscionable standard. He was aided in fact finding by some employees who were frustrated with the conditions under which they were working. The institution was overcrowded. The residents had inadequate clothing. Their personal hygiene was poor. Residents were in restraints for long periods and they were overmedicated.... Woodruff discovered that the dentists were pulling teeth from some residents to prevent self-abuse or harm to others. Many who had been released to the community as part of the state's earlier deinstitutionalization thrust were living in inadequate homes, and they were not receiving adequate habilitation services.... Conditions at Pineland might not have been quite as bad as at Willowbrook [in New York] ... but they were comparable and deplorable. (p. 279)

In an interview, Woodruff explained his decision in more general terms:

> I was working for Pine Tree Legal in the early 70s providing back up legal assistance to inmates at several of Maine's institutions. I started going to Pineland talking to an advocate there who had been pretty successful getting services one on one for individual residents. But I began my visits initially to see how to correct these individual problems. It was a pretty squalid place, and it lacked therapeutic services. After 4 or 5 visits I decided that a class action suit was necessary to really address the problems there. (Woodruff, personal communication, August, 8, 1998)

Maine's class action reflected a changing national strategy in which advocates for persons with intellectual disabilities drew on the civil rights precedents of the 1950s and 1960s to challenge classifications based on mental competence (Minow, 1990, p. 107). The lawsuit directed at Pineland gained national prominence as *Wuori v. Zitnay*, although Margaret Bruns, R.N. was the acting superintendent at the time the lawsuit was filed and had her name initially attached to the case. George Zitnay's name replaced it when he succeeded her as superintendent. It was ironic that Zitnay became the state official most notably linked with Pineland's lawsuit, since reportedly it was he, along with newly appointed BMR director, Kevin Concannon (replacing Baack in 1977), who most observers considered the most helpful of all state authorities (Levine, 1986, p. 279). Appointed superintendent several months after the lawsuit was filed, Zitnay was portrayed as an "experienced, gifted administrator" who saw the opportunity to gain resources, was candid and truthful about conditions at Pineland, and pivotal in convincing the state to settle the case out of court (pp. 279–280).

The lead plaintiff in the class action was a 23-year-old man named Martti Wuori who had resided at Pineland for 13 years, and at the time of the lawsuit was a resident of one of the institution's most notorious buildings—Kupelian Hall. Wuori had worked in the laundry until he was terminated following the *Jorthberg* decision in 1972 (*Jorthberg et al v. the U.S. Department of Labor* et al.). A former Pineland employee called Mr. Wuori a severely mentally retarded man with serious behavior problem, "a very rugged, difficult to manage resident who could get very, very angry. He once broke 135 windows out of one of the buildings" (Herbert, personal communication, April, 23,1999). Woodruff, offered a very different impression, describing Wuori as a capable and likeable man who was unjustly treated and reacted in a predictable fashion, given his background and experiences:

> Martti was ... an interesting person. He was a pretty high functioning fellow who worked in the laundry at Pineland, and the guys in the laundry really liked him.... This job was a big part of who Marti was. He loved working there. Due to some litigation at AMHI [*Jorthberg* decison], the State was required to pay minimum wages for inmate labor. After this ruling Pineland responded by firing all their resident employees, and Martti went berserk, smashing furniture, TVs. He was angry, but could only communicate it this way. (Woodruff, personal communication, August 19, 1998)

Reaction to the lawsuit in Maine varied widely. State officials like Kevin Baack, said they welcomed and supported it, indicating that BMR officials cooperated with the plaintiffs:

> I knew the lawsuit was coming from the day I got here. Andy told me. MARC was pushing for this.... There were the Pineland parents [PP&F] who wanted

> to keep Pineland because they were afraid. But you had this whole other group of parents from the MARC who didn't send their kids to an institution, kept them at home and wanted to see a better life for them.
>
> We were very friendly with the plaintiffs. We helped it [the lawsuit] come.... We were disgusted with institutional conditions and were committed to changing them. We provided any information that we could. I think that the consent decree and class action suit brought a lot of changes and for the better. But it's change and people resist change. (Baack, personal communication, September 5, 1997)

Woodruff agreed that state officials who were unhappy with conditions at Pineland proved to be "amazingly supportive" of the lawsuit and "surprisingly helpful" as he gathered information (Woodruff, personal communication, August 6,1998).

Not all Pineland employees were so supportive. Some like research director, John Hoffman, dismissed the lawsuit as part of the litigious mood sweeping the country in an "era of class action lawsuits on behalf of minorities seen as neglected and mistreated" (Hoffman, 1982, p. 3).

PP&F parents also responded to *Wuori* warily. Some, saw it as a precursor to the massive discharges and deplorable placements witnessed under Peter Bowman's tenure, while also worrying that many parents did not always understand the lawsuit or its implications:

> I don't think we fully understood the suit. They didn't really tell us how it would help our sons and daughters. When the class action suit was filed, the PP&F knew it was coming.... We were not for it because we felt that people would continue to be dumped just as they were under Bowman.... We asked where people were going to go. We were scared about what was going to happen to our kids.
>
> In 1979, I found myself in court against a lawyer who was representing my son against me. They said [son] had "the right" to better quality services than he was getting at Pineland. But they were dumping them into [a] community that was not prepared to accept them. I mean it was a joke. I visited places where there were 15 people in the same building with only a couple [of staff] there taking care of them 24 hours a day 365 days a year. How could they do that? My son ended up in a group home that was filthy.... His room was a mess, and they told me he has a right to live the way he wants.... There was no supervision. If he didn't eat his meals, they said that it's his right whether he eats or not. How can a 4-year old make that decision? Do you ask a 4-year old if they want to clean their room or eat their meals? (Moore, personal communication, August, 19, 1998)

Some initially supported the legal action because they believed it would improve Pineland, but soon became disenchanted:

> What Pineland could have been! That's what we would've liked to see in the class action.... [But] they never really tried to improve it. Yes, they [did] ... for awhile but when they decided they were going to close the institution, I am sure that the greatest objective was, "We are going to make it so miserable for those parents that they are going to beg to have their kid get out. (Choate, personal communication, April 16, 1999)

One couple believed that the lawsuit and consent decree posed an unnecessary danger to their daughter and other residents at a time when conditions within Pineland seemed to be improving:

> We felt Pineland was the proper place for them. By the time that things began to change we felt that we had made improvements there. Residents had more freedom. There was a psychiatric unit. They had a gym, a chapel, a pool. The pens had come down. The whole thing was more open and normal and was more like a residence, and with more money it could be improved more. Dumping was the word of that time I guess.... Communities were not ready. [Another parent] visited a house up in Machias and found people were kept in bed all day, and kept quiet with tranquilizers. These houses had no training, no staff; they were just money making propositions.... We thought they would be better off at Pineland where staff had all the training, and ... knew how to handle them.... We always felt there would always be some who could never leave Pineland. (Murray, personal communication, September 10, 1998)

Maine's class action also attracted widespread attention outside of the state because of its broad legal significance. The Mental Health Law Project (MHLP), a Washington, DC public-interest law firm with considerable experience in such litigation (Levine, 1986, p. 280) became involved in the lawsuit because the case not only focused on establishing standards for improving conditions within Pineland, but more importantly (at least legally) developing standards for assessing community services. *Wuori's* community focus stemmed from the fact that many released residents were officially retained as Pineland residents, and some, like claimant Judith Babb, failed in several community placements, allegedly due to the inadequacy of the settings and insufficient community support, supervision, and counseling. According to Woodruff, without this case, there would have been no opportunity to develop precedent-setting standards for community placements (referred to as Appendix B) in the ensuing consent decree. Appendix A referred to treatment standards applied to Pineland itself. Levine (1986) described the significance of Appendix B:

> The *Wuroi* order affirms for the first time the right of mentally retarded persons released to the community from an institution to receive

> "habilitation" suited to their needs, regardless of age, degree of retardation, or handicapping condition. It is likely that Appendix "B" will serve as a national model for the development of comprehensive community services for mentally retarded persons. (p. 277)

Following the lawsuit, the two sides could not reach consensus for 3 years, despite officials' initial support of the legal action and their early intent to reach an out of court settlement. Woodruff blamed state higher-ups for the delay:

> The state was bent on fighting it. They started out denying that conditions existed.... The second year they made a token response to address the conditions. They suggested changes in an intent draft, and we totally rejected that as a mere charade. Judge Ginoux urged the parties to negotiate something satisfactory, so finally in the third year the state agreed to something meaningful. (Woodruff, personal communication, August, 1998)

Levine (1986, p. 280), concluded that state became reluctant to settle the case after 1977, because it was confident that its newly enacted laws governing the treatment of citizens with intellectual disabilities, with its emphases on client rights, normalization, and community services, clearly signaled a significant change in policy and its constitutional compliance. Maine officials, however, were under enormous pressure to settle due to: (a) the legal strength of the case, secured with the assistance of the MHLP and the candid testimony of state officials; (b) the negative and embarrassing publicity surrounding the wretched conditions at Pineland; (c) the pressure exerted by Judge Gignoux on both parties to resolve the case out of court; and d) the apparent interest that newly elected Governor James Longley had in settling (p. 280).

The parties eventually agreed upon a satisfactory plan for Appendix A in 1978, but remained deadlocked on Appendix B. Commissioner Zitnay and BMR Chief Concannon actively participated in the negotiations, an unusual role for officials in their positions, but, reportedly a critical factor in eventually securing the court's release. Levine (1986) argued that including state administrators "who would have operational responsibility for implementing [the plans]," was an essential ingredient in the state eventually gaining its release from the court's oversight in 1981 (pp. 280–281).

Some characterized Zitnay as overly political and opportunistic, although they also acknowledged that he was an important figure in the revitalized settlement and its long-term effects. Baack called Zitnay's achievements "masterful," adding that:

> we were struggling with Neville [Woodruff] and when George [Zitnay] was appointed Commissioner, he ... became the point man for the consent decree ... [giving] it a lot more visibility and more resources. And he had the ear of the governor ... [who] was getting all this flak from parents in Lewiston. And now along comes Zitnay, who moves the thing from, "Let's close Pineland," to "Let's improve Pineland." Now you can imagine how much support he got for that. They thought he was god-like. And he came up with a pretty comprehensive plan that was pretty liberal in comparison with where we were going. So good things happened to people with MR. And good things happened to George Zitnay. (Baack, personal communication, Septemer 5, 1997)

Woodruff recalled, however, that although Zitnay and Concannon were well intentioned, describing them as "committed to the state doing the right thing," they also

> had orders that they should not cost the state too much money or give up control. It was no give-away.... The negotiations were very hard work. The tendency of the state was to agree to something that would have little binding effect or would be ambiguous. We wanted something clear, mandatory, and capable of measurement. We could spend whole mornings on small provisions. I remember some provision about food-what the residents should eat; what their diet should be. I wanted people to have fresh meat, fresh fruits. They ate pieces of bologna between two pieces of white bread. I didn't think people should have to eat that. Food was certainly not the main issue, but that's the kind of thing we could get into.
>
> Negotiations took a year. I wrote all of Appendix A. Most of it stuck. What I insisted on was basically correct..... I took my role very seriously. I spent a lot of time at the institution. I read the literature [and] talked to staff. (Woodruff, personal communication, August 8, 1998)

In July of 1978, Judge Gignoux approved the consent decree as the state's plan for reforming its mental retardation services. The decree was a detailed mandate to improve conditions within Pineland and develop appropriate community placements. Moreover, it would serve as the standard for creating, expanding, improving, and evaluating services for everyone in Maine with an intellectual disability. Perhaps most significantly, final agreement represented an implicit blueprint for Pineland's closure, although this end was never explicitly mentioned in the consent document. In fact, for the next decade closure became a term that state officials avoided at all costs.

A NATIONAL MODEL OF AN ACTIVIST COURT MASTER: DAVID GREGORY AND THE BATTLE OVER PINELAND'S CONSENT AGREEMENT

Agreeing on a plan was an important step, but implementing it was an entirely different matter that required the oversight of a special court master appointed by Judge Gignoux. The first court master Gignoux appointed was David Gregory, a University of Maine law professor with no background in mental retardation, but extensive civil rights experience at the U.S. Department of Justice. Gregory was succeeded 2 years later by Lincoln Clark, a highly acclaimed mediator with impressive executive and university credentials.

Appointed in the summer of 1978, Gregory used his civil rights perspective to frame the complex, varied roles he assumed throughout his tenure. Gregory became a highly visible, and often inflammatory public figure, embarrassing, cajoling, and bullying the state into what he considered full and fair compliance. He was loved and admired by some, feared and despised by others. In the end, however, Gregory, despite his relatively brief term, became a very influential figure both in establishing an "activist" model for court masters nationwide and changing the perception and treatment of people with intellectual disabilities throughout the state.

From his periodic reports, it was evident that Gregory had become immersed in the legal and professional issues he faced. Along with his assistant, Arthur Dingley, he frequently visited Pineland and community agencies and studied the culture of the institution and its financial, political, professional, and organizational structure. To truly understand the depth of Gregory's involvement and the activist role he played in this case, one needs to understand the political, bureaucratic, and legal maneuvering that surrounded the consent agreement and Gregory's participation in it.

In January 1979, state officials issued a mixed, contradictory report of their compliance progress. In one article BMR director Kevin Concannon expressed delight with Pineland's improvements, pointing out that since July, the facility's census had been reduced by 34, from 450 to 416, and that the state would easily exceed the required reduction target of 400 people by July, 1979 (Roach, 1979, p. A12). Concannon also related that the department had placed 146 people in community settings, exceeding the mandated number of 120.

Zitnay offered a more sanguine view of the state's accomplishments, indicating that "in some instances we have exceeded the time lines, in some instances we're just meeting them, and in some we're having trouble" (Roach, 1979, p. A12). Zitnay also argued that money was not the problem, claiming that Pineland, "was operating in the black" and "was one of the few places where we don't have any financial problems" (p. A12)

Acting Pineland superintendent, Charlene Kinnelly provided the most sobering assessment, noting that although facility staff were "doing everything in our power" to meet the state's compliance goals, they "were unable to meet their deadlines for physical plant construction and "there is a possibility the Bureau may have to request additional funds from the legislature to complete some of the repairs" (Roach, 1979, p. A12).

While state officials reiterated their commitment to the decree, claiming that they were making as much progress as possible given existing time and funding constraints, they were experiencing more serious compliance problems than they were acknowledging. On February 15, Woodruff warned that 100 more staff were needed at Pineland in order to achieve compliance there and the state was "very far behind in three major areas: staffing, quality of programs, and staff training. It's absolutely clear at this point that they cannot do with what they have; staff shortage is rampant" ("Pineland Lawyer Hits Lack of Progress," 1979, p. A27). In response, Concannon admitted that "there are problems in areas dealing with Pineland," and with the addition of only the 50 staff allocated in Brennan's budget, the situation would be "tight" (p. A27).

It was clear that federal assistance would be required for the state to meet its compliance obligations and much depended on receiving Medicaid funding for Intermediate Care Facilities for the Mentally Retarded (ICF/MRs). Calling this funding "the light at the end of the tunnel," Concannon indicated that the ICF/MR program would enable the state to develop three new, 20-person facilities where "severely retarded and multiply handicapped" Pineland residents would be sent, "leaving more time and staff to help with the others" ("Pineland Lawyer Hits Lack of Progress," 1979, p. A27).

Gregory said little publically about the budget debate, but on March 19, he released his much anticipated report, producing banner headlines: "Pineland Praised, Roasted" (Lovell, 1979, p. A1). He praised BMR and Pineland for their serious compliance efforts to improve physical conditions, reduce medication errors, enhance privacy, and increase programming. Although Gregory singled out Concannon for his "tireless efforts to develop new community residences and programs, and to spread the message of the court's decree across the state," he was highly critical of Pineland officials and other state administrators and clearly intended to hold the state to the letter of its consent agreement (pp. A1, A14).

In his sharp rebuke, Gregory unequivocally declared that not only was the state failing to make sufficient progress, but was actively resisting change and flaunting the authority of the federal court. He pointedly criticized Pineland officials for displaying "a worshipful devotion to foolish, cumbersome, convoluted Pineland procedures," avoiding "imaginative problem-solving," and excelling "in producing reasons why things cannot be done" (p A1). Gregory warned that Pineland officials must "waken soon to the fact that it has only one set of supervening instructions: this court's decree; and if necessary may "need to be emancipated from both external and internal limitations on its ability to achieve results quickly and effectively" (Lovell, 1979, pp. A1, A14). Exhibiting sympathy for direct line employees, Gregory observed that "aides in some units are so overworked by the difficulties caused by their residents that they can do little more than keep the lid on, providing essentially custodial care," while officials impose "repressive and unnecessary restrictions on Pineland employees" and "routinely resist opportunities for fundamental change" (p. A14).

Gregory also excoriated "other obstructionist and dilatory" state agencies that were not cooperating with the Department of Mental Health and Corrections, accused them of hindering the state's compliance by holding up federal funds and slowing Pineland discharges, prohibiting the development of group homes, and failing to change its home-licensing regulations that are based on a "nursing home model" (Irwin, 1979, p. A16).

Bureau chief Concannon diplomatically termed the report "mixed ... but fair overall," while emphasizing that the state was making good progress and would require more time to repair "75 years of neglect" (Irwin, 1979, pp. A1, A14). He argued that the state had complied with 150 of the 181 standards in the consent decree, and was committed to accomplishing the remainder. Concannon also pointed to the broadening responsibilities of his department that extended beyond Pineland to include the 4,000 other citizens with mental retardation statewide, 2,500 of whom were "active cases." Finally, he characterized 95% of Pineland's residents as severely and profoundly retarded, indicating that training them for community living was a revolutionary idea that 10 years ago experts considered unthinkable and would require time and additional staff to implement (p. A16).

In April of 1979, the *Maine Times* ran an article entitled "Pineland Is No Longer A Snakepit." The article portrayed Gregory as "riding into the Pineland Center on a white horse," and "jousting with the bureaucracy" but finding instead, "a gigantic turtle, which when cornered, often chose to pull in its head" (Fisher, 1979a, p. 2). Upset by what they considered an unfair portrayal of them as obstructionist, acting superintendent Kinnelly and program director, Mary Crichton, fired back publically. Expressing full support for complete compliance, both denied resisting directives and hiding behind state regulations, arguing that the real power lay above them. Crichton complained that, "the commissioner can cut through the red tape of regulations ... [but] I cannot." Kinnelly called Gregory "naive" in assuming that more than 70 years of custodial treatment could be reversed in just 2 years and wondered if perhaps the court master was "unfamiliar with the bureaucracy" (Fisher, 1979a, p. 5).

In the same *Maine Times* article, Gregory offered his initial vision of what Pineland should be, a view that he would change dramatically in the months ahead. Reverting to the training school idea of the nineteenth century, Gregory portrayed a reformed Pineland as an idyllic community enclave, replete with the moral structure and discipline reminiscent of Seguin's physiological education and the pastoral, rural properties so central to Maine's identity. Harkening back to the images used by former superintendents Bliss, Hedin, and Vosburgh, Gregory expressed his full faith that a reconstituted institution could perform the seemingly

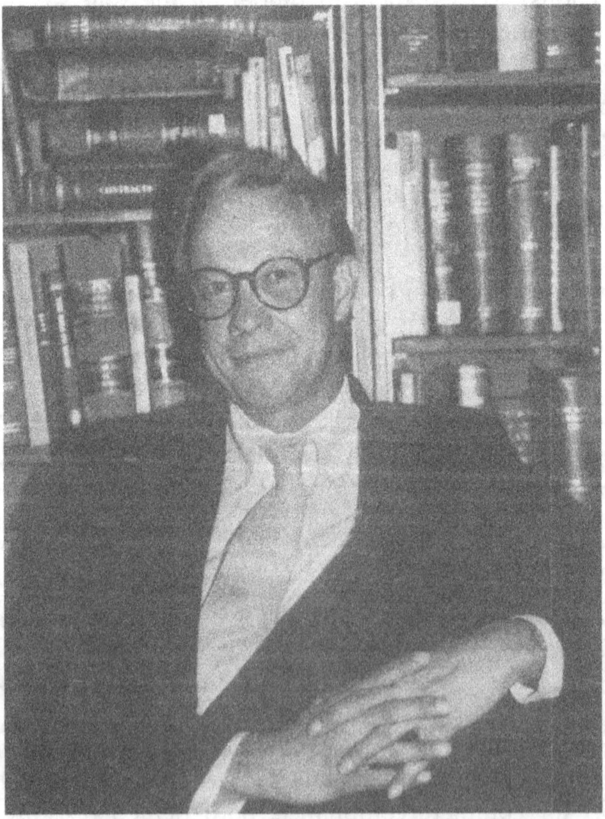

Figure 8.2. David Gregory. *Coping* Interview with David Walker, *Coping*, November, 1985.

contradictory functions of removing people from their communities in order to provide them with the moral training and community exposure they would need to reenter society:

> I think reveille should be sounded every morning at 7:00.... There would be calisthenics, breakfast and then get going. It should be joyous. Instead it's deadening. Pineland has a possibility of being like a little town in the sense that persons who live here could encounter all that a little town could have. They could have nice stores, they could learn to shop. There could be traffic lights to teach them caution crossing streets, there could be various work possibilities. A resident could get up, go to work, take a break, shop, [etc]. (Fisher, 1979, pp. 3–4)

Shortly afterwards, Gregory dramatically revised his views of Pineland and its potential for reform. Although never explicitly calling for it's closing, he became a vocal pessimist regarding its ability to change, and a passionate advocate for its total overhaul.

On November 14, 1979, Gregory wrote his second, and perhaps most critical, report. In it he labeled the state's efforts as "substantial and continuing noncompliance," and charged that "in no major area is Pineland Center meeting the consent decree (*Report of the Special Master*, 1979, p. 2). Gregory's report characterized state officials at all levels as actively resistant, indicating that they were either incapable of reforming themselves, or were flagrantly disregarding the federal court. Acknowledging that some progress had been made in reducing Pineland's census to 400 residents, and expanding community residence placements and day program openings to the required levels, Gregory called these steps inadequate. He charged that conditions within the facility remained "poor," and except for those who were placed in the community, the State's efforts toward compliance had little impact on the lives of Pineland residents (p. 2).

Although focusing primarily on institutional compliance (Appendix A of the consent agreement), Gregory saw institutional reform and community service development (Appendix B of the consent agreement) as integrally related. He looked for institutional reduction as an indicator of improvement, and while convinced that even flawed community settings were superior to living at Pineland, he served notice that the quality of community settings and services must also be ensured:

> In general, new group homes and programs for the retarded while universally underfinanced, often understaffed, under supported, and mis-regulated by the State, are proving the value of the Court's decree in terms of human capacity and aspiration. The problems in the community are older boarding homes and institutions that are not complying with the Court's order, a

> lack of appropriate opportunities for schooling and work, including opportunities for public education and vocational rehabilitation under federally financed programs, and a lack of transportation and other support services. (*Report of the Special Master*, 1979, p. 2)

Gregory's most startling and controversial comments were directed toward what he saw as the deleterious nature and effects of institutionalization and his altered vision of mental retardation and Pineland's future. Departing from his earlier perspective of Pineland as an idyllic enclave with an important role to play in preparing people for community living, Gregory argued that institutions are "inherently abnormal," indefensibly expensive, and "the worst setting in which to teach or learn normal behavior and ordinary skills" (*Report of the Special Master*, 1979, p. 3).

> The problem with Pineland is that Pineland is a custodial institution [that] … exists for the purpose of keeping people away from the community into which they were born. As long as society is willing to pay the cost of pursuing that purpose, then a custodial institution is effectively insulated from reformation or improvement to which it does not assent; institutional residents are hostages to preservation of the status quo. Abnormalities of the person incarcerated … are only the beginning and the least of the abnormalities of the institution itself. Every single task undertaken in a custodial institution is more difficult, and more expensive, and produces worse results than in a more normal environment. The simplest prescriptions of the Court's decree—provide normal clothing, provide normal meals; provide warm, home-like environment; provide privacy, dignity, and comfort; provide toys, games, and learning equipment—cannot be met by a custodial institution.
>
> Not only is a custodial institution incapable of meeting simple needs, but if Pineland is exemplary, it also works a positive evil. Inmates develop uniquely institutional behavior, which comes to constitute a barrier to [societal] assimilation…. Retarded persons become more retarded. Managers and employees exhibit their own modes of institutional behavior. Reasonable persons make unreasonable judgments. Harm is constantly, unintentionally, perpetuated…. Pineland Center has no future as a … place where persons are consigned to live for an indefinite period (p. 5).
>
> For three quarters of a century we have paid to hide retarded individuals…. Fear or misgiving born of our own self-created ignorance, will alone permit us to continue, at extravagant cost, a custodial institution upon our mentally retarded peers…. We cannot justify incarcerating someone simply because they are retarded. We cannot justify confinement on a pretense of providing specialized services which do not exist or could be better provided outside of an institution. (p. 6)

Gregory suggested that the facility should cease to exist as a long term residential institution and begin to function as: (1) an educational facility for people with mental retardation, their families, and agency staffs; and (2) a respite setting, and/or a short term placement for people with serious medical and/or psychological problems (*Report of the Special Master*, 1979, pp. 5-6).

What was particularly significant about Gregory's revised conception of Pineland was that he considered the community "the center of gravity of the Court's decree," (*Report of the Special Master*, 1979 p. 3). In his view, any energy or funding that was diverted from developing and supporting community services to maintaining the institution was an obstruction to full compliance. Interpreting Appendix A and B as essentially incompatible and Appendix B as the priority, Gregory signaled the end of Pineland and virtually guaranteed his early exit from the consent struggle.

Although Gregory's rejection of institutionalization per se and endorsement of community living for virtually everyone, incensed most state officials and institutional supporters, he was particularly angered by the fiscal arguments against compliance raised by his critics. Pointing out that the state was paying approximately $25,000 per year to incarcerate each Pineland resident, Gregory argued that residents were receiving far fewer services than they could buy in the community. He also indicated that new federal laws and policies were now offering and funding institutional alternatives and if Maine's state agencies would stop resisting change, they could secure federal resources to underwrite 70% of the cost of community alternatives (*Report of the Special Master*, 1979 p. 4).

Gregory also charged the state with illegally excluding people with mental retardation from federally funded programs, aiming his sharpest barbs at Maine's Department of Human Services (DHS):

> Officials of state agencies ... are unfamiliar with the needs and capabilities of retarded citizens.... They are content to allow Pineland Center to contain the retarded. They resent being told by a federal court order how the State's conduct ... must be rectified.... The worst offender in this State is the Department of Human Services. It routinely displays only the most elementary conception of law, as a regulatory restrictive, exclusionary, and punitive device; it applies rules purposelessly. (*Report of the Special Master*, 1979, p. 4)

One of the biggest conflicts Gregory had with Maine's DHS involved the agency's refusal to change its Medicaid regulations to allow for the development of ICF/MRs. In addition to requiring improvements in Pineland's physical plant, the consent decree required that by 1980 officials reduce the facility's census from 560 to 350 by developing 130 new community living situations and adding 60 new community living situations per month until all class members had been served. Because Maine had virtually no community component to its mental retardation system, the cost of such development to the state would be high. Changes within the federal Medicaid and Supplemental Security Income (SSI) programs during the early 1970s allowed states to change their Medicaid plans and reduce their large institutions by developing heavily subsidized, smaller ICF/MRs in the community. In fact, ICF/MRs were credited with providing much of the impetus and support for deinstitutionalization and the growth of community alternatives across the country (Lakin & Bruinicks, 1985b, pp. 7–8).

Gregory believed that securing ICF/MR funding would greatly facilitate the state's compliance by reducing Pineland's census, increasing community alternatives, and lowering Maine's costs of deinstitutionalization. Moreover, the savings from transferring these costs to federal sources would free up state funds to develop more of the required nonfederally funded community alternatives. Marie Cribben reported that state officials had come to the same conclusion:

> Pineland's ICF/MR was born around the consent decree … and it was pretty clear to the department staff and the commissioner and Kevin [Concannon] that in order to get a flow of individuals from Pineland to the community we needed to build an ICF/MR program in the community. The first ICF/MR beds were at Pineland, so we decreased the ICF/MR beds there, and increased the beds in the community, and we did that all over the state. (Cribben personal communication, July 3, 2003)

Securing ICF/MR funding was made more difficult because DHS was solely responsible for administering Medicaid funding and geared its funding regulations toward nursing care, a service model at odds with the educational model and normalization philosophy of the consent decree and Maine's mental retardation laws (Levine, 1986, pp. 286–287). Having no experience with this type of program and fearing liability, DHS initially refused to change its regulations. This stance angered Gregory, and due largely to his aggressive advocacy, DHS eventually relented and agreed to develop an ICF/MR program.

Gregory also took the State Bureau of Rehabilitation (BR) to task for its failure to help Pineland residents become employed. Unfortunately for its newly appointed commissioner, BR was also housed within Petit's department, and Gregory was as unsparing in his criticisms of BR as he was of DHS:

> Vocational rehabilitation services ... must be provided in conformity with federal law … that specifies that first priority must be given to persons with the most severe handicaps.… You fail to offer rehabilitation services designed to meet the needs of the most severely handicapped and … such discrimination must end.… Every single case … of rejecting retarded citizens from

> vocational rehabilitation is proof of your department's failure to provide the services they need. (Gregory, personal communication, October 7, 1979)

Gregory defined his authority and directed his criticisms broadly, antagonizing a larger circle that now included some parents and business people who benefitted from Pineland's presence. Seizing on Gregory's remarks about closing Pineland as a custodial facility, the media picked up the story, under headlines such as, "CLOSE PINELAND?" (Fisher, 1979b, p. 16). Closure may have been the issue Gregory's critics seized upon to discredit him as an extreme partisan, but it was his sustained and pointed criticism of public figures that likely sealed his fate. State officials found Gregory intolerable and wanted desperately to be rid of him. As Levine (1986) indicated, David Gregory, as much as the consent decree itself, was becoming the bargaining chip in the increasingly high stakes litigation game (p. 287).

By the winter of 1980, Gregory recommended shifting the authority to administer federal Medicaid funding for persons with mental retardation from DHS to BMR and adding Commissioner Petit's name to the list of lawsuit defendants. Maine's Attorney General, Richard Cohen, responded sharply to Gregory's recommendations. Cohen pointed to specific accomplishments and improvements the state had achieved at Pineland, and now labeled state-approved timetables as "unrealistic" (Fisher, 1980, p. 8). He accused Gregory of aligning with those who wanted to close all institutions and claimed that the failure to achieve compliance was not due to state failures but a flawed special master trying to cover his failings by closing Pineland (p. 8). The state's counterattacks had turned personal.

Not all state officials were so upset with Gregory's actions. In fact, some were praised in his reports and benefitted from his tough criticisms. Gregory served as BMR chief Concannon's and Superintendent Zitnay's biggest ally in changing DHS's Medicaid regulations. Even targets of Gregory's ire, such as Former BMR administrator, Ron Welch, praised his integrity, independence and helpfulness and for saying publically what state officials could not:

> Not only was he a legal advocate but a moral one. He had this little quote on his desk: "To live outside the law, you must be honest." His reports really upset the state … and [the commissioner] really gave it to Concannon. Kevin just said, "Look, Gregory is a court appointed person. I have no control over what he can say." He took us [BMR] on too, and that was fine. It helped when we went to the legislature, in that he was able to put pressure on the legislature for us. He was idealized in the provider community and advocates

> loved him. He and Kevin [Concannon] were seen as sharing the same values. (Welch, personal communication, August, 31, 1998)

Welch also believed that Gregory's tenacious campaign to secure ICF/MR funding was instrumental in eventually achieving compliance:

> The biggest factor in having the court release Pineland from federal jurisdiction was tapping into the Medicaid dollars, and that took some hard negotiations with DHS. Beginning in 1980, this [federal] program allowed for the development of smaller group homes, one half of which were for Pineland people.... Now around this time the state was being embarrassed by Gregory who was saying that the state was not in compliance because the Medicaid agency (DHS) was not flexible enough to meet the consent decree. The state was really taking a pounding from Gregory. (Welch, personal communication, August 31, 1998)

Conversely, the plaintiffs initially saw Gregory as enormously helpful in bolstering their claims of the state's noncompliance. Plaintiff attorney Woodruff considered Gregory tenacious and described the atmosphere under the court master as "exciting:"

> He was able to completely wrap himself around every item in the decree. He had a good idea of what it meant to have the state bound to the agreement, and to successfully establish methods for measuring compliance. He was completely willing to state for the record in frank terms whether compliance was achieved. His writings were marvelous. It was the first time in the life of the decree that someone wrote better stuff than I did. When he made findings around compliance, he would really nail 'em. (Woodruff, personal communication, August 6, 1998)

In March of 1980, Gregory's third report focused on the community side of the consent decree, characterized the state's progress as "slight," and recommended that the court's jurisdiction be extended two more years. Describing most community placements as inadequate, Gregory found model residences within the state that he pointed to as proof that Pineland residents could live full, productive community lives (*Report of the Special Master*, 1980, pp. 62–63). Calling these residences the exception, not the rule, Gregory noted that 60% of former Pineland residents living in the community were assigned to substandard housing (p. 42). He also indicated that there was a decided lack of available support services such as transportation, crisis intervention, and occupational and physical therapy, and that service agencies were not complying with the agreements they made to serve class members (p. 4). Frustrated state officials countered that it is "regrettable that the special master has not assessed and reported recent progress at the Pineland Center" (*Defendant's Memorandum*,1980, pp. 3–4).

In the face of Gregory's insistence on the state's full compliance with a document it had voluntarily agreed to, the state's attorneys concluded that they were losing the battle of public opinion and had little to gain by emphasizing their accomplishments and nothing to lose by returning to court. In early 1980, state officials announced that they were terminating further contacts with the plaintiffs and preparing to prove in court that Gregory was wrong and they had achieved full compliance. They followed this up on June 23, 1980, with another, equally surprising, motion: to terminate David Gregory. Levine (1986) believed that the action to get rid of Gregory was initiated by Governor Joseph Brennan, who saw Gregory as a significant threat to his policy making and budgetary authority (p. 287). In his argument, Assistant Attorney General Laubenstein insisted that the state had made substantial compliance efforts and progress that were unacknowledged by a special master who "exhibits insufficient, if any, sensitivity to bureaucratic obstacles to the changes demanded by institutional litigation ... [and] may in fact impede implementation by failing to appreciate the dynamics of political interaction which produce results" (*Defendant's Memorandum*, 1980, p. 6). In other words, Gregory had become too demanding, punitive, and uncompromising, a charge even some admirers like Ron Welch, began to acknowledge: "Gregory pushed too far ... and would only say that we were not in compliance.... The AG's office, BMR, DHS, and the superintendent were all in agreement that Gregory had to acknowledge what we had accomplished." (Welch, personal communication, August 31, 1998). Plaintiff attorney, Woodruff, also expressed some concerns that, "I was supposedly the radical lawyer out there, and now I had a special master that was more radical ... and was pissing them off" (Woodruff, personal communication, August 6, 1998). Woodruff was also annoyed that the state's focus changed from achieving compliance to jettisoning Gregory, leaving him with the heavy, time-consuming burden of proving the state's noncompliance:

> They [state officials] made the case that they were in compliance and were demanding a trial [to prove it]. I believe ... they did not want to deal with David Gregory.... Judge Gignoux tried to encourage a settlement, but the state ... wanted to discredit his [Gregory's] findings—prove him wrong.
>
> The burden of proof to show that they were not [in compliance] fell on the plaintiffs. Gregory's findings buttressed ... [our position], but we had to prove our case without Gregory's testimony. So we spent an enormous

amount of time preparing for a trial—months, hard, hard months. (Woodruff, personal communication, August 6, 1998)

The anticipated trial never occurred. The parties resumed direct negotiations through what was later described as a purposely staged, but seemingly fortuitous, encounter at a mountain resort. Woodruff described the event and what ensued:

> Mickey B [Boutilier] was holding some [Special Olympics] event at Sugarloaf.... and he invited Kevin Concannon and me to that event. And they turned over an office to us and I spent an hour or so telling him what the plaintiffs felt had to be done, but I acknowledged that the state had made some accomplishments.... Following that meeting there was agreement not to go to trial, and to develop a new work plan to meet the decree. It took 4 months to negotiate a new agreement—the Stipulation Agreement. It consisted of 15 very specific actions that the defendants needed to do immediately. It was a re-direction of focused effort. The consent decree was still fully in effect. The new agreement gave a relatively well defined list.... The list was manageable, and it didn't change the decree requirements. (Woodruff, personal communication, August 6, 1998)

Levine (1986) concluded that the state's desire to get rid of Gregory offered plaintiffs the chance to avoid a lengthy trial and to renew the state's commitment to compliance (p. 287). Woodruff insisted on retaining the special master position, but agreed to support Gregory's termination:

> We agreed not to demand Gregory's re-appointment and to appoint another special master ... because I thought ... Gregory's reports overwhelmed them, and they wanted to get rid of his reports and him. I don't think the state could have succeeded in court, but for the plaintiffs I felt it was more important to reaffirm a commitment to the consent decree.... I loved David Gregory and what he had done, but ultimately the result ... was to alienate the state and undermine their commitment. (Woodruff, personal communication, August 6, 1998)

Ron Welch recounted the meeting when the parties told Judge Gignoux that Gregory was the major obstacle to progress:

> Judge Gignoux called us all in for a conference and asked us point blank if we thought Gregory was the problem in this period. He wanted to know if this was a personality thing. We all said that he was the problem, that he had gone too far in hammering the state. So it was at that meeting that the judge agreed to [end] Gregory as court master. The judge asked for suggestions to replace Gregory, and Laubenstein suggested Lincoln Clark, who he knew was a bridge partner of Gignoux's. The judge said he would take it under consideration. He was able to get rid of Gregory through some

> provision regarding how a court master is appointed.... So at that point we had this 15-point agreement that indicated that we had 15 items to do, and we had done the rest. And we had no Gregory any more. (Welch, personal communication, August 31, 1998)

Kevin Baack offers a different opinion on Gregory's departure:

> I don't think he (Gregory) was moved out as much as he said, "I'm done." Because there were certain goals that were achieved and then it went to a different phase of the consent decree. I have spoken to him about this as recently as a few years ago and the impression I always get is not so much that he was moved out ... but that "I did my part. I don't want to do this anymore." (Baack, personal communication, September 5, 1997)

While the state successfully painted Gregory as an extremist reformer and closure advocate, he was neither. Although he had become clearly disillusioned with long-term institutionalization and the prospects of successfully reforming Pineland, he saw a role, albeit a diminished one, for an improved, reduced, and focused facility. During this period, the national backdrop for the *Wuori* case had changed from one of de-institutionalization to anti-institutionalizaton (Fergler & Boyd, 1980). The most visible class action in the late 1970s was *Haldeman v. Pennhurst* where the intent was to close, not improve, Pennhurst, one of Pennsylvania's largest and most notorious institutions. By the early 1980s, Michigan and other states had moved toward statewide institutional closures, and the movement was spreading to other large states like New York. Clearly, anti-institutional sentiment no longer belonged to the radical fringe.

Although *Wuori's* legal significance stemmed from its community development component, its consent agreement coupled institutional improvement and reduction with new community options and placement. As special master, Gregory demanded tangible evidence of compliance in both spheres, but required nothing that extended the consent agreement beyond its de-institutional framework. The friction between the court master and the state stemmed primarily from political and strategic factors. Through his civil rights lens (which was not unusual during this period), Gregory viewed institutionalization, especially as he observed it at Pineland, as a blatant, historical injustice that persisted for over 50 years with no legitimate rationale. Confronted with policies and practices he considered obstructionist, and armed with a potent and comprehensive consent agreement, Gregory showed little patience for what he considered incremental change and bureaucratic delay. In the end, he concluded that the promise of meaningful reform did not lie with an improved institution but with new community living options. In this regard, he was particularly outraged with the state's slow development of new community facilities and its pleadings for more time and money. By this time, he argued that federal de-institutional funding was available to underwrite the major costs of developing community settings that was far cheaper than continued institutionalization.

Levine (1986) portrayed the state as a generally cooperative party in *Wuori*, and that may have been true compared with other states. Maine officials and politicians saw reform as particularly expensive relative to their overall budget, however, entailing less political risk if undertaken incrementally over a protracted period. Gregory, however, saw compliance as a legal and moral imperative, raising the political stakes and refusing to allow its costs to be diluted or treated as a typical budget item. Without his public whip cracking and legal authority, it is improbable that the state would have moved as quickly or as far toward compliance as it did (Levine, 1986, pp. 287–288).

On January 14, 1981, the Stipulation Agreement was signed by all parties, giving the state what it had long sought: tangible recognition for its compliance accomplishments and relief from a tenacious special master. Gregory was nominally praised in the agreement for his assistance, contributions, and "steadfast insistence on ... implementation (*Wuori v. Concannon*, Stipulation Agreement, 1981, p. 1). The agreement acknowledged the state's achievements on 19 items under Appendix A, and 14 items under Appendix B, some of which Gregory had singled out as deficient. It also included a list of eight deficiencies and corrective actions for 15 items. The agreement fully retained the consent decree, making it clear where the state had not complied, but allowing compliance to proceed without long and costly court proceedings, and making the state's work more manageable by reducing its requirements to specific steps.

On February 14, 1981, Lincoln Clark succeeded Gregory as special master to the apparent pleasure of all parties. Clark was a retired New York University marketing professor with impressive accomplishments. He was a founder of CARE, the world relief organization; the head of Maine's mediation system; and a well-respected negotiator. Clark was not inclined toward inflammatory language and actions, wrote very diplomatic letters and reports, and preferred to do his legal arm-twisting in the private negotiating sessions rather than in the media. Clark was also a friend and bridge partner of Judge Gignoux's, a relationship that gave him added prestige and leverage. Ron Welch described Clark as "a steel fist under a velvet glove, ... a hell of a mediator, who could really knock heads together to get closure" (Welch, personal communication, August 31, 1998). Woodruff termed Clark "a sharp guy" who listened carefully, modified his reports if necessary, and allowed Woodruff to resume the more comfortable role of "moving lawyer," as opposed to following Gregory who "had gotten out ahead of the plaintiffs' lawyers" (Woodruff, personal communication, August 6, 1998).

Gregory's last report, submitted November 24, 1980, was impounded by Judge Gignoux. Released in February 1981, the report reiterated Gregory's previous criticisms regarding the lack of state compliance, in particular that the state was continuing to provide insufficient and inadequate homes, programs and supports for even those whom had been deemed fully capable of community living. According to Gregory, many more Pineland residents could have been living in the community if such services existed (Stevens, 1981, pp. A1, A23).

In response, state officials claimed that Gregory's "desire to close the institution" and his "misunderstanding of the nature and needs of Pineland residents" clouded his judgment. Using images and terms not expressed in years, Assistant Attorney General Laubenstein defended the institution as an enriched, specialized, and appropriate setting of indefinite custody for Pineland's remaining 338 residents who were too cognitively impaired and behaviorally deviant to function anywhere else:

> A sprawling campus like Pineland Center with day and evening programs and leisure activities, specialized medical services, swimming pool, gymnasium, bowling alley, halfway houses and cottages, and off-campus programs and activities may well be less restrictive than a community living arrangement.... Ninety-five percent of Pineland's population is severely and profoundly retarded, and most had suffered brain damage.... At least 70 percent cannot speak, 30 percent suffer seizures, and at least 300 are over the age of 18, which limits their ability to learn. Sensory and motor handicaps further handicap their learning ability. Some have serious behavior problems ... resulting in chronic violence, ... self violence, and property damage.... The state ... has provided a vibrant and comfortable environment at Pineland Center in which the present residents can lead a happy and productive life. Defendants, however, will continue to develop community living arrangements for those few residents who can benefit from life outside the institution. (Stevens, 1981, pp. A1, A23)

In his last report, Gregory pointed out that Pineland officials had themselves recommended community placements for over 90% of the facility's residents, indicating that 313 of the 338 living at Pineland could live in community settings with proper support services (Stevens, 1981, p. A1). Only 2 years before, Kevin Concannon pointed out that, "we all underestimated the capabilities of the mentally retarded" (Fisher, 1979a, p. 5), adding that "properly trained, severely retarded people ... can be placed in a community and function well, given their limitations....

There's been a virtual revolution in professional thinking" (Irwin, 1979, p. A16).

Clearly, state officials had dramatically changed their tune following Gregory's departure. While Lauberstein's reaction was a parting shot at Gregory, it was also a signal that life under Lincoln Clark would be better for the defendants and that the legal pendulum was about to swing in the other direction.

Reviewing the state's compliance claims, Clark concluded that the state was close to achievement on Appendix A, and immediately urged the parties to reach agreement on what would be required to achieve full compliance (Levine, 1986, pp. 288–291).

Administrative musical chairs continued into the early 1980s as George Zitnay returned to Pineland as superintendent. Concannon was elevated to Commissioner of Mental Health and Corrections, and Ron Welch became BMR director. One benefit of this reshuffling was that most of the major players who remained involved had extensive knowledge and experience with the decree and needed no introductions either to each other or the issues facing them. Cooperation was enhanced under Clark's mediation and cited as one reason why Maine was released more quickly than other states from direct court supervision (Levine, 1986, p. 307).

Efforts to achieve compliance within the institution were measurably helped when George Zitnay returned to Pineland as superintendent. A Pineland official in charge of institutional reorganization and quality improvement during the consent decree, remarked, however, that Pineland's reforms started before both the consent decree and Zitnay's return as superintendent. She described a reorganization effort that was developed virtually from scratch, including an institution-wide, staff reallocation that was key to the state's rapid compliance with Appendix A:

> The consent decree technically came into effect July 1, 1978.... But there was so much activity preparing for it, so when July 1st, [19]78 rolled around it was kind of like another day.... From [19]79 through the mid-80s ... our job was to take 480 [residents] and try to give them some structure; organize them to do something meaningful. We had to figure out how to give 480 people 5 hrs of program a day with 80 staff.... Hiring more residential staff and freeing them from doing housekeeping; physical plant construction, hiring clinical staff, putting together the records systems in a way that they were readable and understandable, in my opinion got us out from underneath the [consent decree]. (Cribben, personal communication, July 3, 2001)

In July 1981, Zitnay declared the institution in compliance with Appendix A, meaning that full compliance had been achieved in most areas, and in the others sufficient mechanisms were in place to warrant court approval (Levine, 1986, p. 291). Clark contracted with an outside evaluator to verify Zitnay's claims and following a positive review, and just 7 months after taking over as court master, Clark recommended that Pineland be discharged from the Court's supervision. Judge Gignoux formally signed the order of discharge on September 18, 1981.

The state faced numerous tasks to comply with Appendix B including the review and/or removal of residents from substandard group and nursing homes; and improvement of programming in community residences, vocational programs, and community integration of residents living in community settings. The decree also required better community and technical services and the development of a key component of the new decree—the Consumer Advisory Board. Finally, the state still had to develop more community placements for class members (former Pineland residents), while not violating the equal protection of nonclass members (Levine, 1986, pp. 291–292; *Wuori v. Concannon* 1981, pp. 9–15). In other words, Maine officials had to develop a statewide community services system for *all* Maine citizens with intellectual disabilities, not just those who had lived at Pineland.

Despite his numerous accomplishments, Clark faced the vexing problem of the slow rate at which the state was developing community residences and services. Under enormous pressure from Gregory, DHS reluctantly agreed to change its regulations, allowing state officials to make some progress in starting new federally supported Intermediate Care Facilities for the Mentally Retarded (ICF/MRs). Colburn, Kilbreth, Fortinsky and McGuire (1986, p. 6) reported that between 1979 and 1982 the legislature allocated funding for 35 ICF/MRs that would accommodate 280 people. Despite the numbers, Clark described progress as "agonizingly slow," portrayed existing DHS regulations as "in excruciating need of revision," and termed new ICF/MRs as "seriously delayed" (Levine, 1986, p. 294). Adding to the problem, advocates were now decrying the state's ICF/MR program as outmoded, too institutional and in violation of the consent decree's emphasis on normalized community settings (Colburn Kilbreth, Fortinsky, & McGuire, 1986, p. 6).

Fortuitously, during this time Congress passed the Home and Community Based Services Waiver Authority, a program allowing states to obtain waivers from the U.S. Department of Health and Human Services in order to offer a variety of home and community support services previously offered only in large institutions or ICFs. According to Coburn et al. (1986):

> The principle objective of the [waiver] … is to restrain the growth in institutional long-term care expenditures as a substitute for institutional (nursing home and ICF/MR) care) … [and] allow states to experiment with alternative methods of serving chronically disabled individuals.… Under the waiver program, services such as case management, homemaker, home health aid,

> personal care, adult day care, respite care, habilitation, and respite care may be reimbursed with Medicaid funds. (pp. 1–2)

The waiver appeared to be the state's solution both for addressing major compliance obstacles and eliminating growing criticism of its reliance on ICF/MRs as the state's primary answer to the community living needs of people with intellectual disabilities. Maine's DHS, administrators, however, still had to agree to apply for waivers and, as with the previous ICF/MR proposals, they were resisting. Several state officials believed that overcoming DHS objections (and some hesitation within BMR) and securing the Medicaid waiver was not only the key to gaining release from the court's oversight but to closing Pineland for good. As Ron Welch related:

> The biggest factors in having the court release Pineland from federal jurisdiction was tapping into the Medicaid dollars around 1983.... The Medicaid waiver allowed us to develop more community-based support packages, all individualized ... and was directly connected to the downsizing of Pineland. It offered an intricate formula for reducing ICF/MR beds by waiving the institutional requirements but still receiving institutional federal dollars. Each waiver application targeted a specific number of people, but in order to apply we had to get DHS support.... That took some hard negotiations ... [and] was a tough and prolonged fight.... There was a long standing institutional head-set in the Bureau and DHS. They had to be convinced that they were protected from liability and they were worried that the quality assurances could not be provided outside of the institution where people were living in 4–5 people group settings.
>
> [Once] we won the waivers from the feds more people were assured that the Pineland census was going down. As subsequent waiver applications were submitted, ... and more were accepted, it became obvious that Pineland would have to close. (Welch, personal communication, August 31, 1998)

The waiver was seen as addressing both the spirit and the intent of Pineland's consent decree and producing dramatic cost savings. Analyzing the effects of the waiver in Maine, Colburn et al. (1986) compared the costs and behavioral gains of waiver and nonwaiver recipients 1 year after the waiver program began. The authors concluded that the cost effectiveness of Maine's waiver program was compelling when costs and behavioral gains were examined together and when waiver costs and benefits were compared with those of ICF/MRs alone.

Although numerous former Pineland employees and state officials have proposed that Maine's Medicaid waiver was the magic bullet that produced both compliance and eventual closure, this conclusion would be only partially correct. Consent agreement did not flow from waiver approvals alone. Even after waivers were secured and implemented, significant oversight was required by the newly formed Consumer

Advisory Board, a group that battled the state long and hard to ensure continuing consent compliance and relied on the court's intervention when faced with state intransigence. Regarding closure, Pineland did not close for another 13 years and required numerous other events and parties to accomplish above and beyond the Medicaid waiver.

The Consumer Advisory Board (CAB) was one of the most novel features of Maine's consent decree. Designed to assess the state's continuing compliance after its release from the court master's oversight, the board was comprised of Maine citizens with varied backgrounds who were nominated from throughout the state and selected by the Commissioner of Maine's Department of Mental Health and Mental Retardation. The unpaid Chair of the CAB was Melvin (Mickey) Boutilier, a man described by Levine (1986) as a "strong willed person, [who] dedicated his life to serving the retarded," first as a Pineland recreation worker and later as the Chair of the State's Special Olympics (p. 302).

Reporting on the CAB, Levine (1986, p. 303) called it an effective compliance instrument, a group with "clout" that served as the major force keeping BMR "on their toes" (p. 303). He also argued that the board's long term effectiveness depended on strong leaders with political and negotiating skills, both attributed to Boutilier. But could CAB's effectiveness be sustained? In the 1990s, the group would be tested severely and would prove steadfast but only partially effective in ensuring that the state to meet its consent obligations.

A unique feature of CAB was its use of "correspondents" who were volunteer citizens, referred to by Levine (1986) as "a moral force" serving as the "eyes of the system" (pp. 303, 311). Correspondents were recruited to serve as community friends for current and former Pineland residents who had no family or family contacts. They received training, support, and supervision from CAB and were expected to monitor and report on the treatment and living conditions of the people with whom they are involved. Although the effectiveness and independence of correspondents was unproven, they were heralded as an innovative force who could assist former Pineland residents, monitor the state's services, and develop a nonprofessional political constituency for people classified as mentally retarded. Levine called CAB a promising way "for making the boundaries between professional bureaucracies and the public more permeable" (p. 311) .

In addition to CAB, the state agreed to allow an annual independent and publically disclosed compliance review to be conducted by a professionally qualified person who was not an employee of the State of Maine (Levine, 1986, p. 298). The state was obligated to respond to any documented deficiencies within 3 months. The external review was intended to both bolster and monitor CAB, serving to be sure that the provisions of the consent decree were continued after the court's withdrawal from active oversight.

Before recommending the dissolution of his office, court master Lincoln Clark contracted with three consultants to verify the state's claims of compliance. While each evaluator found numerous areas for improvement, and several noted the need for more performance-based evidence, all concluded either that the state was "on the right track," or had achieved "essential compliance" (Levine, 1986, pp. 295–296). Clark's response to these reports illustrated a major difference between himself and Gregory. Whereas Gregory required that consent decree standards be concretely implemented and assessed before he approved them, Clark was willing to accept organizational plans as the functional equivalent of performance. Although this policy allowed the state to receive a quicker judgment of compliance than it might have under Gregory, it later served as a primary source of ongoing conflict and distrust between the state and CAB.

Following the state's release from court oversight in November, 1983, Levine (1986) and his associates conducted a follow-up visit to assess the effects of the consent decree and the oversight arrangements on the conditions within Pineland (pp. 297–307). At the time, compliance oversight was being conducted by numerous parties, ranging from lay groups like CAB to state funded professionals from the State Office of Advocacy. Visiting several model units, Levine's group was "favorably impressed by Pineland's many new programs, the attractiveness of the rooms, the enthusiastic young employees, and the clean and well-dressed residents, all extending to units housing persons with the most serious disabilities" (p. 299). They also concluded that the oversight groups were functioning well, praising in particular CAB and its citizen correspondents (pp. 298-306).

Ironically, the same year that Levine (1986) and his associates were extolling Pineland's institutional reforms, some disability advocacy groups and the media were criticizing these oversight boards for their regulatory failures and conflicts of interests. The external critics directed particular concern toward Pineland's new intensive treatment program called the Behavior Stabilization Unit (BSU), a specialized locked dormitory designed for current and former residents who exhibited behaviors deemed troublesome, aggressive and/or dangerous. Interestingly, this was an area that state officials declared off limits to Levine and his colleagues because the unit "was having its difficulties and it might prove disruptive to have strangers tour the building" (Levine, 1986, p. 299). State officials would prove correct on both counts. The unit was indeed having difficulties and would soon be further disrupted by the criticisms of "strangers."

CHAPTER 9

COMPLIANCE DEBATES AND CLOSURE WARS

Tension between the state officials and advocacy groups only intensified after the court's release. Community placements lagged and despite the court's declaration of compliance, Pineland residents appeared as vulnerable as ever. Those remaining in the institution faced a deteriorating facility as admissions dwindled. Even state officials acknowledged that Pineland's condition had worsened and would be enormously expensive to repair. In addition, some residents deemed 'troublesome" were often transferred to the newly created and controversial Behavior Stabilization Unit (BSU).

Residents released to the community, continued to face stigma and discrimination and, despite new legal and political clout, residents and their families still lacked sufficient power to control routine "treatment" decisions that would shape their lives, such as where they would live, with whom, and under what conditions. Like most reform efforts that were occurring throughout the country, Maine's overhaul of its mental retardation system was primarily a top-down, technical operation designed primarily to meet its legal obligations and save money.

Voices of Pineland: Eugenics, Social Reform, and the Legacy of "Feeblemindedness" in Maine, pp. 213–244

NEW VOICES IN MAINE

In July 1985, the first of several highly critical articles about Pineland, the state mental retardation system, and the state's protection and advocacy agencies, appeared in *Coping*, a Portland-based monthly magazine, published by an advocacy group called the Maine Association of Handicapped Persons (MAHP). The group described themselves as "a statewide organization of handicapped people, friends, family, and supporters ... that promotes equality and dignity for handicapped people" (*Coping*, 1985a, p. 2). Their periodical achieved considerable notoriety when its editor, Lance Tapley, revealed abusive practices within the state's Baxter School for the Deaf several years earlier.

Under the headline "Death and Abuse at Pineland" Tapley (1985a) alleged that: (a) Pineland staff were physically and sexually abusing residents at an increasing rate; (b) the facility's Behavioral Stabilization Unit (BSU) was the major source of such abuse; (c) incidents of abuse were under-reported and not adequately investigated and staff were rarely disciplined; and (d) the advocacy agencies and monitoring panels set up to safeguard resident safety and rights, were ineffective, inherently compromised, and even in collusion with state officials to obscure abuse allegations and avoid reporting these incidents to the proper authorities (p. 2).

Criticized for bringing such sensational charges, Kathy McInnis (1985), President of MAHP, denied an intent "to shut down places like Baxter School and the Pineland Center or attack dedicated professionals," but to "attack abuse of disabled people," and "to criticize programs and practices that are not serving [individuals'] best interests" (p. 12). As one of MAHP's primary targets, the BSU was called "Pineland's prison, a dumping ground," and a setting where time-out rooms and restraint chairs were physical abuse obscured behind a facade of clinical treatment (Tapley, 1985b, p. 3).

Responding to *Coping's* sharp criticism, the state issued a six-page rebuttal titled, "Behavior Stabilization Unit, Pineland Center," dated August 30, 1985. The document (which listed no author or authorizing agency) described the BSU as an intensive treatment unit established in October 1981 as a cooperative effort "between Pineland Center and the Regional Bureau of Mental Retardation staff, the purpose of which was "to address unmet needs for crisis intervention services for mentally retarded persons in jeopardy" (Behavior Stabilization Unit, Pineland Center, 1985, p. 2). According to this report, the BSU was developed at the request of parents, law enforcement personnel, mental retardation professionals, and the Maine legislature to deal with "a small but troubling number of mentally retarded persons, many of whom were showing up in the law enforcement system in county jails" (p. 1). The report added:

> The Behavior Stabilization Unit has dealt with a full range of "behavioral" problems, including pedophilia, pyromania, suicidal and homicidal gestures, alcoholism, drug abuse, promiscuity, schizophrenia, chronic runaways, various organic syndromes, degrees of character disorders, clients who have broken the law but are not eligible for court edjudication [*sic*] due to incompetency.
>
> The client most often arrives at the BSU after exhibiting behavior that is dangerous to himself or others through an emergency restraint order which is signed by a physician or psychologist, or a community hospital or mental health center. (p. 1)

Superintendent Joseph Ferri referred to the BSU as a place to "cool off" (Nyhan, 1985a, p. 3), while psychologist and clinical director,

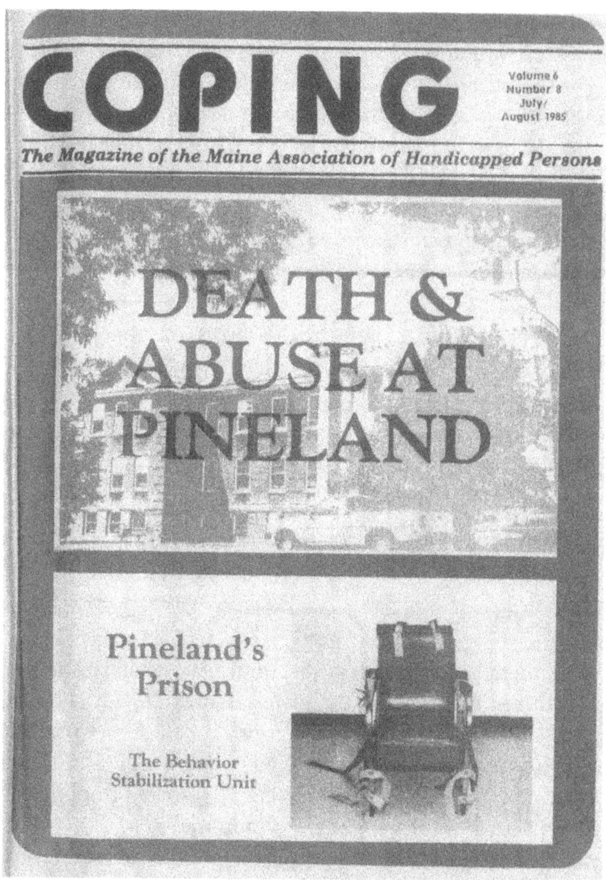

Figure 9.1. *Coping* headline, July/August, 1985. Photographer Anne Marie Bushardt.

Donald Philbrick, described a unit originally designed to serve a small but very difficult group of people, about 85% of whom were "emergency restraints," meaning they were exhibiting violent, aggressive, and/or self-abusive behavior (p. 3). The other 15% who were placed on the unit reportedly were admitted for respite care (Nyhan, 1985a, p. 3), meaning that those caring for them, such as family or paid caregivers, and so forth, were not available for some reason.

The *Maine Times* followed up on *Coping*'s expose` with an article on the BSU titled: "TREATING THE VIOLENT RETARDED PERSON." Included in the coverage was an editorial, in which the BSU was termed a "step backward" and that the state should:

> eliminate the unit, instead of being forced to act, as it was in the past.... Now we find some individuals being strapped into chairs at Pineland again, but this time with a different rationale.... We are a long way from the old Pineland.... On the other hand, there is a link. An institutional viewpoint says that the retarded cannot be treated the same as other human beings. This invariably leads to treatment that is less than human. Those who practice the kind of behavior modification found at Pineland believe that the retarded need same kind of behavioral modification used to train dogs. If you do what your master wants, you are rewarded. If you fail to do what he wants, you are punished. (Cox, 1985, p. 12)

Maine Times reporter, Pat Nyhan who wrote extensively on the BSU and Pineland's consent decree struggles over the years, revealed that more than 70 people were admitted to the BSU each year, with about 70% coming from community group homes and ICF/MRs (Nyhan, 1985a, p. 3). Program officials referred to the unit as a short-term solution, noting that half of its residents remaining no longer than 1 month (53%). Nyhan reported, however, that some remained much longer: 10% for a year; and 8% for up to two years (8%) (p. 3). Nyhan described BSU's treatment activities as follows:

> From the moment a client enters the unit, his actions are monitored, and rewards or punishments are administered in a "token economy" system whereby a client earns S for "Satisfactory" and U for "Unsatisfactory" for behavior such as making his bed, or being cooperative. "S"s, accumulated on a blue card are exchanged for rewards [such] as snacks from the commissary, entrance into activities, or trips to the community.
>
> Philbrick believes in TLC ... and stressed that the ratio of positive to negative reinforcement is 40 to 1.... Dominating the concrete-block main hall are the unit's two symbols of punishment: the "time out" room, an empty room with padded floor where residents are locked in under supervision for peri-

> ods of time up to an hour; and the restraint chair, which looks and feels like an electric chair without the voltage.
>
> Negative reinforcement for non-cooperative behavior ranges from having to stand in the corner for a few minutes to stints in the time out room, to time in the restraint chair. The chair is usually used when someone becomes a danger to himself or others. (p. 2)

BSU's supporters argued that, whatever BSU's deficiencies, they occurred mainly because of its residents. Rose Ricker, a former Pineland employee, chair of the facility's Human Rights and Assurance Committee, and secretary of PP&F called the BSU an excellent idea until it began getting "extremely low functioning people who don't understand it and can't benefit" (Tapley, 1985a, p. 7). Ricker concluded that the unit's primary need and function now was to "take care of behavior problems from the community group homes" (p. 7). Likewise, state officials claimed that individuals placed in the BSU exhibited such violent, self-abusive, and unmanageable behavior that there were no other treatment options that could be employed.

Several staff denied that aversive techniques were used, despite the very aggressive and/or self-destructive behavior of some residents. One approach that was described as particularly effective was the "sitting technique" applied in limited cases where individuals were "completely out of control, like smashing windows;" were "physically aggressive toward themselves others; or were very, very self-destructive." Reportedly the technique was

> used only by "very skilled employees who took the most difficult residents at Pineland and tried to bring their behavior under control.... It really worked and no one ever got hurt, and you'd be amazed that within 5 minutes ... you could bring someone's behavior right under control by sitting on them and talking to them. Now sometimes it would take four to five people. But it eliminated the use of leather restraints and that kind of thing.... Aversive techniques like cattle prods, or withholding cigarettes—anything considered aversive ... were never used; positive techniques, like [offering] food, clothing , special treats, things like that. (Herbert, personal communication, April 23, 1999)

Testing the state's arguments about the need for the BSU to manage particularly troublesome cases, reporter Nyhan selected a community agency for comparison. She chose Creative Work Systems (CWS), a Portland-based program directed by Valerie Landry. According to Nyhan (1985a):

> BSU's philosophy suggests that violence by mentally retarded people is different from that by non retarded people and is best handled by behavior

> modification techniques that include aversive (negative) conditioning.... [CWS's] says that a mentally retarded person usually becomes violent for the same reasons that a non retarded person does, and responds best to a humanistic approach that addresses the causes of the behavior.
>
> CWS, a private, non profit program, [serves] 70 mentally retarded people.... More than a third ... have had behavior problems, ... 10 percent ... with a history of aggressive or assaultive behavior, and 5 percent with self-destructive behavior. Many have been terminated from other programs and have come from the Behavior Stabilization Unit. Yet Landry's organization has never had to send anyone to the BSU. (pp. 3–4)

Landry termed the BSU "artificial and demeaning," and questioned whether people would transfer what they learned there to real community situations (Nyhan, 1985a, p. 2). Another community professional agreed, arguing that "There is no need for so many people to go to the BSU.... Pineland is being used as the boogeyman. [Staff warn residents that] if you do this one more time ... it's back to the BSU" (Tapley, 1985a, p. 7).

Pat Nyhan's and Lance Tapley's articles were damaging to the state, arguing that conditions within Pineland remained deplorable, and an institutional mentality still prevailed there, despite the use of different language and rationales. In addition, contrasting the BSU's and CWS, illustrated how a comparable population of people could be served without resorting to institutionalization or aversive, restrictive treatment. The media accounts also raised doubts about the independence and integrity of advocates who were supposed to serve as watchdogs for resident rights, services, and safety.

State and advocacy officials responded with outraged denials. Commissioner of Maine's Department of Mental Health and Mental Retardation, Kevin Concannon, blasted Tapley's article, calling it "vicious, undeserved, and sensationalized." Referring to MAHP's previous expose of conditions at Baxter, he declared that "[Pineland] is not the Baxter School" ("The Backlash: COPING is Blasted," 1985, p. 9). The Commissioner also defended the BSU as serving "street smart people," adding that, "the aversive or negative conditioning at the Behavior Stabilization Unit is necessary for this population, ... saving them from the county jails" (p. 9).

BMR director Tarpinian called BSU residents "very difficult individuals with aggressive behavior, two thirds of [whom] ... have been successfully placed back in the community" ("Bureau Director Defends BSU," 1985, p. 4), while clinical director Philbrick pointed out that the BSU's stark, dreary appearance was intentional, noting that "the BSU is supposed to be generally negative for people.... My original idea was that people should not like it" (Tapley, 1985b, p. 7).

No matter how the state attempted to reinvent or reframe Pineland, it ran into vocal and diffuse opposition, and was confronted by the media and rehabilitation agencies with examples of successful community treatment alternatives for people the state claimed needed isolation and restriction. The question of, "How can Pineland be improved for the most needy?" was now being gradually replaced with, "Is Pineland really needed for anyone?"

Several tragic events occurred at about the same time that the BSU stories appeared, further fueling the controversy surrounding Pineland and eroding the credibility of those charged with resident protection. In one situation a man was seriously burned after setting himself on fire. In separate incidents, two other individuals died accidentally, one from choking on food, and another after swallowing a safety pin (Nyhan, 1985b, p. 34; "Pineland Deaths," 1985, p. 10). Although none of the incidences occurred within the BSU, and no official misconduct was ever cited, investigators from Advocates for the Developmentally Disabled (ADD) charged that the state's attorney general failed to properly probe reported incidences of abuse in and outside the institution, including the BSU (Nyhan, 1985c, p. 34).

Early the following year, several reports on the BSU were released, one conducted by ADD and another by a Johns Hopkins professor hired by the Department of Mental Health and Mental Retardation (DMHMR). Both concluded that although the BSU could stop aggressive behavior, it was used excessively and inappropriately, accepted people who did not belong there, retained too many residents for too long, and did not adequately explore community based alternatives ("Death Revives Questions," 1986, p. 9).

Again having to defend their policies and actions, state officials ironically cited David Gregory, the man they despised and worked so hard to replace as Pineland's court master, as the source of the BSU idea.

> As Professor David Gregory, former Federal Court Master at Pineland Center, said in his November 14, 1979 report to the court, "There will be a need for some place to provide short-term intensive care for persons suffering from the most perplexing medical and psychological problems." (*Behavior Stabilization Unit Report*, 1985, p. 5)

While Gregory was accurately quoted from 1979, he had quickly reversed himself. Citing his altered perspective, *Coping* published an interview with Gregory several months later, in which the former court master left doubt about what he thought of Pineland in any form:

> The institution is, contrary to popular myth, not a safe place to be ... either for the resident or the employee.... What it finally comes down to is the state of Maine has to provide community homes and community programs for all the people that are entitled by federal court order to be living in community homes and working in the community.... There are incentives built into the institution to impede the right of mentally retarded people to get out of the institution and into society.... You could talk about some kind of unspoken attachment to Pineland as an institution and a desire to keep it running for no other reason than it has been running. You could talk about ... people whose jobs depend upon the continuation of Pineland [who] will necessarily come to realize that as people are placed out of the institution, and into normal community homes that the future existence of the institution is jeopardized. It is natural to expect that there will be resistance within the institution to letting people leave. One form of resistance would be to claim that there are people at the institution whose degree of retardation is so severe that they need to be there. This claim, which I have heard many times, is false as a matter of fact. For every person in Pineland Center, there is someone outside living a better life with the same general characteristics and problems. ("*Coping* Interview: David Gregory speaks on Pineland," 1985b, pp. 6–7)

Perhaps the most notable feature of the BSU expose` was the central, visible, and assertive role played by people with disabilities who emerged as an activist, media-savvy group. The MAHP existed entirely outside of the established monitoring apparatus, defined disability as primarily a sociopolitical issue, and characterized existing institutional treatments as the primary problem rather a viable solution. Outspoken and offering an entirely different image of people disabilities than that portrayed in the media, the MAHP described the consent decree as a conservative document that was rife with compliance shortcomings, treatment abuses, and conflicts of interests that rendered it both inadequate and unenforceable. While MAHP's president Kathy McInnis (1985) denied an intention to close Pineland, she and other group members were clearly skeptical that Pineland could or would ever change and believed that documented changes were mostly cosmetic, related more to self-perpetuation than real reform. MAHP pointed out that there existed well documented, effective treatment alternatives to institutionalization—many operating in Maine—and that the BSU merely served as another way for Pineland to perpetuate itself and justify its continuing existence.

The MAHP was a local branch of the national disability rights movement that modeled itself after the African American civil rights movement that began in the South following World War II and accelerated through the 1950s and 1960s. A grassroots movement, the MAHP defined their issues in primarily political and legal terms, advocating for equity, accessibility, and opportunity, expressing a right to represent themselves and showing distrust of those who claimed to be protecting people with disabilities. Such groups were becoming as activist and sophisticated as other interest groups in using the media to publicize their message and counter the stigma surrounding persons with disabilities—in this case the image of violent offender presented by Maine officials.

Following the end of the court's active oversight in 1983, Pineland's enrollments dipped to under 300, leaving a sparsely populated campus in a rural location with numerous vacant and deteriorating buildings. For some state agencies, however, the location was ideal. The State Department of Corrections, for example, offered to convert the facility to a medium security prison, an idea supported by Commissioner Concannon, who then made the startling proposal to transfer the remaining Pineland residents to "seven, moderately sized, state operated regional institutions" ("Regional Centers Urged to Replace Pineland," 1986, p. A8). Apparently reviving Albert Anderson's regional center idea, Concannon proposed to locate the centers throughout the state from Biddeford in the south to Aroostook County up north, each housing about 50 people at an estimated cost of $25 million, three quarters of which would be reimbursed by federal medicaid funds as ICF/MRs (p. A8). By 1987, the plan was scaled back to five regional centers each of which would include "five homes of seven beds each and one with 15 beds clustered on a campus ... [with] a core building containing offices and services, a recreation building, with therapeutic swimming pool and a playing field" (Nyhan, 1987a, p. 18).

The proposal was immediately attacked from numerous quarters. The *Maine Times* referred to the facilities as "five little Pinelands" and questioned whether the State had learned anything from *Wuori* and its consent decree (Nyhan, 1987a, p. 18). Other critics pointed out that the proposal would perpetuate segregation, incur unnecessary construction and operating costs, and divert state funding from promised community-based projects. As one legislator argued: "If smaller is better and the quality of care is the same, then we should pump 25 million into the community. Shrink that proposal down to a 20 acre Pineland and the only difference is new buildings instead of old" (p. 20).

Some parents feared that the change would make visiting more difficult and eliminate Pineland's employees whom they considered "caring and specialized staff" (Bradley, 1987, p. A17). Community providers strongly protested the plan in part on philosophical grounds, calling it antithetical to the movement away from segregation and toward community services, and in part on financial grounds as potential state-run competition for their own residential programs (Nyhan, 1987a, pp. 18–19). Neighbors of Pineland were also vocal opponents because some were employed at the institution or knew people who were. Some feared the presence of a prison in the neighborhood (p. 17).

BMR director Betsy Davenport defended the regional proposal as the best way for the state to satisfy parents, employee unions, and residents. She also cited the expense of operating a facility designed for 1,500 but housing only 275 and argued that residents would be better served in newer buildings within geographic proximity to their families (Nyhan, 1987a, p. 20). Terming the critics' proposal of diverting the entire cost of the project-25 million dollars-to community services as "naive," Davenport argued that "83 percent of Pineland's current residents are severely or profoundly retarded and the remaining 17 percent have behavioral problems, ... very few of whom could move into regular group homes because of the intensive staffing needs they require" (p. 20).

Assuring people that the state was committed to offering care and programs that were "equal or better" than those offered at Pineland (Bradley, 1987, p. A17), Davenport also argued that the regional plan would enable the state to meet its consent decree obligations, because the proposed centers, although still "operated as institutions ... would be small and 'normalized' " (p. A17).

The media was skeptical of the state's interest in building smaller regional institutions and found examples of successful, less expensive community service approaches serving the populations of people whom the state claimed needed larger, specialized institutional settings. The implication seemed obvious: why do we need any institutions? The closure wars had begun in earnest.

Perhaps to test Gregory's well-publicized contention that all people could live successfully in the community if given adequate supports, *Maine Times* reporter, Pat Nyhan, visited several residential programs run by a nonprofit organization called Opportunity Housing, Inc. (Nyhan, 1987b, p. 2). One setting called the Orrington House was a rambling New England style home surrounded by a low picket fence, and inhabited by six residents classified as "autistic and severely and profoundly mentally retarded" (p. 2). Some individuals had come to the programs from Pineland and some from the Bangor Mental Health Institute (a psychiatric institution) and at the time of their admission were described by staff as eliciting behaviors such as eating rocks and paint, urinating repeatedly, assaulting staff, sexual abuse, arson, stealing, and/or abusing drugs. According to the program's director, Bonnie Brookes, two of the home's current residents had once lived at Pineland's BSU (p. 2).

Nyhan (1987b, p. 4) reported seeing little evidence of destructive behavior, or "any signs of physical restraints or apparent behavior modification techniques." In its 7 years of operation, Orrington House recorded no escape attempts and described its security precautions as minimal, consisting only of gate buzzers on the unlocked gates of the home's surrounding picket fence and a sophisticated fire alarm system. Nyhan also noted that at one point a time-out room had been built, torn down, and rebuilt, apparently at the state's insistence, and over Brookes' objections. According to the director, "crises are best managed in the home, by well trained staff," adding that the BSU was often unsuccessful in changing resident behaviors

> because Pineland doesn't help residents make the transition out of the Behavior Stabilization Unit, with its locked seclusion room and heavy behavior modification atmosphere, to group home life. As for chemical control, all six Orrington House residents arrived on heavy medications. Now three are off altogether, and the other three are on reduced dosages. (p. 3)

Nyhan (1987b, p. 4) contrasted Brookes' treatment philosophy and techniques with those of Pineland staff who believed that "some Pineland residents could never make it in a group home because of such behavior." According to one Pineland employee:

> Pineland has its own engineering and plumbing departments. You need them because residents are destructive.... Pineland is solid. Ordinary sheet rock walls would not hold up.... At least half of Pineland's residents have been tried in the community and failed ... [and] if some residents of this type do succeed in the community "maybe they are drugged up." (p. 4)

Reporter Nyhan raised the question as to whether the state could afford to place all of Pineland's residents in community settings, especially given that places like Orrington House were as expensive as Pineland. Brookes and others argued that only a few places like Orrington House were needed, because this facility, unlike Pineland, had successfully moved people on to less expensive community placements where the annual cost was 40% less than living in a large institution (Nyhan, 1987b, p. 6).

The unmanageable and violent image of persons with disabilities described as severely and profoundly impaired was being challenged through the educational efforts of disability advocates and some professionals. The same groups were also eroding the aura of Pineland as the last bastion for specialized and intensive care for those considered the most troublesome. As reflected in the preceding account of Orrington House, smaller, less restrictive, and less expensive alternatives were increasingly publicized and praised. Along with the erosion of public confidence in even a smaller Pineland, came more serious questions about whether the accompanying and escalating costs of this facility were necessary or desirable. These were also questions state officials began asking. Within a few years they would reverse course and begin arguing against the institution they had vigorously defended since 1908.

By the late 1980s, there were growing signs that the State was again failing to meet its consent decree obligations. In 1988, Nyhan reported that development of new community residences had "all but stopped" (p. B3), and officials were backsliding in other decree obligations. Republishing some shocking photographs from its 1969 Pineland exposé in a special 20 year anniversary issue, the *Maine Times* infuriated state authorities and institutional supporters who saw the publication as an unsubtle hint that conditions within Pineland were continuing to deteriorate and that perhaps the facility was not redeemable after all. They vigorously defended Pineland as a changed and improved facility, and criticized the media for its "inflammatory examples from a dead past" and its "confused, self-serving, recurrent vendettas against what we are accomplishing" (Booth, 1988, p. A13).

Warning signs were emerging, however, regarding conditions within and outside the institution and the state's compliance performance. In September 1988 and again in January 1989, the Consumer Advisory Board (CAB) issued sterner warnings about inadequate progress in areas such as staffing levels, institutional admissions, crisis services, and community placements ("Report Cites Violations," 1989, p. 4). These were followed in March of 1989 by a critical report to the legislature's Human Resources Committee by CAB and the State Advocacy Office, both pointing to serious deficiencies. During the legislative hearings, Richard Estabrook, the state's chief advocate, linked inadequate community crises services to unnecessary institutional admissions and harsh treatment of residents, some of whom were being returned to Pineland "handcuffed or shackled ... like criminals" ("Concern Rises Over Violations," 1989, p. 2).

A former Pineland dietician remembered the conditions in the facility during this time as "abusive," pointing specifically to the use of inappropriate diets to reduce people's weight:

> People [considered overweight] were placed on forced diets.... But when I actually checked them out they were unbelievably underweight—skin and bones.... I can't tell you how many behavior plans—I came to abhor the term— ... were in place to keep people from grabbing other people's food and not stuffing food in [their mouths] too fast and eating things that weren't food. And I was thinking if I was on this starvation regimen you'd be having to knock me down with a stick.... We were able to a complete review of everybody and just undid these god-awful diets. And surprise, surprise

the meal time ... grabbing behaviors ... went away. (Coombs, personal communication, June14, 1999)

One reporter called the state's promised community services "underfinanced and on the brink of breakdown" (Davidian, 1989, p. A1), while parents, service providers, clients, state officials, and advocates argued that proposed cutbacks by the McKernan administration were only delaying development of promised community residences, worsening the low wages and high turnover among community staff, and exacerbating already underfunded services (Nyhan, 1989, pp. 16-19). Sonya White, revealed that she waited ten years for her daughter's community residence that was located near her home (p. A1). Another parent complained that her son "was bounced from one setting to another," as the state attempted to fit him into a series of group homes that were not individualized and therefore resulted in his re-admission to Pineland three times (p. 17). She called for Pineland's closure, arguing for "a community system that builds programs around individuals" (p. 17).

Peter Manning, chair of the legislature's Human Resource Committee, bluntly termed the situation "chaos that would require millions of dollars to fix" and warned that "if we went back into federal court, we would be found in contempt" (Davidian, 1989, p. A10).

Ron Welch, now acting commissioner of the Department of Mental Health and Mental Retardation (DMRMH), acknowledged that "the state was out of compliance with the decree in some areas," citing reduced state and federal funding and an increase in people seeking services as major problems (Davidian, 1989, p. A10).

Criticism by oversight bodies and other consent decree parties triggered scrutiny by the Health Care Financing Administration (HCFA), the primary source of federal Medicaid funding. This agency threatened to cut off 15 million dollars of federal aid that comprised over 70% of Pineland's budget ("Pineland Warned. Medicaid Funds Threatened," 1989, p. 12). The state quickly restored sufficient resources to meet federal regulations. It was highly unlikely that financial help to expand community services would be forthcoming, however, because the state's fiscal health was deteriorating and about to worsen.

In 1989 a separate class action lawsuit was filed against Maine's psychiatric system. This case would eventually be settled in August, 1990, in what became known as the AMHI (Augusta Mental Health Institute) consent decree. While this decree did not apply directly to Pineland, it would profoundly influence the way people classified as mentally retarded were perceived and treated in Maine for many years. The reality was that the AMHI decree distracted officials and lawmakers from their obligations to Pineland and funneled more financial resources to the mental health system. In addition, media accounts tended to merge the AMHI and Pineland decrees, describe residents of both facilities collectively, and criticize what was termed a wholesale release of "mental patients" who used drugs, destroyed property, set fires, and flooded the state's cities with dependents, all justified by the state under the banner of "self-determination" (Fullerton, 1992a, p. A1).

In October 1990, the Pine Tree Legal Services and the State Advocacy Office charged DMHMR with dereliction in enforcing the Pineland consent agreement and threatened to return to federal court in December unless corrective actions were taken ("Pineland: Consent Decree Enforcement is Challenged," 1990, p. 24). DMHMR Commissioner Robert Glover defended his compliance record, but was seeking to narrow his consent obligations to current and former Pineland residents only, and apparently was willing to return to court to do so (p. 24). In December, Glover announced more layoffs at Pineland and acknowledged that projected revenue shortfalls and budget reductions would prevent the state from meeting both its Pineland and AMHI consent requirements (Ferch, 1990, p. A12).

Early in 1991, Superintendent Donald Hartley and acting chief patient advocate, Carroll (Skip) Macgowan, warned that Pineland's census, now totaling 265 residents, had reached its allowable level and more staff cutbacks would again jeopardize its federal Medicaid funding and place the facility further out of compliance ("Cuts to Put Pineland in Tough Spot," 1991, p. A28). Hartley charged that although "it is cheaper to warehouse people ... [it] would literally turn us back ... and put us in jeopardy of legal action (p. A28).

The article's headline read: "Lack of Alternatives Keeps Pineland Open" (Carrier, 1991a, p. B1) and although the article merely reiterated the state's lack of community services and its likely return to court, it was particularly noteworthy because it implied that the state was again seriously planning to close Pineland completely and, unlike 1986, was not proposing to build smaller replacement versions of the facility. While some advocates were arguing that Pineland should close, even the most enthusiastic proponents of closure did not believe it could be accomplished in the near future due largely to the absence of sufficient community living options and services (p. B10).

By 1991, Associate Commissioner Ron Welch could publically embrace the idea of closing Pineland but minimize its immediate prospects: "I think we have an obligation to explore what it would take to achieve that level of independence, ... because we've consistently underestimated what people with mental retardation can do;" adding, however, that closure was "still five to ten years away" (Carrier, 1991a, p. B10). Only 2 months after Welch's estimated timetable, Commissioner Glover made the startling proposal that the state should close Pineland completely in "three to five years" (p. A1). Glover's call was described as "bold and strong" by some, and a "fairy tale" by others like State Representative Donnell Carroll (p. A10). In November, Governor John McKernan made the equally dramatic proposal to privatize the state's major institutions, transfer all residents to privately operated community residences and close Pineland (Fellers, 1991, p. B3). State officials later denied that privatization was related to Pineland's closure, though by now most parties saw the two actions as integrally connected and propelled largely by the need to save money.

Glover's announcement to close Pineland failed to resonate with some influential legislators. In addition to a tumbling economy, and an expensive legal commitment under the AMHI consent agreement, the state was faced with a projected price tag of 16 million dollars for developing sufficient community alternatives to justify Pineland's closing. Of that total, only three million dollars had been included in the governor's proposed budget (Carrier, 1991b, p. A10). A staunch opponent of Pineland's closure, State Representative Carroll of Gray likely expressed the views of many colleagues when he declared that, "the state cannot pour money into community services during a recession" (p. A10).

For state officials, Pineland had few redeeming features or prospects, and was being crushed under its own fiscal weight. Moreover, across the country, community services that were largely federally funded were rapidly expanding for even those individuals previously characterized as appropriate for institutionalization only. Predictably, however, the institution would not go quietly. It still had supporters who would propose new rationales or resuscitate old ones. Ironically, the state now found itself on the other side of the institutional debate, having to unravel what it had constructed, expanded, and defended for nearly a century.

For some, the announcement to close Pineland was interpreted as the State's attempt to deflect attention from its flagging compliance record and probable court appearance. Certainly, one wonders why the State, given its spotty compliance history and difficulty in developing sufficient appropriate community living arrangements, would choose to announce Pineland's closure in this way. Having defended the depleted institution for so long as essential to care for the most impaired and disordered residents, it seems predictable that state officials' claims would come back to haunt them after they so rapidly reversed their position.

In 1990, CAB issued a strong statement affirming its legal commitment to Pineland's consent decree, indicating that it would "take any action necessary to see that the state lives up to its promise to Maine citizens with mental retardation and/or autism to work and play in the most appropriate and least restrictive setting which will meet (their) needs"

(Fullerton, 1992b, p. A8). The Board explicitly stated that it would take no position on Pineland's closing.

CLOSING CONTROVERSIES

In December 1991 and February 1992, newspaper articles aimed a barrage of criticism at state officials, charging that they were secretly closing Pineland "without making a formal announcement" (Fullerton, 1992b, p. A1) or consulting with parents, guardians, consumers, or advocates (Fellers, 1991, p. B3). State authorities had been saying for months that "Pineland has outlived its usefulness" (Fullerton, 1992b, p. A1), although they were careful to characterize closure as integrally bound with compliance and service quality, not just cost savings. Assistant Commissioner Welch described closure as a positive by-product of the state's "new and innovative ways for supportive living approaches in the community, which may and will result in the closing of Pineland" (p. A8). He was quick to add, however, that smaller, privatized community services "would be less expensive than larger state-funded facilities "because private sector wages will be lower, and there will be fewer administrative costs" (p. A8).

Welch's superiors were more blunt, leaving little doubt that the state's highest priority was slashing costs in light of its deepening recession. Defending privatization, the governor and other state officials were not only predicting that privatizing Pineland would save money in next year's budget, but over time would "save millions" (Fullerton, 1992c, p. A1). BMR officials were trying to downplay the idea of large cost savings, due in part to the significant costs that would accompany closure, and in part to fears that opponents would charge them with closing Pineland for purely fiscal reasons. On these points, BMR officials would prove to be prescient.

BMR director, Roger DeShaies, in what appeared to be a risky career move, challenged the governor's claims regarding the cost and timing of closure. Acknowledging long-term savings, Deshaies denied that short term financial gains would result from Pineland's closing, calling the operation "a wash" in that "private care for some residents may cost less. But many other residents with multiple handicaps will need services that could be more expensive than the institution" (Fullerton, 1992c, p. A1). In addition, DeShaies questioned whether Pineland' s closing could occur by December 1994, the governor's deadline for privatizing Maine's mental retardation services, "doubting that there would be enough private services for residents within two years" (p. A8). Deshaies also morally trumped the governor, arguing that closing Pineland would indeed save the state from having to expensively rehabilitate Pineland's old asbestos-laden buildings, but that was the wrong emphasis. According to the director, "closing Pineland is not a financial piece. It is a humanity piece" (p. A8). One cannot question Deshaies' courage or sincerity, especially since the media quickly described him as "undercutting the McKernan administration's main reason for seeking a quick phase-out of the 84 year old institution" (p. A1).

Despite Deshaies best efforts, opposition to Pineland's closure was fierce. Joined by a determined group of parents, institutional employees, union representatives, local business people, community leaders, and some legislators, the media charged the state with trying to save money at the expense of vulnerable, troublesome people who had long institutional histories and who were being releasing into unfamiliar and hostile communities without necessary services and supports. They asked why 250 people were still living in Pineland if the facility was no longer needed.

Following accusations that the state was covertly closing Pineland, public hearings were held throughout the state and packed with angry parents and state employees. Family members stated that their sons and daughters needed the institution because they were too impaired to make personal choices and too vulnerable to participate in community life. One parent argued that the state "is telling us that they are giving our children the right to advocate for themselves in the community.... How can you expect someone with the mental age of 2 to do that? Some of them can't even talk" (Fullerton, 1992b, p. A8).

Parents also believed that communities were hostile and unprepared to deal with their adult children. One parent recalled that "a dog being taken to a vet would be treated better than my daughter was treated at a Portland hospital" (Gadberry, 1992, p. A8). Others reported seeing their adult children handcuffed and driven back to Pineland in police cruisers when their community residence staff could not handle them (p. A8). A parent of a 31 year old man who had lived at Pineland for 17 years exclaimed: "My son today is 6 foot three, weighs 160 pounds and is driven by the mind of a toddler. All of a sudden the state is telling me they have a miracle cures for him in the community. I don't believe it" (Fullerton, 1992b, p. A8).

Parents portrayed Pineland as a desirable, well-equipped community that included security, care, and fun as reflected by the presence of knowledgeable, accepting staff, a safe, spacious environment, and all the recreational facilities and activities any child could want. One parent envisioned an "invisible fence around the center that only [her son] can see and it makes him feel safe" (Gadberry, 1992, p. A8). A mother whose son lived at home and traveled to Pineland for recreation asked why people should leave Pineland to find community activities when "the community comes ... [to Pineland] for services" (p. A8).

Another unhappy group of parents included those whose children lived at home. They were upset that the state's focus on closure during dire economic times diverted funding and attention from the many families whose members desperately needed respite and community services to the relatively few who were still living at Pineland (Carrier, 1991b, p. A10).

Ordinarily, private community agencies would have been strong supporters of closure, if only because it meant more funding for their programs and services. And generally, these organizations favored the state's decision to privatize services, and eventually close Pineland. However, under enormous pressure from the state to provide new community placements and services at minimal cost, they were reluctant to wholeheartedly endorse closure, especially since Maine's fiscal crisis was worsening and the state was failing to meet its consent obligations. One newspaper account reported that "services are already so short that hundreds of mentally retarded people wait months and years for housing, medical care and other services" (Fullerton, 1992c, p. A8). As the pressure to discharge more people rose, and the state announced further budget cuts for community agencies, one private agency director, Richard Tryon, warned that, "We are winding up with a situation that is close to dumping people in the community.... The administration wants to close Pineland to save money. On the other hand, it wants to cut community services to save money. It just doesn't add up" (Fullerton, 1992c, p. A8).

The media continued pummeling the state for closing Pineland for fiscal reasons, hiding its intent, and failing to meet its consent obligations. An article in the *Portland Press Herald* suggested "the notion of choice for the mentally retarded," was merely a guise for saving money:

> Today-in the 1990s-the buzzword is choice.... That notion of choice ... has taken hold in Maine. It is the heart of the plan to phase-out Pineland, Maine's residential facility for the retarded. State officials, under pressure to close an institution that's expensive and considered outdated, are embracing the new philosophy of choice in moving retarded people to the community. (Fullerton, 1992a, p. A14)

The *Lewiston Sun Journal* excoriated the state for blatant disingenuousness, driven by cost savings and the victimization of obviously hapless people:

> Maine has embarked on a cost saving effort couched in terms of self-determination for the mentally disabled. But this justification for cutbacks in mental health care is as transparent as the season's first ice on the pond.
>
> The reasons most of these patients are residents in state institutions is that they do not have the ability to make their own decisions, care for themselves, and act responsibly in society. ("Editorials. Irresponsible Policy," 1992, p. A4)

Combining institutional populations and consent agreements for both Pineland and AMHI, the press, political figures and public safety authorities issued dire warnings that the "mentally disabled" from Maine's largest institutions were being "dumped" into society with inadequate supervision and support, flooding local municipalities with incompetent, sometimes dangerous, people, and bringing with them high costs, crime, degeneracy, and social disorder. According to one Portland city official, "Portland is becoming a mini-institution" (Fullerton, 1992d, p. B1). Closure, self-determination, and cost savings became epithets aimed at the state to characterize their blatant neglect.

Perhaps the most dramatic newspaper accounts were reported by Linda Fullerton who covered Pineland's consent battles and closing controversies for several years. She described the lives of several former Pineland residents living "self-determined" community lives of poverty, neglect, and criminality (Fullerton, 1992e, pp. A1, A14). Fullerton wrote about one man named Steven Gagnon who was living in his own apartment that reeked of "rotting garbage, stale beer, and urine;" alienating his neighbors and landlords so that he was twice evicted; and begging for food so often that a neighbor called the police who drove him to a soup kitchen (p. A14). His personal appearance was described as "dirty,' and "his blue eyes ... glazed [from] ... drugs" while his gestures were termed "spastic" (p. A14). Gagnon was reportedly able to read and write, although he was characterized as childlike and spends much of his time shoplifting, foraging through garbage for food, panhandling cigarettes, prostituting himself for drugs, destroying property, and setting fires (pp. A1, A14).

Gagnon was said to have made excellent progress at Pineland "where close supervision dictated where he ate, bathed, and slept" (Fullerton, 1992e, p. A14). Under the state's "new treatment policy of self-determination," however, officials honored Gagnon's request for discharge, allowing him to care for himself, since "he won't accept help" (p. A14). Following his release, he was assigned a caseworker who saw him daily to give him a \$3.65 allowance, which the social worker limited because of her concerns that he would buy drugs. He was also offered a daily meal, and given \$30 per week for food stamps. Social workers paid Gagnon's rent and any fines he incurred for illegal behavior, found him apartments, summoned medical assistance when needed, and offered him substance abuse counseling and AIDS education. However, juxtaposed with the structure imposed at Pineland, Fullerton reported that the caseworker and her colleagues "don't insist that Gagnon bathe or refrain from committing crimes, like prostitution, [believing] that kind of interference would drive Gagnon away" (p. A14). The article warned that Gagnon's experiences "indicates … how the state plans to manage community care as the 200 residents remaining at Pineland are discharged, and the institution closes for good in 1995" (p. A1).

Gagnon soon became a central image and point of reference in the campaign against closing Pineland and further release of other institutional residents. An editorial in the *Portland Press Herald* called self-determination "high minded words [disguising] … a more sordid reality: the saga of Steven Gagnon." The editors predicted that more releases from Pineland and AMHI would create such an influx of de-institutionalized people that would further overwhelm Maine's cities and already overburdened social services with "mentally ill" ("Life Outside Pineland Falls Short of Freedom,"1992, p. C6). The *Brunswick Times Record* (1992) acknowledged that perhaps Pineland is not needed and that inadequate community services are a major problem, but the headlines read: "Don't Close Pineland," and the editors again raised the specter of Steven Gagnon:

> The state wants to close Pineland to save money. Toward that end Pineland has adopted a new policy of self-determination for residents and is releasing people such as Gagnon … into the community … [without] adequate community-based care programs and facilities … and the supervision they need. (p. A6)

Portland's outspoken Chief of Police, Michael Chitwood declared the state's discharge policy "a total disgrace," "a tragedy waiting to happen" (Fullerton, 1992e, p. A14), and "a public safety issue" (Fullerton, 1992f, p. A1). A few days later, Chitwood and Portland's city attorney, Gary Wood, announce that they would legally challenge further discharges of "mentally ill" residents, and oppose BMR's self determination policy, which allowed the "mentally disabled" to decide how they want to live when they are released from state institutions (Fullerton, 1992e, p. A1). Wood argued that not only had the state reneged on its consent agreement to protect former Pineland residents from harm, but had also placed other citizens at risk since "unsupervised former residents can be dangerous" (Nacelewicz, 1992, p. A14). Officials of Maine's second largest city, Lewiston, also expressed opposition to Pineland's closing and their support for Portland's lawsuit. They argue that shutting Pineland would: (a) create a dire need for people "who have no where to turn;" and (b) place "an unfair and unprepared burden upon residents and taxpayers of local communities" (Gignoux, 1993, p. A13).

Public meetings on Pineland's closing attracted as many as 300 protesters. Parents made very emotional appeals to state officials, while union and business interests cited dire economic consequences that would accompany closure. In 1993, an analysis of the direct and indirect economic impact of the facility's closure was estimated to cost the state 1,311 jobs, amounting to $33.5 in salaries and $43.6 million in sales. Local cities and towns were projected to lose 708 jobs, $18.8 in salaries, and $18.4 in sales tax (Richardson, 1994a, p. B14). One legislator compared the facility's closing with the devastating economic consequences for northern Maine of recently losing the Loring Air Force Base (p. B14).

At the same time, community service providers began to soften their criticism of state policy, expressing conditional support for self-determination and the "end of the era of institutionalization" (Fullerton, 1992g, p. A5). Professionals were quoted as agreeing "in principle with the state's policy of self determination," noting that "the problem is the way it is implemented" One service provider pointed out that "we have gone from telling people with mental retardation that, 'we're going to lock you up,' to telling them they can have whatever they want. Common sense needs to be applied" (p. A5).

There were many reasons to criticize the state's record, including its well documented history of neglect and abuse, exaggerated claims of treatment quality and effects, consistent resistance to its consent obligations, and an absence of collaboration with residents and families regarding depopulating Pineland and developing individualized community living arrangements. It may be argued that Maine's de-institutionalization effort and eventual closure of Pineland represented a classic case of how *not* to conduct such actions. Certainly, in the absence of ongoing collaborative planning and after years of conflict, it is understandable that parents, employees, varied public officials, and the general public would react skeptically when state officials announced their intention to close Pineland and discharge everyone to "humane and individualized" community settings. Most had heard all this before. Doubts were fueled further by fear-inducing news accounts of the allegedly mismanaged community placements, such as that of former resident, Steven Gagnon, where an already worried public is shown more neglect and disorder than supervision and safety in the state's proposal to close Pineland.

Media commentators often claimed they were not opposing closing Pineland, per se, but were against shutting it down for strictly fiscal reasons and before adequate community alternatives were available. That message, however, was often obscured by the more sensational emphasis on former residents whose community lives were particularly troubled.

Largely ignored were the many residents who left Pineland and similar institutions and did not became drug users, prostitutes, or criminals.

In an attempt to blunt some of the fears about discharged residents and counter the image of Pineland as the safe and enriching treatment community described by its supporters, individuals and groups of people with disabilities began speaking out once more. Some like former Behavioral Stabilization Unit resident, Sharon Morse, wrote to the local newspaper:

> I lived at Pineland for a long time and I never want to go back. I hate that place.... I'm not an animal, and I'm treated better out here.... Why don't Channel 13 and the *Portland Press Herald* check out the rest of us who refuse to go back to institutional living. (Morse, 1993, p. A6)

Most former residents, however, did not speak out or write letters unwilling or unable to describe their experiences publically. When interviewed about their experiences at Pineland and after, most expressed strong opinions. Michelle Childress resided at Pineland in the 1950s and emphasized that she tried to get away and would never go back:

> I went in at 9 [years old] and went through there until I was 18.... I got spankings a lot ... ran away; brought back by state troopers. Other people got locked up, naked, in a special room for problems. I seen it. Naked and all drugged. They shouldn't do that. That's abuse. (Childress, personal communication, September 18, 1998)

Betty Thompson remembers Pineland as a bleak and restrictive place where "your mail was censored" and "you had to open presents my parents sent me in the office. The buildings were dark; bars on the windows; doors were locked. You couldn't get out. It wasn't a nice place to be" (Thompson, personal communication, June 17, 2003).

Doreen Reynolds regrets that "they never taught me anything. I had to learn everything myself. They said I wasn't capable of living in an apartment. So I had to fight my way out.. I'm not ashamed of being there but I don't advertise it." (Reynolds, personal communication, June 17, 2003)

Describing the physical and sexual abuse he experienced, Jim Morgan emphasized that he is out now and does "not want to think about it anymore."

> They'd punish me by not giving me food. I'd be hungry and they would tell me there's no food, but I saw the food. I cried and tried to steal food.... They pushed my head into the wall. Pineland was a stupid place.... A lot of abuse.... They would hit me with a wooden stick and a dust pan over the head. They never really told me why. They hit me on my butt many, many

> times.... crotch under the covers. I'd scream. It hurt. A person with a white coat would grab me, tried to kiss me. I had sex with him. (Morgan, personal communication, March 24, 1999)

Ruby Bouchard, 33, describes being furious at being sent to Pineland at age 33 in the 1980s and her determination to get out and never return:

> I was so angry about being at Pineland that I threw a temper tantrum so they ended up sitting on me.... I managed to pull myself together even though I hated it.... I just didn't like being caged in. I felt like the walls were closing in on me, and that's a scary feeling.... I just didn't want to go back into that dump. (Bouchard, personal communication, February 5, 1999)

Some former residents were less critical, citing helpful staff, good friends, and enjoyable experiences and events. Sean Adams describes Pineland as "not a bad place" where he worked with people he liked and enjoyed seeing movies with his friends (Adams, personal communication, January 26, 1999). Although Donald Nevin, recalls the "bars on the windows that makes you think your're in jail," he also remembers "leading the band and all the people in the parade. They knew I was a good conductor. I miss that." He also recalls:

> We used to have a dance at the gym in Pineland. We used to have a party and all that. It was fun.... I was sad when I first came here [to group home], but now I'm not. They've got rules in this place. You gotta wash dishes and you gotta do your own laundry, and all that ... I didn't have to do all that at Pineland. The staff do it. I felt pretty bad about it [closing]. I figure they [Pineland] ran out of business. I think it should've stayed open, yes. I'd go back but I can't because the place is closed. (Nevin, personal communication, April 23, 1998)

In an effort to offer a more optimistic perspective on resident discharges, Fullerton (1992h) reported on the community experiences of a young man under the headline "Former Pineland residents can lead good lives too" (p. A15). She described him as a "loud and aggressive" individual when at Pineland but following his placement in a group home, he "was living a normal life" consisting of a part time job, a community bank account, and the periodic company of relatives and neighbors (p. A15). It was also reported that due to his behavior, the young man was placed under "constant supervision," and the home was surrounded by "a stockade fence" (p. A15).

Clearly, the article offered a more positive and optimistic picture of former Pineland residents living outside the institution, contrasting sharply with the so called "self-determined" lives of people like Steven Gagnon.

Apparently, a new, more nuanced message was being delivered. No longer claiming that all troublesome people required institutionalization, officials acknowledged that most former Pineland residents could live successful, community lives within "highly structured" living arrangements (Fullerton, 1992h, p. 15). The idea of providing structured, "community-based" living circumstances for targeted individuals would apparently linger for years after Pineland closed, returning most overtly as a remarkable proposal in the year 2000 by a well endowed philanthropic organization to elaborately rehabilitate the institutional grounds and re-open part of it for new residents with "multiple handicaps" (Williams, 2000, p. A10).

LEGAL CHALLENGES AND CONSENT REVISIONS

From October 1991 through July, 1994, the State and its oversight bodies engaged in a protracted battle during which the legal standing of the 1978 consent decree was challenged and nearly overshadowed by the controversy over closure. In the absence of a collaborative framework and relying on an adversarial legal process, the parties were plagued by years of poor communication, one-sided decision making, and broken promises. Some of the ensuing distrust was integral to the legal tangle itself and some could be traced to Lincoln Clark's decision to accept the promises of the state for achieving compliance in lieu of actual performance. Signing off on the State's proposed compliance mechanisms, Clark and Gignoux took a leap of faith that the state would follow through. Such promises, however, began to fade as the state's economy sank, other consent obligations emerged, and the pressure of active court oversight receded. In the end, the state resorted to legal maneuvers to escape its compliance commitments. Ultimately these maneuvers failed and in the absence of meaningful communication and negotiation between the parties, the loss to the state went beyond legal defeat, as plaintiffs, advocates, and families became firmly convinced that the State could not be trusted to keep its promises.

Initially the state's decision to challenge the legal standing of its consent agreement seemed to work. Federal court Judge D. Brock Hornby announced on April 30, 1992 that Pineland's consent decree was not valid after 1986, and that federal courts no longer had jurisdiction in the case. According to Hornby, plaintiffs would have to file a completely new class action if they believed their constitutional rights continued to be violated. CAB immediately appealed (Young, 1993, p. A1).

On April 2, 1993, the Federal District Court of Appeals in Boston reversed Hornby's decision, binding the State to its consent agreement and returning jurisdiction to the Federal District Court in Maine which could dissolve the Pineland consent decree only if convinced that its purpose had been achieved or it no longer served the public interest (Fullerton, 1993, pp. B1–B2). Governor McKernan decided to press for dissolution and continue the state's adversarial strategy. On September 30, 1993, the Federal District Court in Maine denied the State's motions to dissolve the 1978 consent decree and dismiss CAB's lawsuit, finding that the state could be cited for noncompliance if proven in court. The state and plaintiff's prepared once again to return to the courtroom in July 1994 as the authority of the decree was re-established, although the state's obligations to it remained in limbo.

In July 1994, the state and plaintiffs elected to settle and accept a renewed consent agreement that came to be known as the Community Consent Decree ("Retarded to Enjoy Range of Support," 1994, p. 2B). The agreement was termed "a new, more relevant document for the 1990s" (*Consumer Advisory Board v. Glover et al.*, 1994, p. 2). In the new agreement the plaintiffs terminated Appendix A of the 1978 decree, focusing only on issues related to community preparation and living situations. The document emphasized ten areas that coincided with CAB's complaints, including (a) requirements for a personal planning process for every individual; (b) provisions for both crisis prevention and intervention; (c) guarantees of professional services; (d) assurances of community development for housing, employment, medical, recreational, avocational, religious, educational, and other professional or therapeutic services; (e) provisions for family-determined respite and supports; (f) right to appeal any grievance arising as part of the decree through both informal and formal means; (g) continuing oversight authority of the consumer advisory board; (h) required annual, public compliance review and report and evidence of corrective action; (i) application of budget surpluses generated by Pineland's closure to development and provision of community services; and (j) assurance of numerous miscellaneous contracts and agreements with private providers, BMR, correspondents, staff, advocates, and other state offices and bodies related to service quality and consent decree compliance (pp. 10–38).

To avoid some of the implementation problems of the 1978 version, the 1994 document contained specific references to the ways in which compliance could be achieved, and how and under what conditions the decree could be terminated. It also contained a set of assumptions that delineated an altered perspective of mental retardation in which people were described as having the same rights as other citizens, including living, working, learning, and recreating in typical community situations; being able to live in a home with necessary services and supports if needed; receiving assessment and planning that included people's active participation (with advocates and family assistance if necessary) in choosing their community living, working, social, and recreational activities in integrated settings and offering "maximum control over their lives" (*Consumer Advisory Board v. Glover et al.*, 1994, pp. 4–5).

Again, CAB specifically noted that they took no official position on Pineland's closing, viewing that development as independent of the state's obligation to develop an adequate community services system. Because the new decree focused explicitly on community opportunities and services, it virtually prohibited institutional options and revealed that the plaintiffs clearly considered closure a positive, though insufficient, sign of victory.

The 1994 document embraced principles such as individual choice, control, and self-determination, all of which were specified throughout the document. These were concepts that had been excoriated in the media only months earlier, rejected as inapplicable and inappropriate for people classified as mentally retarded and characterized as a thin facade for community dumping and state cost reductions.

The new decree also emphasized the importance of acknowledging and enhancing the family as a preeminent, natural source of care and an important recipient of services and supports. In addition, it described the home as a preferential setting, underscoring the value of keeping families together and supporting them with in-home services. An interesting irony surrounded the emerging prominence and power of families and was underscored by lack of enthusiasm many PP&F members had for the reconstituted decree. Although PP&F was likely a major force in enhancing the new roles allotted to families, most members of the group objected as much to the new agreement as they did with previous decrees. As they saw it, family roles and services did increase within the altered decree, but only as long as they supported a community focus. Families supporting Pineland need not apply for consideration.

State officials hailed the new consent agreement as a major step forward. The silence of plaintiffs, however, was deafening. On the day that District Court Judge Gene Carter signed the new consent decree, CAB's chairman, Mickey Boutilier, was "skeptical ... about whether the State will abide by the new decree," adding that "he wouldn't be surprised to see the matter back in court in five to ten years" ("Federal Judge Signs New Pineland Decree," 1994, p. B3). Boutilier was wrong. It wouldn't be that long.

CLOSING UP

Opposition to Pineland's closing continued virtually until the day it shut its doors for good. Some parents continued to speak out publically, while others refused the state's requests for information or approval of their adult children's discharge or community placement (Richardson, 1994a, pp. A1, A7; Vegh, 1995, p. B2). Some parents continued to accuse officials of ignoring their wishes and the best interests of their children by forcing them to accept community placements under threat of a swift closure.

Commissioner Betsy Davenport and Pineland superintendent Paul Peterson defended closing Pineland, first by calling it "the most stable place of last resort " where "much good has been accomplished" (Davenport & Pederson, 1994, p. 4) and then citing their successful placement and cost saving accomplishments. According to the pair, "over 130 people with mental retardation have moved out of Pineland Center and into their home communities in the last two years ... and [are] happier, better adjusted, and manifesting fewer problems than when they lived at Pineland" (p. 4). They also claimed to save over $30 million for capital improvements, and per-year expenses of $160,000 per institutional resident (p. 4).

Despite its claims of successful community placements, the state was again declared out of compliance with their consent obligations. In October 1995, the Federal District Court ordered the state to show evidence of compliance by December 30 or face a contempt charge and daily fines. Specifically, the state failed to achieve sufficient professional-client ratios; develop a person-centered planning manual; and offer adequate crisis services and family supports and resources (Garber, 1995, pp. A1, A9).

In March of the following year, the court agreed to review a negotiated plan, extending the state's deadline for expanding its community services and increasing its funding to improve existing programs. The judge approved the plan but required joint progress reports every 2 months and assured advocates that he would carefully monitor the state's actions.

Concrete signs that Pineland would truly close began to appear. In October 1994, the facility announced its largest layoffs and job eliminations. Announcing that 115 positions would be eliminated, and 90 employees would lose their jobs, Superintendent Rod Bouffard said that "This one really, really hurts in a very big way" (Fellers, 1994, p. A9).

Community providers visited the institution to select among the remaining residents those whom they would admit into their programs. Parental protests subsided and legislative committee meetings where formerly throngs of protestors gathered to oppose Pineland's closing now met in nearly empty hearing rooms. In March 1995, only four family members attended the Legislature's Human Resource Committee meeting (Vegh, 1995, p. B2).

Media attention switched to telling stories about long-time residents successfully leaving Pineland, sometimes escaping never to return like Charlie Wyman in 1928 (Wyman, personal communication, March, 18,

1999); sometimes going reluctantly like 85 year-old, George Giguere, who lived at Pineland for 75 years (Hoose, 1995, pp. G1, G5); and sometimes leaving and getting married like Betty Pinette and her husband, Norman who were admitted to the institution in 1959 and 1972, respectively (Scruggs, 1986, p. 9).

Some employees reminisced about the close relationships they had with residents whom they termed "family," and whom they "fed, bathed, counseled, argued with, and loved" (Vegh, 1994, p. B1). Others talked of taking residents on their family vacations and trips, something they "wouldn't have done ... just for money" (pp. B1, B12). A former supervisor compared the removal of residents from Pineland to taking them from their family's protection and sending them to people who "didn't care about them ... [but] just seemed to have dollar signs in their eyes" (Johns, personal communication, June 28, 1999). Most former employees preferred not to dwell on the negative aspects of Pineland, emphasizing what they considered to be its merits:

> Oh my God, I've seen those pictures. I've heard those stories and that's deplorable. But I think there was certain period of time that it was a nice scene and it was fun. They [residents] had all their services; they had their own laundry, own maintenance, therapists-OT, PT, speech [therapists]. There were nurses, psychiatrists, doctors, and their own clinic. (Wilson, personal communication, April 26, 1999)

Some complained bitterly that they continue to be unfairly maligned by those who never knew what Pineland was really like:

> Sometimes I go to [staff] trainings and I hear things about Pineland and I just get livid. One time ... I heard some young girls and they didn't know anything about Pineland, just what everybody else had told them.... And they had pictures of people just sitting around the institution floor. And then they had pictures of people laughing and they said "this is what happens when they are out in the community".... You know, I've got about a hundred pictures of clients in Pineland laughing. (Johns, personal communication, June 28, 1999)

Former superintendent, Joseph Ferri, however, was unflinching in his recollections, harboring no reservations about the need to close it down: "I can't do it justice in terms of what the conditions were there. It was just disgusting.... It's time for this place [to end]" (Hench, 1996a, p. B12).

Family members reminisced as well, sometimes defiantly, sometimes sadly. Darla Chafin, president of PP&F, noted that Pineland staff helped her daughter feel "like a real person" for the first time. "She was so happy" (Hench, 1996a, p. B12). Sonya White recalled being a 27-year old, overwhelmed and pregnant mother with a 2-year old baby at home, bringing her 7-year old daughter to Pineland, knowing "in my heart that I couldn't care for [her]" (p. 12B).

On April 22, 1996 the last resident, a woman identified only as Ruth Ann, left Pineland, leaving 18 staff members remaining until the closing that was scheduled for June. Eric Gilliam, the last Pineland administrator, was quoted as "feeling a bit of sadness for the employees who have dedicated their lives to the people who lived here, and now some (employees) don't have a place to go" (Hench, 1996b, p. A1). One staff member agreed, remarking that "I'm going to be lost without the clients" while another added that " I learned a lot. Just like the clients blossomed over the years, I did too" (p. A10).

The official closing ceremony was held on Saturday, June 1, 1996 was described as bittersweet, with themes of freedom and change mixed with those of loss and regret. Some in the audience wept. Pineland's Closure Committee placed an engraved stone at Witham Pond, referring to the facility as a "shelter" and a "home" that had become a "wonderful place. … but nobody noticed" (Kimball, 2001, p. 219).

Some in the audience noticed but remained unimpressed. During part of the ceremony, a group of former residents reportedly took over the microphone to represent themselves and define Pineland from their perspective (Kimball, 2001, p. 218). In the end, as it had throughout its history, Pineland symbolized dramatically different things to different people.

CLOSING FACTORS

Despite the controversy surrounding its end, Pineland closed for several reasons. Certainly, large-scale institutionalization was becoming more difficult to defend fiscally, especially as officials were releasing more residents in response to legal mandates, leaving an increasingly empty, deteriorating, and outdated facility badly in need of expensive renovations. More attractive private agencies with lower costs, coupled with heightened federal incentives, offered the state fiscal and legal relief. Money, however, was not the only important reason that Pineland closed. Although Maine and other states have typically underfunded their state institutions, for decades they were willing to initiate, support and expand large-scale institutionalization at considerable cost, even boosting expenses during the most dire economic periods, as long as they believed they had the public's support.

Public and political sentiment toward large-scale institutionalization turned warier following World War II and into the ensuing decades, as scandals revealed overcrowded and abusive conditions, and as organized parent groups such as the National Association for Retarded Children began criticizing state institutions and advocating for facility reforms and community alternatives. By the mid-1960s, media accounts of institutional life, replete with lurid photos, describing Pineland as a "snakepit," shocked ordinary citizens, publically embarrassed public officials, and spawned legal action.

The professional landscape was also changing. Beginning in the late 1960s and accelerating through the 1970s and 1980s, reformist professionals coalesced under the banner of "Normalization," the concept imported from Sweden and Denmark that served as a compelling critique of segregation and discrimination and a call to integrate persons with disabilities into mainstream society. Normalization proponents in Maine, like Albert Anderson, gained prominence and power. Assuming the reins of Maine's fledgling Bureau of Mental Retardation, Anderson also became notorious by advocating for Pineland's closing, galvanizing the opposition, but planting the seed in Maine. Although Anderson became an early casualty in the war over Pineland's fate, he was succeeded by state officials, many of were former staffers and early supporters of his. Following their ascendency to positions of authority, they carefully avoided the subject of closure, but continued Anderson's reform-minded philosophy and policies and initially supported the legal intervention that followed.

The media played an important role in discrediting Pineland, contributing to its eventual demise. Maine Times reporter Hannah Kamber's lurid photographs and graphic descriptions of conditions within the institution and her reporting on Anderson's work in the facility's back wards, followed by John Kerry's follow-up expose' and later the investigative work of Lance Tapley and Pat Nyhan on the Behavioral Stabilization Unit led not only to public awareness about the deplorable conditions within Pineland, but also to questions about whether any new versions of the institution should be considered improvements or were even needed.

Legal action served as the blunt instrument for change, propelling professional and political reforms across the country and in Maine. Class action lawsuits were filed, changing the major issue surrounding institutionalization from one of clinical/medical treatment to that of civil rights, and substituting the authority of medical professionals with that of legal advocates. The lawsuits charged that conditions within state institutions violated residents' constitutional rights, demanding costly reforms, specific discharge policies, alternative community programs, and reduced admissions and enrollments.

By the late 1970s, the movement to close large state institutions gained traction as the plaintiffs in a 1977 Pennsylvania lawsuit, *Haldeman v.*

Pennhurst, transformed a class action from one of institutional reduction and improvement to that of community living and facility closure (Bradley, 1985, p. 84; Fergler & Boyd, 1980). In Maine, the class action lawsuit against Pineland, *Wuori v. Bruns* (later *Wuori v. Zitnay)* gained national notoriety by expanding the court's reach beyond institutional walls, citing the impoverished quality of Pineland's community placements and demanding that higher standards be established for both its institutional care and community-based services.

Dramatic reform in other states did not go unnoticed in Maine. Across the country, professionals were expanding community opportunities for those once deemed capable of only institutional living, nourishing a growing skepticism about the need to institutionalize anyone. When neighboring New Hampshire closed its only institution for persons with intellectual disabilities and nearby Vermont and Rhode Island announced similar policies, Maine officials recognized the growing social and legal advantages of such a decision and were impressed with the prospect of transferring state costs to federal sources and using less expensive private agencies.

The opposing parties in *Wuori* eventually settled, but nowhere was the conflict over the state's required changes and Pineland's eventual fate more clearly dramatized than in the struggles around its ensuing consent decree. And no one person was more influential and infuriating during those legal, political, moral, and fiscal battles than the first court master, David Gregory. Despite his relatively brief tenure, Gregory assumed the role of activist, applying enormous legal pressure, and pushing all parties further than they wanted to go. Gregory, like Anderson, became an early casualty of the closure wars, but despite his relatively quick departure, Gregory shaped the face of the conflict and the subsequent changes to come, making Pineland's eventual closing inevitable.

Perhaps the least discussed, appreciated and documented factor propelling changes in the way persons with intellectual disabilities were viewed and treated was the vocal and vigorous advocacy of persons with disabilities. The active involvement of this group as an organized entity was new, although individual protests at Pineland were not. Resident resistance within the institution began as soon as Pineland opened and continued throughout its history, reflecting a rich tradition of ongoing individual resistance to institutionalization. Escapes were well documented, some of which were carried out by those who merely wanted to return to their family, disappear into the societal woodwork, and remain anonymous and undetected. Other actions demonstrated more anger and resentment, resulting in arson and/or other types of property destruction, and fueling professional characterizations of them as societal deviants. In the 1930s, however, the dramatic stories of former residents like Eleanor

Chase Libby began to emerge, followed later by the detailed accounts of Charles Wyman, reflecting defiance, assertiveness, and wile, and presenting the public with an image of Pineland residents that was far different than that offered by institutional officials.

In the early 1980s, Maine's disability rights movement took center stage as an organized collective, becoming a vocal and influential participant in the Pineland debates and final resolution, counteracting the influence of proinstitutional forces, and representing people who in the past had been largely excluded from such debates. The lead organization was the Maine Association of Handicapped People (MAHP), an organization that waged a well publicized campaign to expose what it considered restrictive and abusive conditions within Pineland's Behavioral Stabilization Unit (BSU) and argue against reestablishing Pineland as a viable therapeutic setting. This effort dramatically illustrated that increasing numbers of people with disabilities had found their voice and could use it effectively in their own behalf.

CHAPTER 10

CONTEMPORARY CHANGE AND CONTINUING LEGACY

MUCH HAS CHANGED

"There are no more imbeciles in America; no more morons or idiots; no more feebleminded of any type or degree. We eliminated them all" (Hayman, 1998, p. 7). Or so it seems. Whether we truly have changed our minds about the nature and importance of human difference or merely modified our language, there are signs that important changes have occurred in the way we perceive and treat persons with intellectual disabilities in the United States.

State institutional enrollments for persons with intellectual disabilities have dropped dramatically across the country from a peak of 194, 650 in 1967 to 34, 670 in 2007 (Larson, Scott, Salmi, & Lakin, 2008, p. 329). Between 1960 and 2004, 174 public institutions or residential units of 16 or more people closed (Prouty, Smith, & Lakin, 2005).

Discharges have also accelerated in nursing homes, the latter showing declining enrollments from 42,164 in 1988 to 29,021 in 2007, from 16% to 7% (Scott, Larson, & Lakin, 2008, p. 242). In addition, Alaska has announced its intent to become the first state to eliminate nursing homes

Voices of Pineland: Eugenics, Social Reform, and the Legacy of "Feeblemindedness" in Maine, pp. 245–256

as a placement for people with intellectual disabilities (Braddock, Hemp, Rizzolo, Parish, & Pomerantz, 2002, pp. 7, 11).

Salmi, Scott, Webster, Larson, and Lakin, (2010, p. 168) called the period from 1988-2008, the "generation of community living" because it showed the greatest net increases in smaller community living arrangements and largest decreases in institutional placements in history. During that time, people living in settings of 6 people or fewer grew from 78,173 (29%) to 321, 025 (73%). That was also the period when residential settings of tree or fewer people encompassed 47% of those living in residential situations with intellectual or developmental disabilities (p. 168).

Coinciding with the decline in larger institutional residences has been a general increase in community living arrangements and services of all types. Spending for institutional services reversed and began declining in 1991 (Rizzolo, Hemp, Braddock, & Pomerantz-Essley, 2004, p. 15). In 1989 public spending for community services exceed institutional funding nationwide for the first time (Braddock et al., 2002, p. 20). By 2002, states were spending an average of 78% of their MR/DD budgets on community services and supports, with more than a dozen states spending more than 90% (excluding nursing facility funding), and only Mississippi spending less than 50% (Rizzolo et al., 2004, p. 15). Within this changing pattern of services, the fastest growing areas includes individual and family supports, consisting of supported living/personal assistance, family supports, and supported employment. In addition, smaller, more individualized community living settings were increasing dramatically.

Funding for family supports (ironically, a proposal first made by Walter Fernald around 1920), including vouchers, reimbursements, and/or direct cash payments to either families or support providers, advanced 85% between 1996-2000 (Rizzolo et al., 2004, p. 28).

Employment initiatives have been enacted to assist persons with intellectual disabilities find community work. One approach called supported employment gained widespread popularity through 1980s, offering job coaching and other supports to employees with disabilities as they performed typical community jobs. Participants in these programs continued to increase after 1988, rising from 11% of those in day and work programs to 19%, in 1993, reaching 24% by 2002 (Rizzolo et al., 2002, p. 27). Between 1996 and 2000, spending on supported, community employment increased 33% and the number of work placements increased 22% (Braddock et al., 2000, p. 31). At the same time, segregated, sheltered employment was eliminated as a legitimate employment outcome by the state-federal vocational rehabilitation system.

Research shows that people with intellectual disabilities, including those classified as "severely and multiply disabled," live successfully in community settings with assistance if necessary, prefer such situations to institutions (Cone, 1998; Gilson, 1998; Ruef & Turnbull, 2002; Shapiro, 1994; Stefan, 2001; Taylor, Bogden, & Lutfiyya, 1995), and benefit measurably from these living arrangements (Craig & McCarver, 1984; Larson & Lakin, 1991).

These national trends are well illustrated in Maine. Pineland remains closed and the state has established a solid reputation for its deinstitutionalization efforts, ranking the highest of all states in reducing its public institutional census and joining eight other states and the District of Columbia in having no state institution for individuals with intellectual disabilities (Braddock et al., 2002, pp. 6–7). The Coleman Institute reports of 2002 and 2004 characterize Maine as establishing an exemplary record of community services, indicating that the state is one of only nine others that spends over 90% of its MR/DD resources on assisting persons with intellectual disabilities live in noninstitutional situations consisting of six or fewer residents (Rizzolo et al., 2004, p. 22). Maine is viewed as a national leader in supported community living and personal assistance, spending over $3,000,000 per 100,00 citizens, far exceeding the national average of $605,896 ((Braddock et al., 2002, pp. 27, 32–33).

CONTINUING LEGACY OF FEEBLEMINDEDNESS

Despite such changes, it would be a mistake to conclude that Pineland's history has little relevance to the present and future. A decade ago, the Supreme Court concluded that despite improvements, "discrimination against individuals with disabilities continues to be a serious and pervasive social problem," in part emanating from a history of societal confinement and isolation (*Olmstead v. L.C,* as cited in Stefan, 2001, pp. 110–111). This conclusion still applies and is reflected in a myriad of ways from continuing segregation in various types of institutional/treatment facilities to abysmally low rates of employment, high poverty, and inadequate community housing and assistance. Thus, despite notably improved community opportunities and services, the legacy of feeblemindedness stubbornly persists in varied and subtle forms, continuing to influence our perceptions and treatment of persons with intellectual disabilities, many of whom are technically living in community settings but often remain isolated and marginalized.

Overall, more than 34,000 people still reside in state institutions for persons with intellectual disabilities (Larson, Scott, Salmi, & Lakin, 2008). As of 2002, 32,333 individuals live in private settings of 16 or more residents, and 30,308 in nursing homes (Rizzolo et al., 2004, p. 3). Fourteen percent of the total U.S. working population is comprised of persons with disabilities who, despite new employment approaches, have a rate of unemployment of about 65% as opposed to around 25% for the general population (Employment of People With Intellectual and Development Disabilities, 2010; Yamaki & Fujiura (2002, p. 136). Those with intellectual/developmental disabilities fared even worse, showing an unemployment rate of 72% (p. 136). Previously cited advances in supported community employment and a diminished emphasis on segregated workshops as legitimate vocational outcomes have leveled off and may be reversing while the poverty rate among people with disabilities remains significantly higher than that of the general population (Employment of People With Intellectual and Developmental Disabilities, 2010).

States vary dramatically in the extent to which they support community access and equity for those with intellectual disabilities. Between 1996 and 2000, all states except Missouri and North Dakota reduced their institutional populations, some states by as much as 86%, others by less than 15% (Braddock et al., 2002, p. 6). While nine states and the District of Columbia have closed all of their state institutions for persons with intellectual disabilities, 13 states have closed none (p. 6). In some states, based solely on the developmental disability label, persons may still be restricted from voting, marrying, and/or parenting. Involuntary sterilization, though rarely applied, remains a legal option in some states (including Maine) if approved by a guardian (Folsom, 1983, pp. 38–39; Pfieffer, 1994, p. 495).

Following Pineland's closing in 1996, columnist Roberta Scruggs (1996, p. C5) exclaimed, "legal battles notwithstanding, Pineland was emptied by the once revolutionary idea that mentally retarded people can make choices about their own lives" (p. C5). Institutional critics might wonder, however, if closing Pineland truly reflects such a dramatically changing discourse about persons with intellectual disabilities, especially since proposals to re-institutionalize this group persist. Even in a reportedly exemplary state like Maine, civic and professional leaders continue to reinvent new and improved versions of Pineland, using stories and rationales that sound eerily familiar. Often obscured by contemporary scientific, technical, economic and humanitarian language, such proposals result in the same ending: societal separation and congregate living.

In 2000, Maine's largest philanthropy, the Libra Foundation, made a remarkable proposal to re-open Pineland to 125 persons with intellectual and developmental disabilities. Libra is a 300 million dollar philanthropic organization that was created by the late Intel heiress, Elizabeth Noyes. Foundation officials proposed to renovate the old Pineland campus at an estimated cost of 40 million dollars, transforming it into a small business park that would also offer recreation, conference, and education facilities, and include a halfway house for people with "mental retardation, mental illness, and behavioral handicaps" (Williams, 2000, p. A10). Libra's president, Owen Wells, described a rejuvenated Pineland as having "spectacular potential ... to meet the needs of the disabled people, both physically and mentally, here in Maine" (p. A10). Ironically, the twenty-first century planners used virtually the same arguments to support their idea as their twentieth century predecessors, proposing to "welcome back" individuals who had been "exiled" from Maine to out-of-state institutions (p. A10). Recall that early in the twentieth century, Maine citizens had been sent to Walter Fernald's Massachusetts facility before the Maine School for Feeble-Minded was built.

Libra officials intended to not only renovate Pineland's buildings and grounds, but also its tarnished reputation, reassuring skeptics that the facility's history was honorable According to Wells, Pineland's history is:

> nothing to be ashamed of in terms of what Pineland was for many years.... Why should all of us shrink from that because of something all of us neglected for a certain period of time?" We all do things that are bad. We don't necessarily try to escape from it. It's part of us .... The history is good. We think it's a history that ought to be acknowledged.
>
> Pineland was "a wonderful farm operation and ... wonderful facility," adding that the renovated campus is place where "beefalo ... will continue to graze," where "hundreds of acres will continue to be hayed," where "fields will be tilled and planted." (Williams, 2000, p. A10)

On the current website of what is now known as Pineland Farms, is a page titled "Pineland's History" that has been compressed into a one-paragraph narrative that includes the following description:

> Pineland Center in New Gloucester, Maine was established in 1908 to serve as a home for the mentally handicapped of Maine. At the time of its official closing in 1996, Pineland consisted of a 28 building campus and 1,600-plus acres. A large part of the acreage consisted of farmland which at one time had been cultivated to sustain the needs of the center's staff and residents. (Pineland's History, n.d.)

In this picture, there exist no eugenics, segregation, sterilization, abuse, or controversy; there are no references to "idiots, imbeciles, morons, feebleminded or defectives." All have been exorcised. What remains for future generations of visitors to contemplate about this historical site is the sanitized and bucolic, Pineland Farms.

In a book that Libera commissioned, its author, Richard Kimball, was asked "to honor Pineland's history," leading Kimball to ask if it is possible to "honestly honor Pineland's past even if part of that past seemed less than honorable" (Kimball, 2001, p. vx). The author proceeds to document Pineland's past as mixed—sometimes very good, and sometimes "appalling" and selects as an epitaph a quote from a former employee for summing up the various perspectives on the state facility: "Pineland did everything bad that every other institution in this country did. It did everything good that every other institution did. Pineland was a product of its time. It needed to be and it needed to end" (p. 239).

It is certainly important to analyze our history and understand that Pineland was a complex organization, a product of a rapidly changing and fearful society. It is also important to remember that the institution was continuously defined and re-defined over time by distinct constituencies for numerous reasons having little to do with human intelligence. Using the phrase "honoring Pineland's history." however, is an unfortunate and misleading way of characterizing such an analysis. This is certainly not a phrase that comes to mind as other states begin responding to the demands of former residents, legal advocates, and professional supporters to apologize for what occurred in their state institutions; not merely to describe and certainly not to honor this history.

In May, 2002, Governor Mark Warner of the Commonwealth of Virginia, home of the infamous Carrie Buck/*Buck v. Bell* case, apologized publically for that state's "shameful effort" in sterilizing Ms. Buck and 7,3324 others from 1924-1980. Later that year, Oregon's governor expressed remorse for "the misdeeds that resulted from widespread misconceptions, ignorance and bigotry" (Stern, 2005, p. 1). Soon after, the governors of California, North Carolina and South Carolina issued public apologies (p. 1). While these officials recognize that many good people worked in state facilities, many good deeds were done there, and many similar institutions operated throughout the country, they also understand that virtuous intentions, kind actions, and general culpability do not exculpate states from acknowledging their injustices.

One of the most forgotten, or least mentioned, facts about Pineland was its central role in sterilizing Maine residents, including individuals transferred from other institutions, such as state asylums and reformatories, for the surgery. Of the 326 eugenic sterilizations documented in Maine, 58% were carried out at Pineland. Of that total, 88 operations (27%) were performed in the state after 1950 and eight (2.45%) after 1960, long after the idea of inherited feeblemindedness was discredited and following the horrific genocide in Europe where the logical extension of eugenic rhetoric became evident to the world.

Contrary to the epitaph cited earlier and the sentiment expressed by some Pineland supporters, it is both insufficient and inaccurate to argue that what occurred at Pineland happened everywhere else, serving as an explanation for our actions. Sterilization, for example, was not inevitable.

There was always some opposition to the surgery and enough uncertainty surrounding its validity that nearby Massachusetts and Rhode Island, along with nine other states, never passed sterilization laws and have no record of coercively sterilizing any of their citizens (Largent, 2008, p. 72). While incidences of eugenic sterilization in Maine were muted somewhat by questions surrounding its constitutionality and the opposition of the Catholic Church, other religious groups, and a few dissident physicians, even relatively modest numbers of surgeries should be considered gross miscarriages of justice and officially acknowledged as such. Perhaps, therefore, Maine should add its name to the growing list of states who are acknowledging publically and apologizing officially for harm they inflicted on a targeted group of their citizens.

Libra's plans have produced a new, vitalized campus complex, although it did not lead to the reassignment of people with disabilities there, largely due to opposition from advocacy and professional groups and a lack of support from state officials. In this instance we appear to have learned from our history, but institutional proposals in Maine did not end there.

In 2004, Spring Harbor Hospital, part of the Maine Medical Center which is by far the largest medical care organization in the state, announced the opening of a new "100 bed psychiatric facility" with an inpatient unit for about 40 children, ages 4–21, who have been diagnosed with multiple disabilities, including "psychiatric illness, autism and mental retardation" ("Spring Harbor: New place, New Autism Unit," 2004, pp. A1; Walsh, 2004, B1). This facility was built with state and private support and, like Libra, is defended as a way to serve Maine people within the state and reduce the number of those who are sent elsewhere for acute specialized care at a cost of $1,300 per day (McPherson, 2004, p. A9; Walsh, 2004, pp. B1, B12). Spring Harbor proponents have argued that an intensive, specialized facility is necessary to temporarily segregate and treat those who have the most disruptive disorders:

> This (autism) is a complex diagnosis to treat … because these youth may also be experiencing speech and language delays, major sensitivity to transitions, and learning issues, all of which need to be taken into account, in addition to the psychiatric illness.
>
> Certainly this population requires a lot more one-to-one [direct professional-client contact] … and behavioral intervention and care than other patients Spring Harbor treats. It is Spring Harbor's intent to … establish a more complete continuum of care that will allow youth to receive treatment in the least restrictive level possible. ("Spring Harbor: New Place, New Autism Unit," 2004, pp. A1, A5)

The article describes the newly constructed hospital as one of "warmth, comfort, safety, and clinical excellence" (Spring Harbor: New Place, New

Autism Unit, 2004, p. A1) that has "a playground, another courtyard with a baseball diamond and basketball court and a gym" (p. A5), and that sits on dozens of acres, abutting a game preserve. Constructed at a cost of $27 million, the facility was "built almost entirely by Maine contractors" according to the chair of the hospital board (p. A5).

Proposing a facility for people described as medically impaired, severely deficient, and/or behaviorally disordered, and describing it as an idyllic therapeutic environment that is economically beneficial to the surrounding community are hauntingly familiar themes from Pineland's history. Although proposals and facilities such as Libra's and Spring Harbor's have diminished with each generation and are applied to a receding population of people, they illustrate what some historians have linked with the ongoing professional needs and interests of technical experts, coupled with the lingering and latent effects of eugenic devaluation.

Consider also the most recent case of institutionalization of a small number of persons with disabilities where three young men from Maine, ages 26, 28, and 33 were placed against their wishes in nursing homes in Maine and Massachusetts because of state budget cuts, the men's deficiencies described as "severe limitations of speech and mobility" and a lack of available residential alternatives (Russell, 2010, p. B2). The ring of historical familiarity is only enhanced when we learn that the men are classified as having cerebral palsy, a developmental disability that once landed people in Pineland. Three people is a very small number and certainly not indicative of a rising trend. In fact, the national trend is in the opposite direction. Recall, however, that around 30,000 individuals with intellectual and developmental disabilities remain in nursing facilities, many of whom, like these three men, are neither old nor ill (two conditions frequently cited as legitimate reasons for such placements).

Unlike previous generations of Pineland residents, the three have access to legal weapons and have sued Maine's Department of Health and Human Services for violating their rights under the Americans with Disabilities Act. They allege that they have been "segregated in nursing homes where they do not receive even minimally adequate training, habilitation, or support services required by law" (Russell, 2010, p. B2). According to their lawsuit, the men "strongly desire to leave the nursing facility and live in a setting that is more integrated in the community" (p. B2). On man, Eric Reeves, said he aspired to be a productive member of society, "and this place is not conducive to that" (p. B2). Another of the plaintiffs, Jake Van Meter, stated emphatically: "I do not want to live here for the rest of my life" (p. B2).

The legacy of feeblemindedness inheres in current practices, proposals, and policies not because we still believe in eugenic ideas and methods, but less tangibly and more enduringly, because we continue to cling to remnants of the assumptions and images that the movement spawned. These ideas, images, and activities persist as reconstituted rationales for social separation and rights restrictions, permeating our social institutions and collective attitudes, echoing Rothman's warning about how difficult it is to change the entrenched and efficient societal practice of removing and congregating troublesome people.

Only thoroughly discredited and denounced since the 1970s, eugenic sentiment firmly established the problem as individual pathology plaguing society and the solutions as individual control and/or care (Carey, 2003, pp. 412–413; Largent, 2008, pp. 138–140; Trent, 1994, p. 4). Eugenic products, including mental testing, segregation, eugenic sterilization, marriage restrictions and discriminatory immigration quotas, embodied what was considered enlightened social progress, a vision that inspired and attracted a large international and interdisciplinary group of scholars, scientists, physicians, wealthy philanthropists, and government leaders who supported and produced massive studies from eugenic centers in Europe and America (Gallagher, 2000, pp. 2–4). Catalogs on human heredity were assembled and infused into schools and university curricula in biology, social work, medicine, and public health and disseminated by churches, patriotic organizations, charitable and welfare organizations (p. 2).

Whether state institutions or facilities like Spring Harbor or nursing homes are needed continues to be debated across the country. Such proposals are made with the best intentions of meeting what experts define as the needs of troubled individuals, are defended as short term, therapeutic for particularly challenging people, and necessary for healthier families, schools, and/or communities. Segregating persons with intellectual and/or developmental disabilities for whatever reasons, however, can never again be discussed in a historical vacuum, considered uncritically, or accepted as self-evidently therapeutic. Gallagher (1999, p. 4) reminds us, disowning our eugenic past requires that we first acknowledge and confront it, recognizing "the enduring power of research findings and the consensus of experts over our perceptions of other people's problems."

The legacy of "feeblemindedness" will likely persist until we reverse our tendency to embed our ideas about who is good and bad, high and low, in the world of nature rather than society (Nourse, 2008, p. 14), changing the stories we tell about people who do not measure up and the assumptions we make about those who do not fit in. Harvard law professor, Martha Minow (1990, p. 80), has observed that the social and physical architecture of our lives was developed and operates without certain people in mind, so that we incorrectly assume their exclusion is natural and just. The answer to social access and equity is not more scientifically sound treatments, no matter how well intentioned or closely monitored they may be. As Burton Blatt concludes:

> Mental retardation is an invented disease, an untrue and unnecessary story about a large group of people ... [that] itself requires the study of our prejudiced inventions about certain people who have loose wires, or who read poorly.... As nothing good obtains from such untrue stories, the treatments for mental retardation are unnecessary inventions and consequently are always abuses.
>
> How can we make sure that we tell "true" true stories about people? Any intervention based on the premise that a person can't learn anything ... that a person's condition is hopeless, or that mental retardation is hopeless ... or genetic (in the same way that Tay-Sachs disease is genetic) are either not at all or not sufficiently true and thus can destroy people.... And abuses are prevented when individuals are given opportunities to contribute to and not merely to cope with society. Abuses are prevented when more of us behave as if people can learn, but even more so when we vigorously support each person's right to his fullest development possible; irrespective of the course of his life or his actual contributions to society. It is with that belief in human educability as well as in our common relatedness and natural rights as human beings that people find ways to prevent abuses. Such stories truly prevent abuse. (Blatt, 1981, pp. 118–122)

Considering persons with intellectual disabilities as first and foremost citizens, and reversing the negative stories and images we have created around them will not be easy. In Maine, now considered an exemplary state, one need only recall Pineland's incredible resiliency, the vigorous and widespread opposition to its closing, the extended need for federal oversight of the state's consent agreement (which finally ended in March, 2010), and the continuing appearance of segregating proposals and policies in which Pineland is re-invented for particular people under various guises and new rationales.

Trent (1994, p. 271)) has observed that a society preoccupied with materialism, production, and competition tends to tell stories about those considered intellectually/developmentally disabled primarily in terms of mindlessness and dysfunction, even while espousing a focus on mental acceleration. Moreover, whatever optimism we may claim for some may not apply to others. In this regard, Minow (1990, p. 215) has suggested that if we hope to achieve equity and inclusion for all, we must go beyond a rights perspective and the legal advocacy that has propelled us thus far. Although a rights-based approach demands that institutionalization be based on the presumption that some people by virtue of their individual traits really are different than others, it prompts an emphasis on discovering who is "really disabled" and should be separated out, and who should be invited into society. In this way segregation, social exclusion, rights restrictions and personal vulnerability continue for some individuals who are defined as the most disabled or most challenging. In addition, securing people's rights without the material and social supports to exercise them, offers only the illusion of inclusion, masking ongoing devaluation and exclusion (Carey, 2009, p. 31).

Assuming a perspective she terms "making *all* the difference," Minow (1990, p. 11) describes human difference not as "the private, internal problem of each individual," requiring some sort of specialized treatment, but a "pervasive feature of communal life" that should be addressed by remaking our social institutions so that they include a wider variety of citizens, students, and employees. Such a social framework means adopting a strong and underlying presumption of human commonality an idea that is not exactly new or radical. In 1866, Samuel Gridley Howe, one of the early Amerian pioneers of the residential school, warned:

> Our people have a passion for public institutions.... They hastily build a great showy building and gather within its walls a crowd of persons with like condition ... and organize a community where everything is run by clock and steam.
>
> Wherever there must be separation of the sexes, isolation from society, absence of true family relation, and monotony of life, there must come evils of various kinds which no watchfulness can prevent and physician can cure.... As much as may be, surround insane and excitable persons with sane people and ordinary influences; vicious children with virtuous people and virtuous influences.... As far as possible they should be treated just as ordinary persons, our equals and friends, are treated. (as cited in Wolfensberger, 1975, pp. 67-68)

Attesting to the changes in thinking that may be required, most of us still find it nearly impossible to see commonalities between persons of widely different physical and/or cognitive abilities, or perceive as typical the needs of people like those considered appropriate for settings like Pineland, Spring Harbor or nursing homes. This, despite the evidence that many individuals classified as "multiply and or severely impaired" demonstrate individuality and capacity, and benefit measurably from typical educational and vocational activities and community participation (Goode, 1994; Linneman, 2001; Nazeer, 2006).

Perhaps Pineland's first court master, David Gregory's simple relational aphorism will enable us to see that much of the human differences we posit is more contrived than we imagine. Gregory came to the job with little background in disability issues. After immersing himself in the subject, he concluded that despite all the political rhetoric, diagnostic labels, and financial arguments, no one belonged at Pineland: "For every person in Pineland Center, there is someone with the same general characteristics and problems outside living a better life. ("*Coping* Interview: David Gregory Speaks on Pineland," 1985, pp. 6–7).

Embedded within Minow's and Gregory's perspective is the daunting challenge of acknowledging and reversing our continuing tendency to identify social inequality as biological inevitability especially during times when public uncertainty and fear run high. Author-biologist, Stephen J. Gould (1996, pp. 60–61), eloquently warns:

> We pass through this world but once. Few tragedies can be more extensive than the stunting of life, few injustices deeper than the denial of opportunity to strive, or even to hope, by a limit imposed from without but falsely identified as lying within.... We inhabit a world of human differences and predilections, but the extrapolation of these facts to theories of rigid limits is ideology. (pp. 60–61)

In calling attention to our continuing policies of social separation and exclusion for some groups, disability activist Harriet Johnson (2003) asks simply, "why not make lock-up the exception" (p. 64). Making lock-up the exception is one option. Eliminating it altogether as Samuel Gridley Howe suggested in 1866, is another.

REFERENCES

$210,000 hospital being built for feebleminded. (1931, January 18,). *Portland Sunday Telegram and Sunday Press Herald*, p. D2.

A few interesting tales of lower Casco Bay. (1927, March 27). *Portland Sunday Gazette and Sunday Press Herald,* p. A1.

An institution of great value. (n.d.). In *Clippings Pownal State School, 1909–1946,* 1989, 22.

Annual Report of the Consumer Advisory Board. (1991).

Annual Report of the Consumer Advisory Board. (1993).

Annual Report of the Maine State School for Feeble-Minded (1920). Pownal, ME: Pineland Hospital and Training Center.

Annual Report of the Pineland Hospital and Training Center. (1960–61). Pownal, ME: Pineland Hospital and Training Center.

Annual Report of the Pineland Hospital and Training Center. (1963). Pownal, ME: Pineland Hospital and Training Center:

Annual Report of the Pineland Hospital and Training Center. (1964). Pownal, ME: Pineland Hospital and Training Center.

Annual Report of the Pineland Hospital and Training Center. (1965). Pownal, ME: Pineland Hospital and Training Center.

Annual Report of the Pineland Hospital and Training Center. (1966). Pownal, ME: Pineland Hospital and Training Center.

Annual Report of the Pineland Hospital and Training Center. (1967). Pownal, ME: Pineland Hospital and Training Center.

Annual Report of the Pineland Hospital and Training Center. (1968). Pownal, ME: Pineland Hospital and Training Center.

Annual Report of the Pineland Hospital and Training Center. (1969). Pownal, ME: Pineland Hospital and Training Center.

Annual Report of the Pineland Hospital and Training Center. (1970). Pownal, ME: Pineland Hospital and Training Center.

Annual Report of the Pineland Hospital and Training Center. (1971). Pownal, ME: Pineland Hospital and Training Center.

Annual Report of the Pineland Hospital and Training Center. (1972). Pownal, ME: Pineland Hospital and Training Center.

Annual Report of the Pineland Hospital and Training Center. (1973). Pownal, ME: Pineland Hospital and Training Center.

Annual Report of the Superintendent Pownal State School. (1939). Pownal, ME: Pownal State School.

Annual Report of the Superintendent, Pownal State School. (1951). Pownal, ME: Pownal State School.

Annual Report of the Superintendent, Pownal State School. (1953). Pownal, ME: Pownal State School.

Annual Report of the Superintendent, Pownal State School. (1954). Pownal, ME: Pownal State School.

Annual Report of the Superintendent, Pownal State School. (1955). Pownal, ME: Pownal State School.

Annual Report of the Superintendent, Pownal State School. (1957). Pownal, ME: Pownal State School.

Ashe, W. H., Martin, J. T., & Thrall, C. L. (2004). Living in the community: options for people with complex medical needs. *TASH Connections, 30,* 3/4, 27–30.

Austin, P. (1972, February 8). Senator charges sexual promiscuity at Pineland. *Portland Press Herald*, p. A24.

Babcock, R. H., Frenette, Y., Scontras, C., & Eagan, E. (1995). Work and workers in the industrial age. In R.W. Judd, E.A. Churchill, & J.W. Eastman (Eds.). *Maine. The pine tree state from prehistory to the present* (pp. 448-479). Orono, ME: University of Maine Press.

Barondess, J. A. (1998). Care of the medical ethos: Reflections on social Darwinism, racial hygiene, and the holocaust. *Annals of Internal Medicine, 129,* 891-898.

Barry, W. R. (1980, November). The shameful story of Malaga Island. *Downeast Magazine*, 53-58, 83-84.

Bassuck, E., & Gerson, S. (1978). Deinstitutionalization and mental health services. *Scientific American, 238,* 46-53.

Bateman, L. C. (1912, November 9). Maine's home for feeble-minded. *Lewiston Journal*, Illustrated Magazine Section, p. 8.

Behavior Stabilization Unit, Pineland Center. (1985, August 30). New Gloucester, ME: Pineland Center.

Becker, H. (1973). Labeling theory reconsidered. In *Outsiders: Studies in the sociology of deviance* (pp. 177-208). New York, NY: The Free Press.

Bishop McCarthy urges parishioners to protest. (1941, April 14). *Lewiston Daily Sun*, p. A1.

Black, E. (2003). *War against the weak. Eugenics and America's campaign to create a master race*. New York, NY: Four Walls Eight Windows.

Blatt, B. (1981). How to destroy lives by telling stories. In *In and out of mental retardation* (pp. 115-135). Baltimore, MD: University Park Press.

Blatt, B., & Kaplan, F. (1966). *Christmas in purgatory*. Boston, MA: Allyn & Bacon.

Bogdan, R., & Taylor, S. J. (1994). *The social meaning of mental retardation. Two life stories*. New York, NY: Teachers College Press.

Booth, W. (1988, October 28). Other voices. *Maine Times, Section 1,* p. A13.

Bowman, P. W. (1956). *Memorandum to His Excellency Governor Edmund S. Muskie.* New Gloucester, ME: Pownal State School.

Bowman takes over. (1953, April 4). *Portland Press Herald*, p. A1.

Braddock, D., Hemp, R., Rizzolo, M., Parish, S., & Pomerantz A. (2002). *State of the states in development disabilities.* Boulder, CO: University of Colorado Coleman Institute for Cognitive Disabilities and Department of Psychiatry.

Bradley, V. (1985). Implementation of court and consent decrees: Some current lessons. In R. H. Bruinicks & K. C. Lakin (Eds.), *Living and learning in the least restrictive environment* (pp. 67–80). Baltimore, MD: Paul H. Brookes.

Bradley, T. (1987, March 11). Pineland prison plan raises concerns. *Portland Press Herald*, p. A17.

Breed, A. (2006). No longer a reproach: The story of Malaga Island. In H. H. Price & G. Talbot (Eds.), *Maine's visible Black history.* (pp. 69-74). Gardiner, ME: Tilbury House.

Bruinius, H. (2006). *Better for all the world. The secret history of forced sterilization and America's quest for racial purity.* New York, NY: Knopf.

Brunnelle, J. (1972, April 9). Pineland "normalization" better termed humanization. *Maine Sunday Telegram*, p. A20.

Buck v. Bell, 274 U.S. 200 (1927).

Bureau director defends BSU. (1985, July/August). *Coping, 8,* 4.

Care of feeble-minded big problem for Maine. (1914). Unknown newspaper, p. A2. In *Clippings Pownal State School, 1909-1946,* 1989. New Gloucester, ME: Pineland Center.

Carey, A. C. (2003). Beyond the medical model: A reconsideration of "feeblemindedness," citizenship, and eugenic relations. *Disability and Society, 18,* 411–430.

Carey, A. C. (2009). *On the margins of citizenship: Intellectual disability and civil rights in twentieth century America.* Philadeplhia: PA: Temple University Press.

Carrier, P. (1991a, February 17). Lack of alternatives keeps Pineland open. *Portland Sunday Telegram,* pp. B1, B10.

Carrier, P. (1991b, April 12). Mental health chief wants Pineland shut within 5 years. *Portland Press Herald*, pp. A1, A10.

Castles, K. (2004). "Nice, average Americans": Post-war parent groups and the defense of the normal family. In S. Noll & J. W. Trent (Eds.), *Mental retardation in America: A historical reader* (pp. 351–370) New York, NY: New York University Press.

Charges of neglect at Pownal State School to be filed. Connolly says (1938, March 6,). *Sunday Telegram and Sunday Press Herald*, pp. A1, A7.

Clippings Pownal State School, 1909–1946. (1989). New Gloucester, ME: Pineland Center.

Colburn, A. F,, Kilbreth, E. H., Fortinsky, R. H., & McGuire, C. A. (1986). *The impact of the home and community-based Medicaid waiver for the mentally retarded in Maine.* Portland, ME: Human Services Development Institute, University of Southern Maine.

Concern rises over violations. (1989, March 31). *Maine Times*, p. 2.

Condemn home for feeble-minded. (1913, January 28). *Daily Eastern Argus*, p. A1.

Condon, R. H., Eastman, J. W., & Allin, L. C. (1995). Maine in depression and war, 1929-1945. In R. W. Judd, E. A. Churchill, & J. W. Eastman (Eds.), *Maine. The pine tree state from prehistory to the present* (pp. 506–529). Orono, ME: University of Maine Press.

Cone, A. A. (1998) Self-advocacy in the United states: Historical overview and future vison. In P. Wehman & J. Kregel (Eds.), *More than a job* (pp. 25–46). Baltimore, MD: Brookes.

Connor, S. E. (1937, January 6,). $2,000,000 spent on Maine institutions-does not eliminate waiting lists-operating costs up. *Lewiston Sun-Journal* (Annual Review Edition), p. A16.

Connor, S.E. (1944, September 16). State must provide more room at Pownal. *Lewiston Evening Journal*, pp. A1-A2.

Consumer Advisory Board v. Glover et al., No. 91-321-P-C (D. Maine, September 28, 1994).

Coping. (1985a, July/August) p. 2.

Coping Interview: David Gregory speaks on Pineland (1985, November). *Coping, 9,* 6-7.

Court battle over bride begins. (1937, February 13). *Portland Evening Express*, pp. A1-A2.

Cowan charges abuse at state insane hospital. (1944, December 30). *Lewiston Evening Journal*, pp. A1, A5.

Cox, P. (1985). Opinions. What is acceptable for a retarded person? *Maine Times*, p. 12.

Craig, E. M., & McCarver, R. B. (1984). Community placement and adjustment of deinsititutionalized client: Issues and findings. In N. Ellis & N. Bray (Eds.), *International review of research in mental retardation* (pp. 99–152). Orlando, FL: Academic Press.

Cuts to put Pineland in tough spot. (1991, January 1). *Lewiston Sun Journal*, p. A28.

Davenport, B., & Pederson, P. (1994, May 7). Families a part of Pineland shift. *Your Views*, 4

Davidian, G. (1989, October 29). Pineland accord coming up short. *Maine Sunday Telegram*, pp. A1, A10.

Davies, S. P. (1959). *The mentally retarded in society*. New York, NY: Columbia University Press.

Death revives questions (1986, March 21). *Maine Times*, p. 9.

Degler, C. N. (1991). *In search of human nature*. New York, NY: Oxford University Press.

Deutsch, A. (1949). *The mentally ill in America* (2nd ed.). New York, NY: Columbia University Press.

Don't close Pineland. (1992, December 17). *Brunswick Times Record* [editorial], p. A6.

Dowbiggin, I. R. (1997). *Keeping America sane. Psychiatry and eugenics in the United States and Canada, 1880–1940*. Ithaca, NY: Cornell University Press.

Dr. N. S. brands Connolly's charges as being absolutely false. (1938, March 7). *Portland Press Herald*, p. A1.

Dr. S. E. Vosburgh, Supt. Of Pownal dies (1937, Dec 24). *Lewiston Evening Journal*, pp. A1-A2.

Dr. Tyson opposes Sterilization Bill—No Opposition to Juvenile Court. (1931, March 12). In *Clippings Pownal State School, 1909–1946*, 1989, 275.

Dr.Vosburgh describes work of state school at Pownal. (n.d.). In *Clippings Pownal State School, 1909–1946*, 1989, p. 392

DuBrule, D. (1999). How the state of Maine destroyed a "different" community. *Island Journal*, 48–53, 90–91.

Edgerton, R (1967). *The cloak of competence*. Berkeley, CA: University of California at Berkeley Press.

Irresponsible policy [Editorial]. (1992, December 9). *Lewiston Sun-Journal*, p. A4.

Educating boys in farm work featured at Pownal State School. (1943, January 2). *Lewiston Journal* [Magazine Section], p. A-11.

Eighth Annual Report of the Maine School for Feeble-Minded. (1916). Waterville, ME: Sentinel.

Eleventh Annual Report of the Maine School for Feeble-Minded. (1919). West Pownal, ME: Maine School for Feeble-Minded.

Elkins, T. E., & Anderson, H. F. (1992). Sterilization of persons with mental retardation. *The Journal for Persons with Severe Handicaps, 17*, 19–26.

Employment of people with intellectual and developmental disabilities: Key points and data (2010, January). Retrieved from United Cerebral Palsy website: http://www.ucp.org

Farber, B. (1968). *Mental retardation: Its social context and social consequences*. Boston, MA: Houghton Mifflin.

Eugenics: Compulsory sterilization in 50 states.

Federal judge signs new consent decree. (1994, September 29). *Portland Press Herald*, p. B3.

Feeble-minded not a great threat to society-Myerson. (1930, October 17). *Lewiston Evening Journal*, pp. A1, A16.

Fellers, E. (1991, December 1). Pineland's closing looms. *Lewiston Sun-Journal*, p. B3.

Fellers, E. (1994, October 21). Pineland cutting 90 people, 114 jobs. *Lewiston Sun-Journal*, pp. A9, A10.

Fergler, D, & Boyd, P. A. (1980). Anit-institutionalization: The promise of the Pennhurst case. In R. Flynn & N. Nitsch (Eds.). *Normalization, social integration, and community services* (pp. 141–166). Baltimore, MD: University Park Press.

Ferch, D. (1990, December 20). Commissioner: Budget crisis imperils mental health decree. *Portland Press Herald*, p. A12.

Ferguson, P. M. (1994). *Abandoned to their fate. Social policy and practice toward severely retarded people in America, 1820–1920*. Philadelphia, PA: Temple University Press.

Ferguson, P. M. (1987, summer). The social construction of mental retardation. *Social Policy*, 51–56.

Ferguson, P. M., Ferguson, D. L., & Taylor, S. J. (Eds). (1992). *Interpreting disability: A qualitative reader*. New York, NY: Teachers College Press.

Fernald, G. (1918). Maine's defective delinquents and backward children. *The Journal of the Maine Medical Association, IX*(5), 105-119.

Fifth Annual Report of the Maine School for Feeble-Minded. (1913). Waterville, ME: Sentinel.

Filling up the state hospitals. (1925). In *Clippings Pownal State School, 1909–1946,* 1989, p. 71.

First Report of the Maine School for Feeble-Minded. (1910). Augusta: Kennebec Journal Print.

First steps taken to form a Pownal parents' club. (1953, November 11). *Portland Press Herald,* p. A1.

Fishell, D. (2010), September 13). Reconciliation reins on Malaga Island. *The Times Record.* Retrieved from: http://www.timesrecord.com/

Fisher, P. (1979a, April 13). Pineland is no longer a snakepit. *Maine Times,* pp. 2–5.

Fisher, P. (1979b, November 30). Close Pineland? *Maine Times,* pp. 17–18.

Fisher, P. (1980). Pineland. The state replies. *Maine Times,* pp. 7–8.

Folsom, L. (1983). *Maine's due process in sterilization act of 1982 and the sterilization of mentally handicapped persons.* Portland, ME: University of Maine Law School.

Foucault, M. (1973). *The birth of the clinic. An archeology of medical perception* (A. A. M. Sheriden Smith, Trans.) New Yor, NY: Pantheon Books.

Foucault, M (1976). *Mental illness and psychology.* New YorK, NY: Harper & Row.

Fullerton, L. (1992a, December 6). Retarded man free to choose his life. *Portland Press Herald,* pp. A1, A14.

Fullerton, L. (1992b). Pineland phase-out under way. *Portland Press Herald,* February 5, A1, A8.

Fullerton, L (1992c, February, 28). Pineland won't result in short-term savings, officials says. *Portland Press Herald,* pp. A1, A8.

Fullerton, L. (1992d, December 9). City wants information on closings. *Portland Press Herald,* pp. B1, B2.

Fullerton, L. (1992e). State wants retarded adults to decide how to live. *Portland Press Herald,* p. A14.

Fullerton, L. (1992f, December 29). Chitwood says arson suspect didn't get proper supervison. *Portland Press Herald,* pp. A1, A10.

Fullerton, L. (1992g, December 12). State lacks system to replace AMHI, Pineland services. *Portland Press Herald,* pp. A1, A5.

Fullerton, L. (1992h, December 20). Former Pineland residents can live good lives, too. *Portland Press Herald,* pp. A15

Fullerton, L. (1993, April 3). Appeals court orders services for retarded. *Portland Press Herald,* pp. B1, B2.

Gadberry, S. (1992, March 2). Crowd tells state to save Pineland. *Portland Press Herald,* pp. A1, A8.

Gallagher, N. L. (1999). *Breeding better Vermonters. The eugenics project in the Green Mountain State.* Hanover, NH: University Press of New England.

Gallant, M. (1981). *Pineland Center. Past, present and future.* Unpublished manuscript.

Garber, A. (1995, October 26). Pineland decree penalties face state. *Portland Press Herald,* pp. A1, A9.

Gardiner deplores crowded conditions at Pownal school. (n.d.). *Portland Evening News,* August 14, "in *Clippings Pownal State School, 1909–1946,* 1989, p. 176.

Gignoux, G. (1993, April 9). City offers support in Pineland suit. *Lewiston Sun-Journal*, pp. A13.

Gilson, S.F.(1998). Choice and self-advocacy: A consumer's perspective. In P. Wehman & J. Kregel (Eds.). *More than a job* (pp. 3–24). Baltimore, MD: Brookes.

Goode, D. (1994). *A world without words. The social construction of children born deaf and blind*. Philadelphia, PA: Temple University Press.

Gordon, S. (1914). Sterilization of the unfit. *Journal of the Maine Medical Association*, *5*, 168–170.

Gould. S. J. (1996). *Mismeasure of man*. New York, NY: W. W. Norton.

Greenleaf sees expansion. (1941, April 17). *Lewiston Daily Sun*, A1.

Gregory, D. (1979, October 7). Letter to Commissioner Michael Petit. U.S. District Court, Portland, Maine.

Greico, J. (2004). Shudder Island. *Portland*, *19*, 26–30.

Grob, G. (1983). *Mental illness and American society, 1875–1940*. Princeton, NJ: Princeton University Press.

Had varied program. (1910, March 24). *Lewiston Evening Journal*, p. A11.

Haldeman v, Pennhurst State School and Hospital, 446 F. Supp. 1295 (E.D. PA. 1977).

Hayman, R. L. (1998). *The smart culture. Society, intelligence. and the law.* New York, NY: New York University Press.

Hedin, C. (1914). State care and training of the feeble-minded in Maine. *The Journal of the Maine Medical Association*, *IV*, 1894–1898.

Hench, D. (1996a, March 22). Final days of Pineland stir memories both good and bad. *Portland Press Herald*, pp. B1, B12.

Hench, D. (1996b, April 23). Pineland Center stands empty after 88 years. *Portland Press Herald*, pp. A1, A10.

Hoffman, J. L. (1969a, September 30). *An investigation of factors contributing to successful and non-successful adjustment of discharged retardates.* Report on Project RD-1606-P. Social and Rehabilitation Service, U.S. Department of Health, Education, and Welfare, Washington, DC.

Hoffman, J. L. (1969b, September 30). *Tabular Supplement to an investigation of factors contributing to successful and non-successful adjustment of discharged retardates.* Report on Project RD-1606-P. Social and Rehabilitation Service, U.S. Department of Health, Education, and Welfare, Washington, DC.

Hoffman, J. L. (1982). *A brief history of the Pineland Center.* New Gloucester, ME: Pineland Center.

Hood, P. (1968). Pineland's 60 years, 1908–1968. *The Pineland Observer*: New Gloucester, ME: Pineland Hospital and Training Center.

Hoose, S. (1995, July 16). Leaving Pineland. *Maine Sunday Telegram*, G1, G5.

Horacek v. Exon, 357 F. Supp. 71 (d. Neb. 1973).

House agrees to rule out sterilization. (1941, April, 15). *Lewiston Evening Journal*, p. A1.

Ingalls, R. J. (1978). *Mental retardation: The changing outlook.* New York, NY: Wiley.

Irwin, C. T. (1979, March 21). Programs for retarded move toward goals. *Portland Press Herald*, pp. A1, A16.

Inspect home for feeble-minded. (1914, November 6). *Portland Evening Express*, p. A7.

Jacobs, A., Weingold, J., & Dubrow, M. (1965). *The sheltered workshop. A community rehabilitation resource for the mentally retarded.* New York: New York Association of retarded Children.

Johnson, H. M. (2003, November, 22). The disability gulag. *New York Times Magazine*, 59–62, 64.

Johnson, K. (1998). *Deinstitutionalising women. An ethnographic study of institutional closure*. Cambridege, England: Cambridge University Press.

Johnson, K., & Traustadottir, R. (Eds.). (2005). *Deinstituionalization and people with intellectual disabilities: In and out of institutions*. London: Jessica Kingsley.

Jones, K (2004). *Education for children with mental retardation: Parental activism, public policy, and family ideology in the 1950s.* In S. Noll & J.W. Trent (Eds.), *Mental retardation in America: A historical reader* (pp. 322–350). New York, NY: New York University Press.

Jorthberg et al., v. U.S. Department of Labor, James D. Hodgson, Secretary of Labor, Augusta State Hospital, and Roy Ettlinger, Superintendent, No. SD (D. Maine, July 14, 1972).

Kaelber, L. (Ed.). (2009). *Eugenics: Compulsory sterilization in 50 states.* Retrieved from University of Vermont website: http://www.uvm.edu/~lkaelber/eugenics/

Kamber, H. (1969a, January 31). Inside Maine's snakepit. *Maine Times*, pp. 2–3.

Kamber, H (1969b, March 21), What hope for the hopeless? *Maine Times*, pp. 8–9

Kamber, H. (1969c, May 16). Is the end near for Pineland? *Maine Times*, pp. 8–9.

Kerry, J. (1972). The plight of Maine's mentally retarded. *The Church World* (Special issue). Portland, ME: Roman Catholic Diocese of Maine.

Kevles, D. J. (1985). *In the name of eugenics*. Cambridge, MA: Harvard University Press.

Kimball, R. (2001). *Pineland's past. The first one hundred years*. Portsmouth, NH: Peter E. Randall.

Kiwanians elect officers and listen to scholarly address by Judge Sanborn. (n.d.). In *Clippings Pownal State School, 1909–1946*, 1989.

Kleinberg, J. (1974). *History of Pineland (Maine School for the Feeble-minded).* Brunswick, ME: Bowdoin College.

Kupelian, N. S. (1939, February 8). 1072 mental cases attend state school. *Daily Kennebec Journal*, pp. B1, B15.

Lakin, K. C., & Bruinicks, R. H. (1985a). Contemporary services for handicapped children and youth. In R. H. Brunicks & K. C. Lakin (Eds.), *Living and learning in the least restrictive environment* (pp. 3–22). Baltimore, MD: Brookes.

Lakin, K. C., & Bruinicks, R. H. (1985b). Social integration of developmentally disabled persons. In K. C. Lakin & R. H. Bruinicks (Eds.), *Strategies for achieving community integration of developmentally disabled citizens* (pp. 3-26). Baltimore, MD: Brookes.

Landesman, S., & Butterfield, E. C. (1987). Normalization and deinstitutionalization of mentally retarded individuals: Controversy and Facts. *American Psychologist, 22*(8), 809-816.

Langley, L. (1972, September, 29). Under the controversy lies a political morass. *Maine Times*, p. 28.

Langley, L. (1973, January, 12). Pineland: behind the controversy. *Maine Times*, pp. 2–3.

Largent, M. A. (2008). *Breeding contempt. The history of coerced strilization in the United States.* New Brunswick, NJ: Rutgers University press.

Larson, S., & Lakin, C. (1991). Parent attitudes about residential placement before and after institutionalization. A research synthesis. *Journal of the Association of Persons with Severe Handicaps, 16,* 25-38.

Larson, S., Scott, N., Salmi, P., & Lakin, K. C. (2008). Changes in the number and characteristics of people living in state institutions. *Intellectual and Developmental Disabilities, 47,* 329–333.

Laski, F. (1985). Right to habilitation and right to education: The legal foundation. In R. H. Brunicks & K. C. Lakin (Eds.). *Living and learning in the least restrictive environment* (pp. 66–80). Baltimore, MD: Brookes.

Laubstein, W. H. (1980, June, 23). Defendants' memorandum in opposition to motion to reappoint Special Master. Filed in U.S. District Court, Portland, Maine, ref. *Wuori, et al. v. Concannon, et al.*—Docket No. 75-80 SD.

Lazerson, M. (1975). Educational institutions and mental subnormality: Notes on writing history. In M. J. Begab & S. A. Richardson (Eds.), *The mentally retarded and society: A social science perspective.* (pp. 33–54). Baltimore: MD: University Park Press.

Levine, M. (1986). The role of special court master in institutional reform litigation: A case study. *Law & Policy, 8,* 275–321.

Life outside Pineland falls short of freedom. (1992, December 13). *Maine Sunday Telegram*, p. C6.

Linneman, R. D. (2001). *Idiots: Stories about mindedness and mental retardation.* New York, NY: Peter Lange.

Lombardo, P. A. (2008). *Three generations, no imbeciles. Eugenics, the Supreme Court, and Buck v. Bell.* Baltimore, MD: Johns Hopkins Press.

Lord, A. (1930, December 3). Salvaging wrecked humanity is one of the tasks set for Pownal State School, where notable work is being done. *Lewiston (Evening?) Journal*, Magazine Section, p. 1-A.

Lord, A. (1933, November 18). From inside looking out at Pownal State School today. *Lewiston Evening Journal Illustrated* (Magazine Section), pp. 2–A, 4–A.

Lovell, J. (1979, March 19). Pineland, praised, roasted. *Portland Evening Express*, pp. A1, A14.

Ludmerer, K. M. (1972) *Genetics and American society.* Baltimore, MD: Johns Hopkins University Press.

Macklin, R., & Gaylin, W. (1981). *Mental retardation and sterilization: A problem of competency and paternalism.* New York, NY: Plenum Press.

Maine Home for Feeble-Minded at West Pownal, ME (n.d.). In *Clippings Pownal State School, 1909-1946*, 1989, p. 7.

Maine's problems in sub-normals. (n.d.). In *Clippings Pownal State School 1909–1946*, 105.

McInnis, K. (1985, November). A letter to parents of Pineland residents. *Coping, 9,* 12.

McPherson, P. (2004, February 9). Ill children near home is goal of professionals. Letters to the Editor. *Portland Press Herald*, p. A9.

Mental and old age cases confront city with problem. (1943, December 22). *Portland Press Herald*, pp. A11–A12.

Metzel, D. (2004). Historical social geography. In S. Noll & J. W. Trent (Eds.), *Mental retardation in America: A historical reader* (pp. 420–444). New York, NY: New York University Press.

Miller, H. W. (1913, Jan, 6). Eugenics. *The Journal of the Maine Medical Association*, pp. 1125–1150.

Minow, M. (1990). *Making all the difference. Inclusion, exclusion, and American law.* Ithaca, NY: Cornell University Press.

Mitchell, D., & Snyder, S. (2003). The Eugenic Atlantic: Race, disability, and the making of an international Eugenic Science, 1800-1945. *Disability & Society, 18,* 843–864.

Morse, S. (1993, March 8,). Independence. Ex-Pineland resident glad she left [Letter to the editor]. *Portland Press Herald*, p. A6.

Mosher, J. P. (1991). *No greater abomination: Ethnicity, class and power relations on Malaga Island, Maine, 1880–1912*. Portland, ME: University of Southern Maine.

Mrs. Libby released after compromise is reached. (1937, February 20). *Portland Evening Express*, p. A1.

Much being accomplished for the feeble-minded of this state. (1909, March 19). *Portland Evening Express*, p. A15.

Nacelewicz, T. (1992, December 10). City seeks partners in suit against state. *Portland Press Herald*, p. A14.

Nazeer, K. (2006). *Send in the idiots*. New York, NY: Bloomsbury.

Need accommodations for mentally defective. (1940, June 19), *Lewiston Evening Journal*, p. A14.

New York State Association for Retarded Children, Inc., v. Rockefeller, 357 F. Supp. (E.D. N.Y. 1973).

Ninth and Tenth Annual Report of the Maine School for Feeble-Minded. (1917–1918). Waterville, ME: Sentinel.

Nirje, B.(1980). The normalization principle. In R. J. Flynn & K. E. Nitsch (Eds.), *Normalization, social integration and community services* (pp. 31–50). Baltimore, MD: University Park Press.

Nirje, N. (1969). The normalization principle and its human management implications. In R. Krugel & W. Wolfensberger (Eds.), *Changing patterns of residential services for the mentally retarded* (pp. 179–195). Washington, DC: President's Committee on Mental Retardation.

Noll, S. (1995). *Feebleminded in our midst. Institutions for the mentally retarded in the South, 1900–1940.* Chapel Hill, NC: University of North Carolina Press.

Noll, S., & Trent, J. W. (Eds.). (2004). Introduction. In S. Noll & J.W. Trent (Eds.). *Mental retardation in America: A historical reader* (pp. 1–22). New York, NY: New York University Press.

Nourse, V. F. (2008). *In reckless hands: Skinner v. Oklahoma and the near triumph of American Eugenics*. New York, NY: W. W. Norton.

Nyhan, P. (1985a, October 4). The behavior stabilization unit. *Maine Times*, pp. 2–5.

Nyhan, P. (1985b, December 6). Coping is vindicated. *Maine Times,* pp. 34-35.

Nyhan, P. (1985c, November 29). Trouble at Pineland. *Maine Times*, p. 34.

Nyhan, P. (1987a, May 1). Serving Maine's retarded citizens. *Maine Times*, pp. 18–20.

Nyhan, P. (1987b). Success stories. *Maine Times*, pp. 2-6.

Nyhan, P. (1988, October, 28). Out of the snakepit. *Maine Times* (Special 20th Anniversary Issue), Section 2, pp. B1–B4.

Nyhan, P. (1989, December 15). Broken promise to mentally retarded citizens. *Maine Times*, pp. 16–19.

Olmstead v. L.C. 527 US 581 (1999).

Our imbeciles and insane. (n.d.). In *Clippings Pownal State School, 1909–1946*, 1989, p. 96.

Outspoken Pineland superintendent out of job. (1971, July 21). *Portland Press Herald*, pp. A1, A16.

Paul, J. (1965). *"Three generations of imbeciles are enough ..." State eugenic sterilization laws in American thought and practice.* Washington, DC: Walter Reed Army Institute of Research.

Pfieffer, D. (1994). Eugenics and disability discrimination. *Disability and Society*, *9*, 481–500.

Philbrick, S. (2001, Summer). From the collections. Richard Turcotte collection. *Maine History*, *40*(2).

Pickens, D. K. (1968). *Eugenics and the Progressives*. Nashville, TN: Vanderbilt University Press.

Pineland: Consent decree enforcement is challenged. (1990, October 19). *Maine Times*, p. 24.

Pineland deaths. One probe complete. (1985, December 13). *Maine Times*, p. 10.

Pineland Hospital and Training Center. (n.d.) [Brochure] New Gloucester, ME: Pineland Hospital and Training Center.

Pineland lawyer hits lack of progress. (1979, February 15). *Portland Evening Express*, p. A27.

Pineland warned. Medicaid funds threatened. (1989, May 27). *Maine Times*, p. 12.

Pineland's history (n.d.). Retrieved from http://www.pinelandfarms.org/visitors/history.htm

Portland clergy differ with Pope on birth control. (1931, January 9). *Portland Evening News*, pp. A1, A16.

Pownal school, fish station work urged. (1944, September 19). *Daily Kennebec Journal*, pp. A1, A8.

Pownal school improves services for weak-minded. (1932, November 10). *Lewiston Evening Journal*, p. A6.

Pownal State School head sued for $25,000. (1937, March 2). *Portland Evening Express*, pp. A1–A2.

Prouty, R. W., Smith, G., & Lakin, K.C. (2005). *Residential services for persons with developmental disabilities: Status and trends through 2004*. Minneapolis, MN: University of Minnesota Institute on Community Integration, Research and Training Center on Community Living.

Racino, J. (1993). *The closing of Laconia: From the inside out.* Syracuse, NY: Syracuse University Center on Human Policy.

Rafter, N. H. (1997). *Creating born criminals.* Urbana, IL: University of Illinois Press.

Rapley, M. (2004). *The social construction of intellectual disability*. Cambridge, England: Cambridge University Press.

Regional centers urged to replace Pineland. (1986, September 11). *Portland Press Herald*, p. A8.

Reilly, P. R. (1991). *The surgical solution: A history of involuntary sterilization in the U.S.* Baltimore, MD: Johns Hopkins University Press.

Remarkable progress made in work at state's new home for feeble-minded at West Pownal, ME-half a hundred inmates already there. (1909, July 10). *Lewiston Saturday Journal*, p. A11.

Rep. No. 1925, c. 208, p. 198 .

Rep. No. 1931, c. 275, p. 308.

Report cites violations. (1989, January 27). *Maine Times*, Section 1, p. A4.

Report of the Maine Commission for the Study of the Feebleminded and of the Survey by the National Committee for Mental Hygiene. (1918). Augusta, ME: Maine Commission for the Study of the Feebleminded.

Report of the Maine School for Feeble-Minded (1912). Waterville, Me Semntiel.

Report of the Special Master to the United States District Court for the District of Maine. (1979, November 14). Part I: Conclusions of the Special Master. Filed U.S. District Court, Portland, Maine.

Report of the Special Master to the United States District Court for the District of Maine (1980). Filed U.S. District Court, Portland, Maine, ref Martti Wuori v. George A. Zitnay. Civil no. 75-80-SD.

Retarded to enjoy range of support (1994, July 29). *Portland Press Herald*, p. 2B.

Richardson, J. (1994a, March 13). Pineland decays as future debated. *Maine Sunday Telegram*, pp. B1, B14.

Rizzolo, M. C., Hemp, R., Braddock, D., & Pomerantz-Essley, A. (2002). *The state of the states in developmental disabilities.* Washington, DC: American Association on Mental Retardation.

Rizzolo, M. C., Hemp, R., Braddock, D., & Pomerantz-Essley, A. (2004). *The state of the states in developmental disabilities.* Washington, DC: American Association on Mental Retardation.

Roach, E. (1979, January 27). State officials pleased with progress at Pineland. *Portland Press Herald*, p. A12.

Rothman, D. (1971).*The discovery of the asylum.* Boston: Little, Brown and Company.

Rothman, D., & Rothman, S. (1984). *Willowbrook wars. A decade of struggle for social justice.* New York, NY: Harper & Row.

Ruef, M. B., & Turnbull, A. P. (2002). The perspectives of individuals with cognitive disabilities and/or autism on their lives and their problem behaviors. *Research ands Practice with Persons with Severe Disabilities*, *27*(2), 125–140.

Russell, E. (2010, January, 4). Disabled men sue for home of their own. *Portland Press Herald*, p. B2.

S. Rep. No 6, 1905, January 12, 1-7

S. Rep. No 6, 1905, January 12, 1905, 11.

S Rep. No 6, 1905, April 20, 9-12.

S. Rep. No 44, 1907, 336-337.

Salmi, P., Scott, N., Webster, A., Larson, S., & Lakin, C. K. (2010). Residential services for people with intellectual or development disabilities at the 20th anniversary of the Americans With Disabilities Act, the 10th anniversary of

"Olmstead," and in the Year of Community Living. *Intellectual and Developmental Disabilities, 48,* 168–171.

Sanborn, B. (1904, April 20). Address to the legislative committee relating to the feeble-minded. In Report of Committee on Home for Feeble-Minded. S. Rep No 6, 1905, Jan 12, 9-12.

Sanborn, B. (n.d.). The care of feeble-minded. *Transactions of the Maine Medical Association*, pp. 45–52.

Says state needs second institution for feeble-minded. (n.d.). In *Clippings Pownal State School, 1909–1946*, 1989, p. 441.

Scheerenberger, R. (1983). *A history of mental retardation*. Baltimore, MD: Brookes.

School at Pownal.(n.d). In *Clippings Pownal State School, 1909–1946*, 1989, p. 22.

Scruggs, R. (1986, Summer). On their own. *Coping*, p. 9.

Scruggs, R. (1996, April 28). A once revolutionary idea empties Pineland. *Maine Sunday Telegram*, p. C5.

Scull, M. (2005). *Madhouse: A tragic tale of megalomania and modern medicine.* New Haven, CT: Yale University Press.

Senator Bishop proposes sterilization of the "defectives at large." (1941, Jan. 25). *Lewiston Daily Sun*, p. A1

Seventeenth and Eighteenth Annual Reports of the Pownal State School.(1926). Pownal, ME: Pownal State School.

Seventh Annual Report of the Maine School for Feeble-Minded. (1915). Waterville, ME: Sentinel.

Shakespeare, T. (1997, August). [Review of the book From idiocy to mental deficiency: Historical perspectives on people with intellectual disabilities by D. Wright and A. Digby (Eds.). London: Routledge]. *Disability and Society, 12,* 658–660.

Shapiro, J. P. (1993). *No pity. People with disabilities forging a new civil rights movement.* New York, NY: Times Books.

Shoultz, B. Walker, P. Hulgin, K., & Taylor, S. (1999). *Closing Brandon Training School: A Vermont story.* Syracuse, New York, NY: Syracuse University Center on Human Policy

Sixth Annual Report of the Maine School for Feeble-Minded. (1914). Waterville, ME: Sentinel.

Smith is against prize fighting films … Dr. Tyson opposes sterilization bill. (1931, March 12). *Lewiston Daily Sun*, p. A6.

Snyder, S. L., & Michell, D. T. (2006). *Cultural locations of disability*. Chicago, IL: University of Chicago Press.

Sofair, A. N., & Kaldjiian, L. C. (2000). Eugenic sterilization and a qualified Nazi analogy: The United States and Germany, 1930–1945. *Annals of Internal Medicine, 132,* 312–319.

Spring Harbor: New place, new autism unit. (2004, Spring). *One in Five, 3*(2), A1, A5.

Standing Committee Report (1912). In *First Annual Report, Maine School for Feeble-Minded,* pp. 19–23.

Staples, W. G. (1990). *Castles of our conscience*. New Brunswick, NJ: Rutgers University Press.

State may drop its "gold brick." (1913, January 28). *Daily Eastern Argus,* pp. A1.

Stefan, S. (2001). *Unequal rights*. Washington, DC: American Psychologial Association.

Sterilization bill is aired. (n.d.). In *Clippings Pownal State School, 1909–1946*, 1989, 746.

Sterilization of Maine defectives is advocated by doctors, professor. (1941, March 21). *Lewiston Daily Sun*, p. A1.

Sterilization bill rejected. by Maine senate, 28 To 4. (1941, April 14,). *Portland Press Herald*, pp. A1, A11.

Stern, A. M. (2005). *Eugenic nation*. Berkely, CA: University of Califirnia Press.

Stevens, E. (1981, February, 11). Impounded Pineland reports released. *Portland Press Herald*, pp. 1A, 23A.

Sundram, C. (2000, April). Report of the Independent Audit Compliance with the Consent Decree "Consumer Advisory Board v. Duby.

Superintendent's Annual Report of the Pownal State School. (1939). Pownal, ME: Pownal State School.

Superintendent's Annual Report of the Pownal State School. (1940). Pownal, ME: Pownal State School.

Superintendent's Annual Report of the Pownal State School. (1942). Pownal, ME: Pownal State School.

Superintendent's Annual Report of the Pownal State School. (1945). Pownal, ME: Pownal State School.

Superintendent's Annual Report of the Pownal State School. (1946). Pownal, ME: Pownal State School.

Superintendent's Annual Report of the Pownal State School. (1947). Pownal, ME: Pownal State School.

Superintendent's logs (1930, October 9, p. 14); New Gloucester Historical Society, New Gloucester, Maine.

Swift, H. (1914). Sterilization of the unfit. *Journal of the Maine Medical Association, V,* 161–170.

Switzky, H. N., & Greenspan, S. (Eds.). (2003). *What is mental retardation? Ideas for an evolving definition*. Washington, DC: American Association on Mental Retardation.

Tapley, L. (1985a, July/August). Death and abuse at Pineland. *Coping*, pp. 1–2

Tapley, L. (1985b, July/August). Pineland's prison: The behavior stabilization unit. *Coping*, p. 3.

Taylor, S. J., Bogdan, R., & Lutfiyya, Z.M. (1995). (Eds.). *The variety of community experience*. Baltimore, MD: Brookes.

The backlash: COPING is blasted in September press conference. (1985, November, 9). *Coping*.

The home for feeble-minded at Pownal. (1913, January 30). *Portland Evening Express and Advertiser*, p. A15.

Thompson, C. H. (1975, April 7). Mental health chief denies Pineland closing. *Portland Press Herald*, pp. A1, A7.

To stamp out crime. (n.d.). In *Clippings Pownal State School, 1909–1946*, 1989, p. 459.

Traustadottir, R. (Eds.). (2005). *Deinstitutionalization and people with intellectual disabilities: In and out of institutions* (pp. 93-107). London: Jessica Kingsley Publishers.

Trent, J. W. (1994). *Inventing the feeble mind. A history of mental retardation in the United States*. Berkeley, CA: University of California at Berkeley Press.

Turkel, T. (2001, June 24). What really happened at Malaga Island? *Maine Sunday Telegram*, pp. B1, B8.

Twelfth Annual Report of the Maine School for Feeble-Minded. (1920). West Pownal, ME: Maine School for Feeble-Minded.

Twenty-fourth Annual Report of the Pownal State School. (1932). New Gloucester, ME: Pownal State School.

Twenty-fifth Annual Report of the Pownal State School. (1933). New Gloucester, ME: Pownal State School.

Twenty-sixth Annual Report of the Pownal State School. (1934). New Gloucester, ME: Pownal State School.

Twenty-third Annual Report of the Pownal State School. (1931). Pownal ME: Pownal State School.

Two men and two women are held as a result of unusual triangle. (1937, February 13). *Portland Press Herald*, A1, A2.

Urges sterilization of the feeble-minded. (1925, March 5). *Lewiston Evening Journal*, p. A2.

U.S. Census Bureau (n.d.) *State and county quickfacts.* Retrieved from U.S. Census Bureau website: http://quickfacts.census.gov/qfd.

Vegh, A. (1994, October 30). Partings tug at Pineland staffers. *Portland Press Herald*, pp. B1, B12.

Vegh, S. (1995, March 31). Families concerned about future after Pineland. *Portland Press Herald*, pp. B1, B2.

Vincent Clukey. (1991, January 29). [Obituary] *Kennebec Journal*, p. A8.

Vosburgh, S. (1926). The problem of the sub-normals in Maine. *Journal of the Maine Medical Association, XVIL*, pp. 43–49.

Walsh, B. (2004, January 22). Hospital opening new unit for autistic children. *Portland Press Herald*, pp. B1, B12.

Welsch v. Likins, 373 F. Supp. 487 (D Minn 1974).

Williams, C. (2000, July 23). Exorcising Pineland. *Lewiston Sun-Journal*, pp. A1, A10.

Williams, P., & Shoultz, B. (1982). *We can speak for ourselves.* Boomington, IN. Indiana University Press.

Wolfensberger, W. (1975). *The origin and nature of our institutional models*. Syracuse, NY: Human Policy Press.

Wolfensberger, W. (1972). *The principle of normalization in human services.* Toronto, Ontario: National Institute on Mental Retardation.

Woodard, C. (2010, August). *A quiet apology. Down East.* Retrieved from: http://www.downeast.com/

Work among the feeble-minded in Maine. (1930, October 30). *Lewiston Evening Journal*, p. A4.

Wuori v. Bruns, No. 75-80-SD (D. Maine, July 3, 1975).

Wuori v. Concannon, No. 75-80-P (D. Maine, January 14, 1981). Stipulation Agreement.

Wuori v. Zitnay, No. 75-80-SD (D. Maine, July 4, 1978).

Wyatt v. Stickney, 344 F. Supp. 373 and 387 (M.D. Ala. 1972).

Yamaki, K., & Fujiura, G. T. (2002). Employment and income status of adults with developmental disabilities. *Intellectual and Developmental Disabilities, 40,* 132-141.

INDEX

www.ingramcontent.com/pod-product-compliance
Lightning Source LLC
LaVergne TN
LVHW052257200926
848481LV00002B/389
9781617354144